Medical Anthropology

World Anthropology

General Editor

SOL TAX

Patrons

CLAUDE LÉVI-STRAUSS
MARGARET MEAD
LAILA SHUKRY EL HAMAMSY
M. N. SRINIVAS

MOUTON PUBLISHERS · THE HAGUE · PARIS
DISTRIBUTED IN THE USA AND CANADA BY ALDINE, CHICAGO

Medical Anthropology

Editors

FRANCIS X. GROLLIG, S. J.
HAROLD B. HALEY

MOUTON PUBLISHERS · THE HAGUE · PARIS
DISTRIBUTED IN THE USA AND CANADA BY ALDINE, CHICAGO

General Editor's Preface

Modern medicine concerns itself with the physical and mental welfare of individuals in their respective family and social contexts — and anthropology adds a cross-cultural and whole-species perspective to this concern. As a result, medical anthropology encompasses vast areas: much of human biology and epidemiology, physical and mental illness and curing, nutrition, reproduction, family planning, problems of all age groups, and even the delivery of health care. All these aspects must be studied historically and comparatively, relating individual and cultural, diachronic and synchronic. This book samples the widely-varied concerns of medical anthropologists over the world as they write for and participate in an unusual international congress.

Like most contemporary sciences, anthropology is a product of the European tradition. Some argue that it is a product of colonialism, with one small and self-interested part of the species dominating the study of the whole. If we are to understand the species, our science needs substantial input from scholars who represent a variety of the world's cultures. It was a deliberate purpose of the IXth International Congress of Anthropological and Ethnological Sciences to provide impetus in this direction. The *World Anthropology* volumes, therefore, offer a first glimpse of a human science in which members from all societies have played an active role. Each of the books is designed to be self-contained; each is an attempt to update its particular sector of scientific knowledge and is written by specialists from all parts of the world. Each volume should be read and reviewed individually as a separate volume on its own given subject. The set as a whole will indicate what changes are in store for anthropology as scholars from the developing countries join in studying the species of which we are all a part.

The IXth Congress was planned from the beginning not only to include as many of the scholars from every part of the world as possible, but also with a view toward the eventual publication of the papers in high-quality volumes. At previous Congresses scholars were invited to bring papers which were then read out loud. They were necessarily limited in length; many were only summarized; there was little time for discussion; and the sparse discussion could only be in one language. The IXth Congress was an experiment aimed at changing this. Papers were written with the intention of exchanging them before the Congress, particularly in extensive pre-Congress sessions; they were not intended to be read aloud at the Congress, that time being devoted to discussions — discussions which were simultaneously and professionally translated into five languages. The method for eliciting the papers was structured to make as representative a sample as was allowable when scholarly creativity — hence self-selection — was critically important. Scholars were asked both to propose papers of their own and to suggest topics for sessions of the Congress which they might edit into volumes. All were then informed of the suggestions and encouraged to re-think their own papers and the topics. The process, therefore, was a continuous one of feedback and exchange and it has continued to be so even after the Congress. The some two thousand papers comprising *World Anthropology* certainly then offer a substantial sample of world anthropology. It has been said that anthropology is at a turning point; if this is so, these volumes will be the historical direction-markers.

As might have been foreseen in the first post-colonial generation, the large majority of the Congress papers (82 percent) are the work of scholars identified with the industrialized world which fathered our traditional discipline and the institution of the Congress itself: Eastern Europe (15 percent); Western Europe (16 percent); North America (47 percent); Japan, South Africa, Australia, and New Zealand (4 percent). Only 18 percent of the papers are from developing areas: Africa (4 percent); Asia-Oceania (9 percent); Latin America (5 percent). Aside from the substantial representation from the U.S.S.R. and the nations of Eastern Europe, a significant difference between this corpus of written material and that of other Congresses is the addition of the large proportion of contributions from Africa, Asia, and Latin America. "Only 18 percent" is two to four times as great a proportion as that of other Congresses; moreover, 18 percent of 2,000 papers is 360 papers, 10 times the number of "Third World" papers presented at previous

Congresses. In fact, these 360 papers are more than the total of ALL papers published after the last International Congress of Anthropological and Ethnological Sciences which was held in the United States (Philadelphia, 1956).

The significance of the increase is not simply quantitative. The input of scholars from areas which have until recently been no more than subject matter for anthropology represents both feedback and also long-awaited theoretical contributions from the perspectives of very different cultural, social, and historical traditions. Many who attended the IXth Congress were convinced that anthropology would not be the same in the future. The fact that the next Congress (India, 1978) will be our first in the "Third World" may be symbolic of the change. Meanwhile, sober consideration of the present set of books will show how much, and just where and how, our discipline is being revolutionized.

Other volumes in this series deal with medical problems as they relate to physical anthropology and human biology, nutrition, population problems, mental health, shamanism, drug use, differences of ethnic groups and of sex, age, and economic class, and public health and the practice of medicine. Taken in conjunction with this volume, they probe some of the most interesting aspects of this immense field.

Chicago, Illinois   SOL TAX
March 12, 1976

Welcome Address to the Pre-Congress Conference on Medical Anthropology

Colleagues and Scholars:

I am indeed grateful to have the opportunity to welcome this contingent of the IXth International Congress of Anthropological and Ethnological Sciences to Loyola University and to Chicago. In a day when international congresses are multiplying in numbers, scope, complexity, and comprehensiveness, there is probably no discipline other than anthropology which affords a greater opportunity to draw on a long tradition of practical investigation and theoretical development (through fieldwork) of a worldwide scope. This vision is reflected in the theme of your Congress: "One Species, Many Cultures." This vision is reflected in the medical anthropology program to which you are contributing your thoughts, reflections, fieldwork, and scholarly memoranda and papers. I am impressed.

I have read with interest the proposal that this Congress will contribute permanently to the world's information and inspiration the transactions of the Congress in a series of some eighty volumes — a series that will update anthropology. I wish you well in your deliberations and await the publication of your volume, *Medical anthropology*: your contribution to the *Acta* of the Congress. May God bless you and prosper your work. I am happy to say to you this word: WELCOME.

President, Loyola University   RAYMOND C. BAUMHART, S.J.
Stritch School of Medicine
Chicago, Illinois
August 31, 1974

Preface

To Dr. Sol Tax and his persistent urging of the desirability of a session devoted to medical anthropology in the IXth International Congress of Anthropological and Ethnological Sciences must go the credit for the final production of this volume. On August 11, 1972, he invited Dr. Dorothea Leighton to organize a "volume/session on the 'Developments in Medical Anthropology.'" For a variety of personal reasons the invitation was declined and other potential organizers/editors were suggested.

In his next invitation, Dr. Tax wrote on August 21, "It occurs to me that since acupuncture has now begun to diffuse from East to West, a systematic review of other non-Western medical practices of all kinds and from all cultures might be of interest and importance to the medical profession. In addition to whatever else is done, we might interest somebody in developing a research conference to precede the Congress and report on it."

Dr. Janice A. Egeland accepted the invitation and with Dr. Hazel H. Weidman developed a splendid tentative program on the proposed theme, but they came to realize that it would take some years to produce such a program and the accompanying handbook reviewing developments in medical anthropology. It could be ready for the 1978 ICAES. Dr. Tax agreed that they were "perfectly right to wait for the 'definitive' review on medical anthropology," but pleaded (November 6, 1972) for action for the 1973 Congress: "Doing something COULD include even a small group of excellent position papers or even outlines done soon to be sent abroad for systematical comment, to serve as the basis for the Chicago session. ANYTHING that is creative . . . will attract and bring colleagues for a major discussion and review of the content, conclusions, and tasks ahead in the broad field" of medical anthropology. This point of view was not accepted; medical anthropology was again an orphan.

The Society for Medical Anthropology met with the American Anthropological Association in Toronto in the latter part of November, 1972. At this meeting the invitation to organize such a session/volume was offered to the Society. The executive committee and the officers declined to accept the invitation, but presented the invitation to the meeting of the membership for discussion. A volunteer was called for, but as Dr. Steve Polgar wrote to Dr. Tax, "No one came forward."

In a letter (December 4, 1972), volunteering to attempt the organizational and editorial work, I wrote to Dr. Tax concerning the Toronto discussion, "It was not an acrimonious discussion, rather the hope was that with new information participation could be achieved. The question was really open and it was only the lack of a volunteer to direct the work that allowed the reconsideration to confirm the executive committee's [negative] decision. There was a strong undercurrent of agreement with your position that Medical Anthropology should be presented in the Congress. . . . One of the main problems expressed in the discussion was the dire need for a presentation of a body of organized THEORY for Medical Anthropology (as opposed to the proliferation of more mere case studies of Medical Anthropology), and the inadequacy of the time now left to get this material together." Having felt so strongly the need to have medical anthropology represented in the Congress, Dr. Sol Tax was willing to encourage something rather than nothing; we hope that he is not disappointed.

Since the topic obviously involves the fusion of the two fields of medicine and anthropology, it was equally obvious that the burden should be borne by representatives of both disciplines. It is seriously doubted if the co-organizer/editor, Harold B. Haley, M.D., ever realized how much of the burden he was volunteering for when he so graciously agreed to be a partner in the project. Not the least of his contributions were the many trips he made from Roanoke to Chicago for editorial conferences. In recognition of his contribution, it is fitting that he has been given the "last word" on the subject.

The medical anthropology contribution to the Congress rapidly became a reality. With the help of Harold Haley, a Pre-Congress Conference was planned and executed through the generous cooperation of the Stritch School of Medicine of Loyola University of Chicago. We believe it appropriate to include in this volume the brief welcome message of the Rev. Raymond C. Baumhart, S.J., president of the University.

The Pre-Congress Conference on Medical Anthropology was held on August 31, 1973, at the Stritch School of Medicine of Loyola University of Chicago. The Chairman was Harold B. Haley, M.D., Professor of Surgery and Associate Dean of the College of Medicine of the University of Virginia at Roanoke; the co-chairman was Francis X. Grollig, S.J., Professor and Chairman of the Anthropology Department at Loyola. The day was divided into four work sessions in which no paper was read by anyone, but the papers were organized, distributed, and discussed under four themes: (1) Native Cultural Aspects of Healing; (2) Specific Subject Papers; (3) Interaction of Traditional and Western Medical Practices; and (4) Theoretical Aspects of Medical Anthropology.

Out of each one of these work sessions came a summary position paper. These four position papers were presented and officially tape-recorded by the Congress at the opening of Session 423 on medical anthropology, of the IXth ICAES. A transcription of this material was produced by the editor and co-editor of this volume on medical anthropology. With only a small amount of editing, these four position papers are reproduced here as the statements introducing each of the first four sections of the ICAES papers in this volume. These four statements are the products of four individuals. The chairman placed no restrictions on their preparations. In the first and second chapters the threads of thought contained in the respective work sessions are presented in the form of a brief commentary on the papers discussed; in the third chapter the themes that surfaced in the discussions of the papers are presented; the questions raised in the Pre-Congress Conference discussion form the introduction to the fourth chapter.

As planned, this position-paper part of our session took about one-half of the allotted time. The balance of the time was devoted to discussion from the floor which was also recorded. This section of the tape — again, only slightly edited — is the important fifth chapter of this volume.

The co-editors of this volume have consciously refrained from extensive "revisions" of the manuscripts and transcriptions because we believe that no good purpose can be served by straining the thoughts of the whole world through a Western (ethnocentric!) screen: we respect the individuality of our colleagues and their scholarly contributions to the volume. It was our duty to develop themes out of the proffered papers — to provide a forum for the enjoyable interaction of these participants.

There is no bibliography for the field of medical anthropology added here because this would be merely to duplicate the already splendidly organized and well-known bibliography of Dr. Horatio Fabrega.

In addition to those already mentioned, there are certainly many more persons deserving of individual recognition, but we feel particularly obligated to the following for making the Pre-Congress Conference, the Congress Session, and this volume possible: the staff at the Chicago headquarters of the Congress office, in particular Kathleen Cushman, Enid Fogel, Roberta McGowan, Gay and Neil Neuberger, and especially Karen Tkach, who has been in The Hague patiently helping the volume through to publication; Dean J. A. Wells, our host at the Stritch School of Medicine; Dean Ronald Walker of the College of Arts and Sciences of Loyola University who provided the Pre-Congress Conference with transportation and hospitality; Drs. Julius Goldberg, Dana Raphael, John Pfifferling, and the Associate Dean of Northwestern's School of Medicine, Richard Kessler, for their notable contributions to the Pre-Congress Conference; Virginia Balnius and Rael Slavensky of the Congress Service Corps, who covered innumerable details; Patricia Keenan, Research Associate and secretary of the University of Virginia School of Medicine at Roanoke, and Bonnie DeZur, Anthropology Department secretary at Loyola University, who were responsible for most of the typing; and Sharon Renkosiak, my Research Assistant who spent an entire semester on editorial details for this volume. To these and to many more we owe our gratitude and our thanks for the success of this presentation. I will accept the blame for the omissions and shortcomings.

Loyola University   FRANCIS X. GROLLIG, S.J.
Chicago, Illinois
June 15, 1974

Table of Contents

SECTION ONE

Native Cultural Aspects of Healing

Introduction

FRANCIS X. GROLLIG, S.J.

The topic which we discussed first in the Pre-Congress Conference on Medical Anthropology was native cultural aspects of healing. I find it very interesting that materials for the medical anthropology conference and this session come, literally, from all over the world — the United States, Switzerland, Peru, Malawi, Mexico, southeast Arabia, India, Hawaii, Kenya, Italy, Cuba, Nigeria, Canada, Yugoslavia, the Philippine Islands, Japan, Brazil, and Colombia. In a sense we have here among these papers a splendid cross section of the types of native cultural aspects in healing to which we addressed ourselves. David Frisancho Pena, a medical doctor from Puno, Peru, provided us with a vast amount of background in his published volume, *Medicina indígena y popular*. He speaks of, among other types of remedies, vegetable, animal, and mineral remedies including herbs, magical procedures, and amulets.

Dr. Alifeyo Chilivumbo reports on the physical and psychological bases of illness and the *nganga*, the native physician. He also comments on some of the largely mystical cures which are used. No treatment of the native cultural aspects of healing would be complete without a discussion of folk medicine. In her presentation, Miss Janet Belcove from Southern Methodist University discusses the primary curative agents in the pharmacopoeia in Spanish-American traditional medicine in Taos, New Mexico, and includes herbs that are used by the *curanderos*. These herbs are used for scientific disorders, cancer, influenza, etc. She also discusses folk illnesses — *mal de ojo* and *susto* — to name just two of them. Kenneth Taylor, Ph.D., of the University of Brasilia, introduces another new concept: the use of assistant spirits that must be reckoned with in the diseases among the Sanumá Indians of Brazil, in cases involving both indigenous and Western medicine. In his paper, Kivuto Ndeti, Ph.D., the Chairman of the Department of Sociology at the University of Nairobi, condemns the "bad" and puts a perspective on the "good native aspects of healing," as he calls them. In the Pre-Congress Conference a very heated discussion followed this presentation and involved the very concepts of "good" and "bad" as applied to medicine. Michio Tsunoo, M.D., from Japan emphasizes the cultural differences involved in the psychological reactions toward advanced Western surgical techniques including heart transplants. He also comments on the traditional Japanese use of acupuncture for neurological pain. As he looks into the future, Dr. Tsunoo sees the developing of "different approaches to medicine among different people." Joseph Gagliano, Ph.D., an historian, Professor of History at Loyola University of Chicago, placed coca (whence comes, of course, cocaine) and the use of coca and popular medicine in Peru in an historical setting. Harvey Doorenbos, M.D., from the Caliphate of Oman, south Arabia, gives an interesting picture of some of the challenging situations in medicine which are a carry-over, as he puts it, "from the prescientific era." He describes, for example, the post-partum salt-packing procedure which causes many and serious surgical situations.

In addition to the papers here commented upon, we have included two more papers. Francis Clune, Jr., Ph.D. (State University of New York at Brockport), "Witchcraft, the shaman, and active pharmaco-poeia," asks the question, why were the drugs originally used by the shaman and/or witchdoctors? And in his (shortened) paper, Franklin Loveland, Ph.D. (Gettysburg College), looks at snakebites through the eyes of a Nicaraguan Indian and discusses "Snakebite cure among the Rama Indians of Nicaragua."

Witchcraft, the Shaman, and Active Pharmacopoeia

FRANCIS J. CLUNE, JR.

Medicine has been practiced one way or another since man became a cultured animal. There even is some evidence that a first-aid technique derives from our primate ancestors, as in the picking and cleaning of wounds observed by DeVore among baboons (Sahlins 1969: 4). There is evidence in Shanidar Cave that a member of the Neanderthal group living in that cave seems to have suffered and survived an amputation of the hand and forearm, which would call for at least a rudimentary knowledge of bodily structure and first aid (Coon 1962: 563).

Ethnographic evidence indicates that the usual person to call to the aid of an injured or sick person has been the shaman or "witch doctor." We will not get into the argument over variations in this treatment system but merely note that in most cultures there is a specialist who treats illness, injury and disease and quite frequently this person corresponds to the leader of religious practices, whatever he or she may be called. In many cultures the medico-religious practitioner is also considered to be a practitioner of magic and witchcraft. The amount of knowledge of curing by a shaman in a culture is recognized by the culture as possibly dangerous. The basic attitude is that if he can cure disease then he can cause disease. In medieval Europe doctors were often killed because they were considered to have started the plague (Haggard 1929: 501–505) to get more patients. This of course ignored the fact that the doctors had a higher than average death rate due to treating the sick. In many religious systems the method of treating a disease is to treat the individual by special magical processes and concoctions that are supposed to bring back the spirit of the sick person. Again, if the shaman has the power to retrieve the spirit, it is quite reasonable to consider that he would also have the power to destroy a person by taking the spirit away.

When the Europeans arrived in the New World they ran into a very different sort of medical system and a very different view of what ought to be the proper treatment of disease. From various sources the European medical view can be summed up as a system of treating the symptoms of disease. (It must be noted that European medicine was still in the barber-blood-letting stage, along with the doctor.) This was in direct contrast to most of the medicine practiced by the medical practitioners of the New World in which the American Indians treated the person and not the symptoms. European doctors were not too interested in the mental attitude of the individual patient except that they admitted that the best cure for a patient is the best doctor — here we have faith-healing, faith that the doctor will cure the patient. The medicine men of the New World were much more worried about the mental attitude of the patient and not the symptoms. Here faith-healing was practiced. However, both also used various drugs to aid the patient in his recovery, or to cure the symptoms, depending upon which theory of treatment was being used.

At this point it is necessary to discuss the pharmacopoeia of the New World medicine man. Erwin H. Ackerknecht, one of the outstanding experts in medical anthropology and the history of medicine, estimates that the medicine men of various tribal groups throughout the world had a pharmacopoeia that consisted of 25 to 50 percent active drugs! That is, drugs which produce some sort of effect (Ackerknecht 1942; reprinted in Lessa and Vogt 1958). This is not to say that the drug is always used in the proper manner with the proper dosage.

Ackerknecht was quite surprised at the high percentage of active drugs and hard put to explain this fact, given the basically non-scientific, if not irrational reasoning behind the treatment used. He therefore suggested:

Just as the ill man and the ill animal still instinctively choose their food, just as the ill animal eats herbs and performs other reflex-like healing measures . . . in the same way man or preman chooses his herbs (1958: 350).

This is an extremely heavy load to place upon "instinct," particularly when man is acknowledged to have the fewest directions given to him by his instincts.

What alternative is there to instinct? Ackerknecht had worked with primitive tribal groups and had examined the pharmacopoeia of many such groups. As a result of these studies he had seen no evidence of experimentation with new drugs and thus he ruled this out as a possible manner of selecting drugs. Here the problem is the history of the drug itself. In the Old World and the New World almost every available narcotic with psychogenic properties has been found and experimented with: coffee, tea, tobacco, yerba maté, peyote, marijuana, opium, alcohol, hallucinogenic mushrooms, and several other drugs (Cooper 1949). The earliest use of any of these drugs is buried in the past and in the mythology of the group. Any drug used is almost certain to have a long mythological background even though there may be evidence in the archaeological record that the use is recent. In many cultures of the world the innovator is viewed with suspicion if not alarm; the old ways are being changed and only in recent times have any cultures viewed the constant change of modern American and European societies as something that has a positive value. The result would thus be that anyone asking questions about an item in the cultural inventory is quite likely to be given an equivocal answer, or even a spurious one.

All of the above is to indicate that the investigators into the question — How did a medically unsophisticated aborigine come up with an effective drug? — could have been asking the wrong questions and been given the wrong answers.

In my investigations I have found that there is more than enough evidence to indicate that experimentation in the old-fashioned trial and error system is not unique to Western European societies, or even to "civilized" societies.

An entire area of interest in the field of anthropology has sprung up because of this special interest: ethnobotany — the uses of plants in aboriginal populations. The reason why Ackerknecht, and others, have not been able to show evidence of this experimentation is because the actual case histories and experimentors have long since been forgotten; the experimentation took place a long time ago.

Notwithstanding this time factor there is still evidence of testing. It is to be found in some few rare instances of the use of a drug by aboriginal populations, earlier than they were used by European medical men. Two rare instances are given: 1. Quinine as a treatment for malaria was developed in Peru by an unknown "witch doctor" and, since it was effective, was then used by Europeans to whom the medicine was being prescribed by sympathetic natives. (Malaria was a disease introduced in the New World.) Finally the European "medical profession" took up the drug (Garrison 1913: 290). 2. Curare, a rather unusual poison, was used by the Jívaro Indians of the Ecuadorian jungle. Matthew W. Stirling (1938: 84) gives a reasonable presentation which indicates the poison was first used during the seventeenth century and was unknown prior to that time. The effects of the poison were considered useful to European medicine only in the late 1930's and became an accepted but dangerous muscle relaxant in the 1940's and later.

Another drug which is not from an aboriginal population but again was treated with an amazing lack of understanding by the bulk of the medical profession is reserpine, a tranquilizer which had been used for centuries in India but was not accepted into the European pharmacopoeia until the late 1940's (it was the basis for Miltown).

One area of experimentation which was present but not available to researchers in primitive medicine was the use to which the drugs were ORIGINALLY put.

The author contends that the experimentation in much of the world was taken up in the attempt to find a secret potion that would kill one's enemy. If in addition to that it made him uncomfortable and he died in agony or embarrassment so much the better. Later came the realization that if a lot of a given drug brought certain death then maybe a little would produce effects but not cause death. Let us examine some of the plants that are effective drug plants in the Philippines to see if this idea has a reasonable chance of fitting. In the book, *The medicinal plants of the Philippines* (De Tavera 1901), a listing of all of the medicinal plants along with usages and dosages was made by a medical man trained in Europe but a native of the Philippines. In the listing of hundreds of plants with hundreds of different uses an amazing quantity turn out to be rather violent in their actions. Roughly one-third of the drugs are dangerous if taken in large dosages, many are emetics or cathartics, a few are vesicants. The normal use for most drugs was for vermifuges, emetics and cathartics. (The Philippines seem almost as bad as televisionland with respect to things to cure you.) The problem of efficiency in the use of the drug is compounded by the fact that units of measure are not accurate; few were even as accurate as the "pinch" of spice in modern recipes. Another feature is the circumstance that plants vary in their concentration of drugs. In most plants that have a drug effect the seeds carry a concentrated dosage, but this is modified by the wetness of the climate, the age of the plant, and the season. In addition, when dry it may not be as usable as when fresh. All of these problems were readily seen by those early investigators of drugs used in different parts of the world. They are passed on at this time to indicate that research was done but, due to the difficulty of such studies they did not produce much acceptance of native remedies (one might say they did not bear fruit).

As far as the native use of certain drugs, for example, poisons, we have the following: chopped-up whiskers of large cats such as leopards, tigers and jaguars are rumored to be used in charms. Sanderson (1937: 69) reports an experiment in which he fed chopped-up leopard whiskers to a monkey in its mush and, although the monkey did not like it he finally ate it. A few weeks later he died and autopsy revealed a "great number of small cyst-like inflammations deeply buried in the lining of the stomach wall. Upon opening these, I was most astounded to find a single chip of the leopard whisker (never two or more) quite unaltered, as on the day it was swallowed." The immediate cause of death, however, was bronchial pneumonia. In humans this material would produce an absolutely marvelous case of peritonitis and probably cause death.

The presence of arrow poisons (fish poisons are a different problem) such as aconite, curare, and strychnine is evidence of the fact that effective poisons are available in many areas of the world. Curare in fact is restricted to use with blow gun darts. Its use against humans is tabooed (Steward and Métraux 1948: 84ff; Stirling 1938). The rather ineffective arrow poison made with rattlesnake venom which is used by the Paiutes is likewise tabooed for use against humans. The belief in this case is that if it is used against humans it will lose its effectiveness against animals (Robert F. Heizer, personal communication). Southeast Asia and tropical Africa (the Pygmies) use arrow poisons against humans. In the tropical forest and montaña areas of South America a very large quantity of drugs was used and from the history of the area it would appear that they experimented with drugs (Steward and Faron 1959: 347) although until the breakdown of the culture the uses were restricted to the shamans (ibid.; see also Cooper 1949).

This latter piece of information fits in with the general hypothesis the author has attempted to develop — that the native populations of the world experimented with drugs and found those that were active and those that were dangerous poisons (in some instances these were the same drugs except the dosage was different). This experimentation was carried out by the shaman and the probable reason for the experimentation was the attempt to develop a new and better poison to be used to silence those selected for one reason or another.

REFERENCES

ACKERKNECHT, E. H.
  1942 *Bulletin of the history of medicine,* 11:503–521. (Reprinted 1958 in *Reader in comparative religion: an anthropological approach.* Edited by William A. Lessa and Evon Z. Vogt, 343–353. Evanston, Illinois and White Plains, New York: Row, Peterson.

1949   "Medical practices," in *Handbook of South American Indians*, volume five: *Comparative anthropology of South American Indians*. Edited by Julian H. Steward, 621–643. Bureau of American Ethnology Bulletin 143. Washington, D.C.: Smithsonian Institution.

COON, CARLETON S.
1962   *The origin of races*. New York: Knopf.

DE TAVERA, T. H. PARDO
1901   *The medicinal plants of the Philippines*. Translated and revised by J. B. Thomas, Jr. Philadephia: P. Blakiston's Son.

DRIVER, H.
1961   *Indians of North America*. Chicago: University of Chicago Press.

GARRISON, FIELDING H.
1913   *History of medicine with* . . . (reprinted July 1967). Philadelphia and London: W. B. Saunders.

HAGGARD, HOWARD W.
1929   *Devils, drugs and doctors*. New York and London: Harper & Bros.

HEIZER, ROBERT F.
1953   Aboriginal fish poisons. *Anthropological Papers* 38:225–283. Washington, D.C.: Smithsonian Institution.

SAHLINS, MARSHALL D.
1960   The origin of society. *Scientific American* (September): 2–13.

SANDERSON, IVAR T.
1937   *Animal treasure*. New York: The Viking Press.

STEWARD, J., L. C. FARON
1959   *Native peoples of South America*. New York and London: McGraw-Hill.

STEWARD, J. H., A. MÉTRAUX
1948   "Tribes of the Peruvian and Ecuadorian montaña," in *Handbook of South American Indians*, volume three: *Tropical forest tribes*. Edited by Julian H. Steward, 535–656. Bureau of American Ethnology Bulletin 143. Washington, D.C.: Smithsonian Institution.

STIRLING, MATTHEW W.
1938   *Historical and ethnographical material on the Jívaro Indians*. Bureau of American Ethnology Bulletin 117. Washington, D.C.: Smithsonian Institution.

The Relevance of African Traditional Medicine in Modern Medical Training and Practice

KIVUTO NDETI

It would seem inconceivable for any group of people, no matter what level of cultural development they may have attained, not to have empirically tested knowledge of medical science. The mere fact that they have lived in their environment for a prolonged period suggests that they have, to a certain extent, acquired enough homeopathic adaptation to enable them to survive. The factors of time and space are crucial variables in man's struggle to overcome the selective pressures exerted by the pathology of his environment. This point cannot be overemphasized when one realizes that human knowledge on the whole is acquired by the processes of trial and error. In other words, so long as people living in a particular territory are selected out by "mystical forces" (variously known as demons, diseases, spirits, germs, parasites, and viruses) it would seem most nonhuman not to discover some remedies to ward off these challenges to existence and the perpetuation of the species. Experience of any nature is man's best teacher; hence time and space provide a laboratory in which man experiments with reality in order to perpetuate his kind in the dynamic struggle for existence.

An attempt is made here to show the evolution of the types of men who, while believing mortality is the natural end of all living organisms, still challenge the causes and attempt to give rational explanations for its occurrence. The methods used in explaining the existence of these men draw from the physical, social, and humanistic sciences. These people are known by various designations in African societies (see Table 1).

From Table 1 several contrasts can be made based on some features of the surface structure of the languages (the terms "deep" and "sur-

Table 1.   Sample of African languages contrasting wisdom, sorcerer, and witch doctor

Informant	Language	Wisdom (W[1])	Sorcerer (S)	Witch doctor (W[2])
Maloba	Kiluhia	Obu-kesi (β)	Omu-losi (θ)	Omu-lesi (γ)
Muga	Dhaluo	Ri-eko (β)	Ja-jouk (θ)	Aju-oga (γ)
Bujra	Kiswahili	Bu-sara	M-chawi	M-ganga
Joroge	Kikuyu	U-ugi (β)	Mu-rogi	Mundu-mugo (γ)
Elsie	Luganda	Ma-gezi	Mu-logo	Muganga
Ndeti	Kikamba	-ui (β)	Mu-oi	Mundu-mue (γ)
Elaso	Kumamu	Ry-eko	Aj-wok	Emu-ron
Gutosi	Lumasaba	Kama-khula	Umu-wosi	Umu-sawu
Onyonka	Ekegusi	Ehi-semi	Mu-rogi	Omonya-mosira
Cecilia	Kisagara	—	Mh-awi	Mla-guzi
Yasufu	Arusha	—	—	Olo-ibon
Msaki	Chagga	Mh-re	Ms-awi	Mw-anga
Mblambuka	Matumbi	L-unda (β)	Mw-abi	F-undi (γ)
Masongo	Nyamwezi	Ma-sara	Ml-ogi	Mf-umu
Kingoria	Meru	U-ume	Mu-rogi	Mu-gaa
Keriasek	Maasai	Eng-eno (β)	—	Olo-iboni (γ)
Musikari	Bukusu	Bu-kesi (β)	Omu-losi	Omu-ng'osi (γ)
Msawi	Kirombo	—	Ms-avi	Mw-anga
Makama	Lusoga	Ama-gezi (β)	Omu-sezi (θ)	Omulu-guzi (γ)
Ejiogu	Ibo	N-zu	Omu-su	Di-bia
Vanda	Kikinga	Ama-aka (β)	Mh-awi	Ug-anga (γ)
Akiiki	Rutoro	Om-gezi	Omu-rogo	Omu-fumu

face" structures are used to characterize two very important components of a language). Deep structure in this sense means the semantic aspect of language while the surface structure applies to the phonological aspect. The two components are the most basic characters of a natural language (Lenneberg 1968: 397). For the sake of analysis W[1], S and W[2] are used where W[1] = Wisdom, S = Sorcerer and W[2] = Witch doctor. Also β, Θ and γ are used corresponding to the W[1], S and W[2] to indicate the categories of overlapping. The contrasts are as follows:

1. W[1] versus W[2] = 40.9 percent overlap of the basic components marked by β and γ respectively
2. W[1] versus S = 13.6 percent overlap of the basic components marked by β and Θ respectively
3. W[2] versus S = 13.6 percent overlap of the basic components marked by γ and Θ respectively

Column S, on the basis of the surface features, seems to fall into three broad categories. The morphemes of category [-o-i $_{(o)}$] consist of 45.5 percent of the total column entries. The second morphemic category of [a $_{(e)}$ -il] consists of 31.8 percent of the total. The rest fall in the third category which for convenience will be indicated by [-n], meaning a different language family or a prolonged separation which lacks obvious contrast. The morphemes in this category consist of 22.7 percent of the total. Although the writer depended entirely on the orthography of the informant in writing down these morphemes, the fact that such nice morphemic categories are not obvious in W^1 or W^2 suggests the uniqueness of S in the cultures represented by the sample. The factor of the language family in the sample does not seem to play a significant role in establishing the overlap correlations of W^1, S and W^2.

However, the table was used to establish the fact that there is a basic correlation between the terms "wisdom" and "witch doctor" in many traditional African languages. Although this sample takes only a few Sudanic and mainly East African Bantu languages, it shows conclusively that there is a 45.5 percent overlap between W^1 and W^2 on surface structures and to a certain extent on deep structures. Thus the name of a witch doctor in the majority of African languages coincides with wisdom. He was always a man with wisdom based on practical knowledge. Unlike his counterpart, the sorcerer (a sinister character or night runner), he practiced his work in public. In the majority of cases, there was little mystery surrounding his art. It was an open secret that anyone could scrutinize.

On the other hand, lower percentages of overlap between S and either W^1 or W^2 may be attributed to chance or uncritical orthography of the informant. This means that, while most African medical practices have been identified with S, there is little or no empirical evidence which supports the identification. Whatever functions S may carry out in a given African society, there is little or no correlation with either wisdom or the art of healing. At least this is true for the sample given above. However, no one should be under the impression that this sinister character has no function in African society. He has his place, mysterious as it may be.

Let us now take another aspect of the art of the traditional doctor. He is often accused of being "Jack of all trades but master of none" by his professional colleagues in modern medicine. Like a philosopher, he knows everything about all diseases but nothing about any particular one. His diagnoses are marred by the aura of mystery and so are some of his therapies. Furthermore, he has no formal scientific training in modern medical science. Most of his work is guesswork. He does not understand the magnitude of things like germ theory, or cause and effect of disease dynamics. His surgical practices, to say the least, are very primitive and backward. Although he may give an herbal prescription, in the majority of cases this is nonscientific. He is a clever rascal and to a certain extent an extortionist. He is a barrier to the progress of modern medical practice in the rural areas of the developing countries and at least a threat to progress as a whole. He relies too much on the spirits of ancestors when diagnosing obvious cases such as diarrhea, malaria, gonorrhea, syphilis, goitre, schistosomiasis, trypanosomiasis, pains, or just the common cold. For most of these diseases, cases can be effectively cured if scientific methods are properly applied.

Many of these accusations do apply to some traditional doctors. Not all witch doctors are good doctors or are motivated by alleviation of human suffering. Some of them, like some modern doctors, can be racketeers and exploiters who overcharge their patients in exchange for very mediocre medical services. This is an accusation which can be leveled against professionals in other areas as well. There are those who enter a profession with specific motives of material gain. These characters are interested in their profession as a means to an end rather than as an end in itself. There is no doubt that in the profession of traditional medicine, which carried so much honor and prestige in African societies, such amateur native doctors existed. Even now, some are still around, human nature being what it is.

The allegations against them apply largely to some part-time witch doctors, and no intelligent person would condone the barriers they put in the way of progress in medical science and public health programs in the developing countries. In some cases they are so notorious that the government is called upon to curb their activities. In this way the government protects its citizens against fanatic ideas, practitioners who are emotionally disturbed, and the exploitation of certain traditional medical arts as a convenient means of personal aggrandizement.

On the other hand there are individuals who enter a profession in response to a vocational call. They take their vocation with seriousness and purpose. They take the training in the same way. Such vocational dedication seems to come from the individual's serious consideration of the meaning of the human condition and its relation to general schemes of human destiny. It is even possible that some individuals might be motivated by selfishness but still work for noble ends insofar as they consider the welfare of humanity. Others might be motivated by sheer honesty and tenacity of purpose. In such cases vocation is conceived of as a realization of man's fulfillment in human spirit.

In traditional "medicine-man-ship" there were many individuals with such a noble view of their vocation. Thus, in Table 1, there are various terms describing the qualities of the witch doctor. In Kisagara he is called *mlaguzi* [diviner or person who possesses the ability to divine]. In Kirombo he is known as *mwanga* [light]. In other words, he is a leading star of his community. In Luganda he is described as *muganga* [curer, healer, remedy]. In Ekegusi he is known as *omanyamosira* [he who posesses power to treat any organism]. In Kikuyu he is known as *mundu-mugo* [wise man, seer, diviner]. In Kikamba he is called *mundu-mue* [diviner, seer, rainmaker, wise man]. In Bukusu he is called *omung'osi* [cultural hero, big powerful man]. In Maasai he is called *oloiboni* [he who performs good acts and has no counterpart anywhere else].

All these designations point out clearly that a native doctor in traditional African societies was a man of critical mind endowed with many abilities and he was dedicated to his vocation. He was well informed about the problems of his environment and possessed practical knowledge of botany (herbistry), pathology, psychology (divination), surgery, animal and plant curative agents, climatology, cosmology, sociology, and psychiatry. He was a man renowned for his critical abilities. Thus criticisms leveled against him by his modern professional colleagues do not apply in all cases. It is true that questions can be raised concerning his medical education. But no one should forget that the native doctor worked within the means and provisions of his culture. Lack of effective media of communication such as writing and the proper keeping of professional records limited the transmission of professional ideas to the following generations.

This, however, does not mean the traditional doctor was not professionally competent in any given generation. Oral history, folktales, stories, and folklore kept alive many important ideas for generations. These means of keeping ideas and records of the significant events in the history of a community may not seem effective and accurate because of our own biases. It is known, however, that events recorded orally can be as authentic as historical documents (Vansina 1968). Limited though the media of transmission may have been, important ideas still managed to filter through. Also in many cases the witch doctor had an apprentice or an heir apparent. He guarded and carried the medicine man's herbs, divining apparatus, and all the other items involved in the art of healing. Upon the death of the witch doctor, the apprentice or his close follower always inherited his healing arts.

Let us now turn to another matter raised by criticisms of the native doctor, some of which bring up a very fundamental problem in medical science. The medicine man was thought of as one who employs all types of techniques and therapies in the treatment of his patients. The handling of patients in this manner, however, takes into consideration the phenomena of pathology and the nature of the human body, and the witch doctor's therapeutic techniques stem from these considerations. Disease will be discussed both from the witch doctor's and the patient's point of view. The following cases, observed some time ago, represent various efforts in understanding the concept of disease dynamics. The cases were observed in villages in Tanzania and Kenya.

The first incident took place in 1953. The case involved a little girl who had recurrent illnesses including abscesses, malaria, measles and eye infections. The uncle in charge of this little girl was undoubtedly familiar with these diseases. But what he could not account for was the fact that these illnesses followed one after another; and even after the cycle was completed some of them reappeared. In the second cycle the eye infection had progressed to a bleeding stage. At this point the uncle decided to break away from modern medical practice which so far had proved ineffective. He was convinced by then that there was a spiritual force behind the patient's illnesses which had not been taken care of by the drugs. He therefore decided to offer a special prayer to the ancestral spirits, asking them for an explanation of this misfortune and also for a remedy. While the prayer was being said, flour and water were sprinkled on the patient as if to cleanse her from the wrath of the ancestors. The chanting of the prayer was as follows:

Mvose mwe akena Nhelua na mwe kena Anatoli mkagone. Nagwee Nhelua mwenyego haukanilongela nimsole ayumwana. Sambi ni choni mala ino ni maipu, mala ingi ni mtwe mtwe mala ingi ni meso negano meso gasambi ninhali kugaona na damu yangulawa umo! Mkagone mwvose, akina Mwambalile, mlekeni mwana asome.

The uncle was talking to his dead father and mother requesting them to leave this child alone. He reminded them of their decision, when they were on this world, to give him (the uncle) charge of this girl. He urged them to rest in peace. To his greatest satisfaction and in accord with his belief, this alternative therapy worked. Eventually the girl got well.

Another case took place in 1966 and involved a sixteen-year-old girl who was attending a girl's boarding school. The headmistress reported to her parents that she was ill. When the parents arrived at the school they found she had somewhat lost her mind. She was taken to a hospital where a physician diagnosed a case of cerebral malaria. She was treated for a while and finally recovered. However, she developed other complications later. She began to bleed in the eyes, a condition which continued for almost two years. During this time she was taken to several eye specialists including some in Kenyatta Hospital. The doctors examining her eyes could not diagnose any defect whatsoever. The girl was sent home. The parents, who are modern in their ways and education, decided to try traditional medicine. They called a traditional medicine man and secretly asked him to treat the girl.

One of the first things the medicine man did in diagnosing the case was to consider at great length the geneological history of the girl on the mother's and father's lines of descent. To the surprise of everyone it was found that some of the dead ancestors in the mother's line had cases of eye disease. The native doctor told the patient's parents it was the ancestors of the girl who wanted some blood. He ordered that they kill a goat and have the girl wash her face and eyes with warm blood. The witch doctor went into the bush and fetched some herbs which he later mashed. He added some soup from the goat meat and asked the girl to drink it. The following day he brought in another herbal medicine in the form of powder and applied it to the patient's eyes. He advised the parents to make arrangements for a traditional dance where the girl would be invited to participate. The native doctor's orders were carried out and to the amazement of the parents the girl was cured and since then she has gone back to school.

The third case took place in 1967 in a small village in Kenya. The incident involved a man of about thirty-five years. He had been complaining for a long time of pains in the chest, headaches and aching knees. A native doctor was called and he diagnosed the case as being caused by witchcraft. Someone in the village had introduced some little organisms which caused the pains that he was experiencing. The pains and aches resulted from the fact that the little organisms moved like grazing cows from the head through the chest to the knees. The native doctor told the patient that he was going to arrest the organisms while they were migrating into different areas. He made incisions in the aching parts of the head and covered the bleeding parts with a cow's horn, called *chuku/mbibi*. By drawing out air from the horn chamber he caused blood to flow from the head through the incisions. He repeated the same process with other aching parts. In all cases coagulated blood came out. He then applied a thick liquid-like herbal concoction on all the incised parts. He then took some of the coagulated blood from different areas and asked for a live chicken. He forced the chicken to swallow the blood. He took both the chicken and the patient with him to a place where several paths converged. He released the chicken at that spot ordering it to take the patient's illness to the person who caused it. He came back with his patient and a few days later the man was cured. The patient had a child of about six years of age who had a swollen leg. The witch doctor examined it and said it was a case of a boil situated near the bone, adding that he would prescribe a specific medicine that would draw the boil from the bone area to a particular spot on the surface of the leg. He went out to collect the medicine and came back with roots and leaves of various plants. He crushed them in a mortar and pestle until they formed a paste. He then located a place on the leg where he wanted the boil to come through. He applied the paste and a few days later the boil appeared on the spot. He pierced the boil with a sharp point and a lot of pus flowed out. Then he washed the wound with an herbal solution and in a few days the child was cured.

These incidents, although observed in different parts of East Africa, raise a profound and fundamental problem in medical science as conceived by African traditional practitioners. From the citations and the general understanding of the operations of the native doctor, several theories or ideas of disease emerge. There is no doubt in the mind of a native doctor that disease is an external force which enters a human body in a specific way and interferes with the normal bodily functions. For the sake of analysis these external forces will be divided into two classes.

In African medicine, the concept of disease first takes into account the role of the spirits of dead ancestors. This concept cuts across almost all African societies. Because of the organic and psychological relations that exist between the living and the dead, the spirits of dead ancestors seem to take keen interest in the affairs of the living. They mysteriously regulate the general conduct of individuals in African societies. Those who deviate from the normal activities in the culture, such as refusing to offer sacrifice to ancestors, disobeying cultural ethics, doing injustice to others, refusing to cooperate with others for the general good or ignoring one's responsibilities to himself and others must pay the price individually. The spirits do not discriminate in their attacks. Their victims include both adults and children. Their activities, however, are concentrated on the adults. Children are hardly ever possessed as adults are. The attack on the children seems to be a consequence of negligence on the part of adults in maintaining peaceful coexistence with ancestral codes. Animals and plants also follow suit because of this general ignorance.

This concept of disease as originating with mischievous and dangerous spirits takes into consideration the cultural reality of human life. The fact is that the memory of the dead ancestor haunts human reality. Culture helps one to rationalize the reality of death as an inevitable ending of human life. Although man is a mortal being, as the maxim states, fundamentally and emotionally man is afraid of death. The fact that death is the greatest shock is deeply rooted in human consciousness. This psychological shock constantly reminds man in the African culture that the only conceivable relationship that exists, after the disintegration of the dead body, is in an intangible reality. The encounter between the living and the dead must therefore be through spirits. Also the fact that after death only spirit remains raises the question of the power of spirit. If spirit cannot die then it must be above the power of death and consequently it must control death. This is a logical construct, but when one considers the whole phenomenon, including the theology of death, one cannot help feeling that a native doctor's involvement of spirits in his therapies is not as foolish as it might seem from superficial analyses by modern doctors. Perhaps the concept of disease could be further clarified by taking another line of approach. That is, the psychological myths of African experience bind the living to the dead through the spirits. The living are a culmination of a long historical chain tracing back to the beginnings of things. This is what every culture in fact teaches its followers. Hence why would a modern doctor find it so difficult to understand the native doctor's method of incorporating the psychological and cultural realities of African experience in therapy? It would seem, human nature being what it is, that all diseases, real or imaginary, are to a large extent psychosomatic. Physiological malfunctions which occur in a human body will undoubtedly have an effect on the psychological orientation of the individual or *vice versa*.

Let us move to the second concept of disease. Unlike the first, this concept reduces the cause of the disease to the organic level. This is quite evident in all citations. The fact that special effort is made to treat the human body with herbs or by any other means of organic nature indicates the assumption that sickness in a human body has an organic basis. These organic antagonists interfering with normal bodily functions can be conceived as antigen-antibody reactions in modern medicine, or *Nyamu/Nhamu* in the native doctor's terminology. In medical science today the antigen-antibody reactions are due to the fact that when foreign bodies enter a "normal" human body the natural resistance of the body mounts an attack to counteract foreign organisms. The native doctor recognizes these foreign objects and he names them

Nyamu or *Nhamu* which, according to some Bantu languages, literally means "vicious little organisms" which cause death and can be passed from one person to another. These organisms as understood from the witch doctor's language seem to adhere beneath the human nails and when swallowed with food or drink cause illness and consequently death. Among the Akamba there is an old saying: *vai utinda na mukundu ndakunduke* [he who stays around a person suffering from skin rash is also likely to get it]. From these remarks it is untrue to claim that a witch doctor did not understand concepts such as those of germ theory, infectious disease, and disease dynamics. It is very likely that he did not understand the biology of the organisms. He did not categorize them into viruses, bacteria or parasites. Nonetheless, his healing technique and use of drugs leave no doubt about his knowledge of organisms as the cause of some diseases. On the whole, one can strongly argue that the native doctor understood clearly the psychological and organic basis of diseases.

The standard technique of modern medicine is the use of physicochemical means for controlling pathology. Remarkable strides have been made in this approach to human disease. Indeed the area has grown so fast since the beginning of this century that it has been almost imposible for any physician to keep up to date with literature on production of drugs. Because there are many full-time scientist-physicians engaged in pure research in such areas as nuclear medicine, space medicine and the technology of medicine, we may expect more startling medical discoveries in the future. The tendency now is to have some specialists who keep up with these advances in medicine and who can advise the general physician on the use of these new drugs and techniques. The specialist's advice, however, is not always immune from human error. When the advice is uncritical, it can have a serious consequence, as in the case of thalidomide. This drug was widely used in many Western countries as a means to relieve tension and pain in pregnant women. But the drug proved to be mutagenic; women who had been taking it for some time gave birth to deformed children. Because of professional cults and private financial interests it took some time to convince medical practitioners and entrepreneurs that the drug was responsible for deformation of children. Consequently there is now a whole thalidomide generation. Similar mistakes have been made in other areas of scientific activity as well. Nonetheless, this is the price that man must pay for his scientific activity if precautions are not taken.

The discovery of antibiotics is another landmark in the progress of medicine. They are used to boost the energy of resistance factors to fight many pathological agents in the body. Surgery is another area which recently has caused mixed reactions because of heart transplants. Although still in dispute by some physicians because of its inability to produce effective drug therapies, psychiatry is another active area of modern medicine. The impact of psychiatry is felt in the area of mental health which to date is a serious problem in the technologically advanced countries. According to some experts there seems to be a correlation between the incidence of mental illness and fast technological change in some countries.

In many of these countries social institutions have not kept up with rapid and vast changes brought about by innovations in science and technology. Because the need for industrial development has become a matter of urgency in the underdeveloped countries if they are to survive, the incidence of mental illness is also like to increase. Hence, facilities for psychiatric treatment become a necessary corollary. For instance, in educational institutions such as universities or colleges, in addition to having a physician to take care of specific diseases there is also a psychiatrist who takes care of the mental health of students. In the law courts as well, prior to a trial for murder or any other serious crime, a psychiatrist is consulted in most cases to ascertain whether the criminal was in good mental condition when the crime was committed. Thus whether this aspect of modern medicine is scientific or not, its importance cannot be overemphasized. If he fails to recognize it, a physician's work is half done.

The native doctor is not as sophisticated as his modern counterpart. His training is not as formal as that of a modern doctor. However, he follows closely what seems to be the ideal practice of a physician. He recognizes the important role that culture plays in the phenomenon of human diseases. He refuses to accept the simple-minded philosophy that a diseased human body is a collection of pathological states. Or rather, he accepts that philosophy but goes beyond factual information. The physico-chemical approach to disease in the form of liquified or powdered herbs is a clear indication of factual cognition of the basis of human disease. It is in this physico-chemical approach to the treatment of disease that most triumphs have been realized in modern medicine, and nobody doubts that greater triumphs are yet to come. Advances in molecular medicine for the treatment of human diseases are currently a popular idea among many practitioners of modern medicine. Indeed this seems to be one of the reasons put forward for more emphasis on biochemistry, physics and molecular biology in most of the curricula of medical education. This emphasis helps to upgrade medical education from its present status as a "service science," for ideas discovered in other branches of science, to a positive science.

The witch doctor is a part of this belief insofar as he is an herbalist. But he transcends the limits of the molecular approach. He takes into account the powerful influences and interplay of an individual with his family, his culture and his environment. All these affect his bodily states. Also he recognizes the fact that human beings are constituted of psychic and physical realities which are distinct but not separate. They interact and influence each other in all conscious and subconscious acts. For example, the unhealthy body threatens the existence of the soul which forms the principle of life. On the other hand, psychic derangement is easily translated into physical acts. In view of these two realities constituting the phenomenon of man, no treatment or therapy would be complete if it considered only one of the two. The native doctor is extremely aware of the two distinct aspects of man and they form his philosophy of medical practice:

The shaman, like the physician, tried to cure his patient by correcting the causes of his illness. In line with his culture's concept of disease, this cure may involve not only the administration of the therapeutic agents, but provision of the means for confession, atonement, restoration into the good graces of the family and tribe and intercession with the world of the spirit. The shaman's role may thus involve aspects of the roles of physician, magician, priest, moral arbiter, representative of group's world view and agent of social control (Kiev 1964: vii).

The above statement regarding the work of the shaman would be quite appropriate in defining the functions of a good modern doctor. There is a lot of psychology involved in the doctor-patient relation in medicine. While a doctor must use objective methods in evaluating the patient's health complaints, he should also pay serious attention to other factors such as the patient's verbal self-diagnosis. In order to understand and interpret the patient's health problems it seems absolutely essential for a good doctor to know his client's background. This issue raises a very important point in the training of a doctor. In older countries medical education strongly emphasizes curative medicine. In fact, great advances in medicine are found in this area. Although the cliché that "prevention is better than cure" is still kicked around among medical men, not much allocation of money or staff is given to preventive medicine. This is particularly so in developing countries:

Mr. Chairman, one thing you said which I find difficult to accept, is that there is an over-emphasis in Africa between preventive services and curative services, and that the emphasis is in favour of preventive services. I will agree with you that in the last 10 years there have been unfortunate repetitious statements about the need to emphasize preventive medicine, but the emphasis has not been reflected in actual services. . . . If there is an over-emphasis, let it be reflected in the allocation of staff or funds (Sai 1968: 34).

This area of medicine is also most difficult because so much of its success depends on understanding of cultures and behavior of the people on whose behalf the health programs are being implemented. Thus, training of a doctor must give serious consideration to all factors relevant to human behavior. Thus, the introduction of social and behavioral sciences into a medical curriculum is not just an additional unnecessary burden for medical students but extremely useful knowledge which will prove most effective in their professional practice. This call for a rethinking of medical education, especially in the underdeveloped countries, is heard in many medical encounters. The old, orthodox approach to medical training has lately come under severe attack by some critics, as reflected in the following statement:

The "biological principles" bandied about by an earlier or older generation of physicians are, most of them, nonsense — among them the deep-seated and all but ineradicable belief that natural dispositions and adaptations are well-nigh perfect, and that sickness and other disabilities are part of a long-drawn-out expiation for leaving nature and leading unnatural lives. A case can be made for thinking out medical education anew and building it upon a foundation of human biology. . . . As matters stand, human genetics makes its appearance, if at all, as a supernumerary course fitted somewhere into the clinical years; demography is mixed up with sanitation, and human ecology is treated as something which, though it may help us to understand the medical predicaments of foreigners, is barely relevant to our own cosy domestic medical scene (Medawar 1964: vi).

The British Medical Association recently announced the inclusion of behavioral sciences in medical training curricula, possibly in response to calls similar to the one cited above by Medawar.

Needless to retort that the native doctor knew all along that human diseases of whatever nature were psychosomatic. By psychosomatic it is meant that health problems of whatever magnitude are likely to affect the "normal functions" of an individual on both physical and psychological levels. Because of this realization he made sure that the diseased body got its share of herbs, and psychological imbalances were restored. The psychotherapies took the forms of divination, confession, restoration of faith in the dead ancestors, offerings and "bibliotherapy." The native doctor prescribed dances in accordance with traditional culture. The dances were meant to entertain the spirits so that they would keep away all the afflictions which cause human suffering. Voodoo and *Zambi*, found in many African cultures, are in this category of dances. In addition, the dances formed an excellent base for group therapy. It provided a free climate for catharsis.

In sum, a witch doctor treated effectively the three broad categories of diseases recognized in modern or scientific medicine:

1. SPECIFIC DISEASES: The diseases in this class were fairly well known to the witch doctor. He knew specific herbs that he could administer and get the expected result. In modern medicine diseases in this category are not many.

2. SYMPTOMATIC DISEASES: The diseases in this group involved both herbal treatment and a psychological result. In other words the witch doctor gave an herb which reduced the symptom of disease in the patient without necessarily changing his pathological state.

3. PSYCHOLOGICAL DISEASES: The witch doctor gave psychological therapies in addition to bibliotherapy. In this way he was able to improve the feeling of the patient without necessarily changing his pathological condition. A good doctor in the modern sense has to be more or less like the traditional native doctor. He is not a specialist who treats only specific diseases but also one who treats nonspecific diseases, that is, symptomatic and psychological ones which make up as much as 90 percent of all known diseases.

Finally, the art of healing, whether modern or traditional, cannot escape the paraphernalia which surround the mystery of curing agents. There is a great deal of scientific emphasis in modern medicine and this is well and good in all fairness to science. However, in view of the quackery and mystery of healing agents, human nature being what it is, scientific medicine would do better and would advance its professional goals if it recognized the legitimacy of the so-called nonscientific approach to human healing. This nonscientific approach seems as if it will always be there in one form or another. To date, beliefs such as Christian Science, divination, palmistry, superstition, occultism, fortune-telling, magic, soothsaying, miracle healing, exorcism, possession, witchcraft, will of God, fatalism, shamanism, juju and voodoo, are still in existence. These beliefs are as old as man. They figure very much in the inner reality of human life. So far they have been a hindrance to the progress of so-called scientific medicine in many parts of the world. Modern medicine would do better if it stopped adhering to the cult of science and professionalism. Even the most ambitious program geared to eradicating a specific disease is doomed to failure if the planner fails to recognize the complexity and relevance of cultural institutions in the matter. An example of such failure was the effort made by the World Health Organization to eliminate schistosomiasis in the countries along the Nile Valley where the disease is endemic. One of the barriers to complete eradication of schistosomiasis is the Islamic tradition. The religious rite of washing the genitalia after excretion acts as a medium of transmission of the disease. In order to institute an effective control of the parasite, modern medical men would have to ban the rite. Yet it does not seem likely that devoted Muslims would give up an age-old holy rite in response to medical advice. It would be a wise move for scientific medicine to meet tradition half-way in such matters.

This also applies to the relation between the witch doctor and his modern counterpart. In view of its activities, powers, limitations and the very nature of the subject, modern medicine must accept and recognize the reality of the native doctor. He is a very important part of the medical scene and possesses legitimate knowledge essential for medical science. Professional jealousies, cults and god-complexes surrounding modern medicine should be shunned, and all the hypocrisy thereof. Therapies and treatments performed by witch doctors should be examined critically and the relevant elements should be adopted into modern education. They touch many vital areas which are beyond the imagination of the present medical education and they are wholesome in approach. This is a virtue which modern medical science cannot afford to condemn.

REFERENCES

HARRISON, G. A., J. S. WEINER, J. M. TANNER, N. A. BARNICOT, *editors*
    1964   *Human biology: an introduction to human evolution, variation and growth*. New York: Oxford University Press.
INTERNATIONAL PLANNED PARENTHOOD FEDERATION
    1968   *The role of family planning in African development*. Hertford: Stephen Austin and Sons.
KIEV, A., *editor*
    1964   *Magic, faith and healing studies in primitive psychiatry today*. London: Collier-Macmillan.
LENNEBERG, E. H.
    1967   *Biological foundations of language*. New York: John Wiley and Sons.
MEDAWAR, P. B.
    1964   "Foreword," in *Human biology: an introduction to human evolution, variation, and growth*. Edited by G. A. Harrison, et al. v-vi. New York: Oxford University Press.

NDETI, K.
1972a *Elements of Akamba life.* Nairobi: East African Publishing House.
1972b Socio-cultural aspects of tuberculosis defaultation: a case study. *Journal of Social Science and Medicine* 6:397–412.
SAI, F. T.
1968 "Useful entry points for preventive medical services," in *The role of family planning in African development.* Edited by International Planned Parenthood Federation, 34–36. Hertford: Stephen Austin and Sons.
VANSINA, J.
1968 "The use of ethnographic data as sources for history," in *Emerging themes of African history.* Nairobi: East African Publishing House.

Body and Spirit among the Sanumá (Yanoama) of North Brazil

KENNETH I. TAYLOR

This paper is a discussion of one aspect of the supernatural beliefs relating to the shamanism of the Sanumá Indians of the upper Auaris River valley in the northwest of Roraima Territory in northern Brazil.[1] This has to do especially with the nature of the relationship between one category of the assistant spirits used in Sanumá shamanism — the faunal *hekula* — and human society.

The Sanumá are tropical forest slash-and-burn horticulturalists who also depend considerably on the results of regular hunting of game birds and animals and the gathering of wild forest products. Their main crops are bitter manioc, plantains, and bananas; their more important game animals are tapir, peccaries, monkeys, paca, agouti, and armadillos. They are still an isolated group, their only regular contact with outsiders being with missionaries and Makiritare Indians (known as Maiongong in Brazil). They are one of four main subgroups (Yanomami, Yanomam, Yanam, and Sanumá) of the Yanoama[2] of north Brazil and south Vene-

[1]   My understanding of shamanism as practiced in the upper Auaris region shows a number of differences of detail from that reported for other subgroups of the Yanoama, and even for other Sanumá. It should be understood, then, that this paper is based on my own data and observations. My information was collected primarily in two settlements (Auaris and Kadimani) and is based on regular observation throughout a twenty-three-month period of fieldwork (between April 1968 and September 1970), including five months during which I devoted some half of my interview work to certain aspects of shamanism.

The fieldwork was conducted jointly with that of Alcida R. Ramos, and I am much indebted to her for useful comments on this paper. Some preliminary results of our research are: Ramos (n.d., 1972); Taylor (1971a, 1971b, 1972).

The research was financed by a National Science Foundation doctoral dissertation grant, which support is gratefully acknowledged.
[2]   Also known in the literature as Waika, Shiriana, Guaharibo, Shamatari, etc.

zuela. This is a linguistic division, each subgroup consisting of the speakers of one of the four closely related languages of the Yanoama language family (Migliazza 1972).

The shamanism of the Sanumá of the upper Auaris region is based entirely on the use of assistant spirits (*hekula dibi*) to act on the shaman's behalf. Shamanism is used primarily in curing, which involves the destruction or chasing away, by the shaman's *hekula*, of those other spirits (which can be of several different types) which have caused or which intend to bring about sickness and death. It can also be used to ensure hunting success. Another possibility is to "shamanize," that is, to ask certain *hekula* (which can also be used in curing, etc.) to attack and kill the enemies of one's group. In each case the shaman's role is simply to call the appropriate *hekula*, from the many at his disposal, and present them with the problem at hand.

The relationship between the *hekula* and their shaman, and that between the people of his village and allied villages, is one of benevolent, helpful cooperation. With certain qualifications this seems to be true of all *hekula*, but it is particularly so in the case of those which are the spirits of dead animals.[3] It would not, however, be correct to say that these faunal *hekula* exist simply to serve mankind. In fact, by no means do all faunal *hekula* do so. The demography and life spans of animal and human populations are such that there are always more faunal *hekula* available than there are shamans to use them. This remains the case even after allowing for the fact that older shamans often have several *hekula* of a given animal species living in their chests — one, or one pair, from each of several specified distant territories. When it comes time for a shaman to call a *hekula* to his service, to come and live in his chest, there is always a plentiful supply of faunal *hekula* in any given house of their species. Nevertheless, those faunal *hekula* which do function as assistant spirits to a shaman do so in a highly cooperative, helpful way.

I am describing the faunal *hekula* of Sanumá shamanism as essentially helpful and cooperative. This can be compared with the equivalent information, where available, as contained in other researchers' reports. Zerries (1955:81) mentions use of the *hekula* only in terms of their being induced "to bring mishap and sickness to the enemies of the village." Wilbert (1963) speaks of both the killing and curing powers of the *hekula*, but explains that he has the impression that the actions of the *hekula* are

---

[3]   The Sanumá category which I refer to here as "animals" — *salo bi* — may be more accurately glossed as 'edible fauna'. It includes birds, mammals, fish, amphibians, some insects, snakes, etc. For a more detailed discussion of the concept, see Taylor (1972:217–220).

only in response to the wishes and direction of the shaman. De Barandiaran, who criticizes other missionaries for calling the *hekula* demons or evil spirits, says that they are at all times on the watch and waiting for the shaman's call for help. His account deals almost exclusively with curing shamanism, though he does include the introduction of a "hostile" *hekula* into the body of the patient, by an enemy shaman, as one possible cause of sickness (1965:26).

Chagnon emphasizes the contribution of the *hekula* to the pattern of inter-village hostility, in their causing sickness and death. Their function in curing he mentions only in passing, and evidently considers the *hekula* to be essentially evil, calling them "demons" and "evil spirits" (1968:24, 45, 51, 52, 90). The incidence of inter-village raiding and associated hostile relations is very much lower for the Sanumá than for the Yanomami of the Mavaca River area. Thus the enemy-killing function of the *hekula* can be expected to receive less emphasis among the Sanumá. Nevertheless, I would insist that the difference must be one of emphasis only and the general nature of the *hekula* (helpful and cooperative, whether in curing one's kinsmen or in killing one's enemies) remains the same for both the Sanumá and the Yanomami. Whatever evil is involved is human. The *hekula* simply oblige by doing what the shaman asks of them.

In the soundtrack to the film *Magical Death* (1971), Chagnon gives a more satisfactory impression of the *hekula*. The film is, of course, specifically about a session of shamanism for the purpose of killing enemy children, but in the soundtrack full recognition is also given to the curing function of the *hekula*, and it is also made clear that their action in either curing or killing is entirely at the behest of the shamans. Goetz (1969) gives a well-balanced account of the *hekula* as assistant spirits which help the shaman both in attacking and interfering with the food supply of his enemies, and in protecting, helping, and curing his own people. Helena Valero's information on Yanomami shamanism, in Biocca (1971), also tells of the *hekula* as spirits which are used by shamans both against enemies and in curing fellow villagers. Thus, in spite of differences of detail and fullness of information, and with the exception only of Chagnon (1968), there is general agreement that (at least for the Sanumá and Yanomami subgroups) the *hekula* act only at the request of the shamans and in such a way as to cooperate with them in their intra- and inter-village relations.

My purpose is, then, to attempt an explanation, within the terms of the Sanumá belief system itself, for the especially cooperative character of the faunal category of *hekula*. The explanation I shall suggest is not expressed as such by the Sanumá, but it is implicit, and can be readily discerned, in the series of beliefs concerning the mythological status, and the present-day life cycle of the faunal beings. In mythological times the ancestors of animal species, just as the other beings of that time, were corporeal, humanoid in both body and spirit, and indestructible. When they were transformed into animals they lost this condition, becoming animaloid and destructible. The cooperative nature of the faunal *hekula* can, then, be understood as part of an attempt on their part to re-establish, to the extent that present-day circumstances permit, the situation of their mythological ancestors, i.e. that of humanoid appearance, indestructibility, and corporeality.

GENERAL CHARACTER OF SANUMÁ SHAMANISM

The Several Types of Shamanism

I have data on five principal types of shamanism. These are:
(1) curing shamanism;
(2) protection from evil spirits, etc.;
(3) festival hunting shamanism;
(4) other hunting shamanism; and
(5) shamanism to attack enemies.

CURING SHAMANISM   A Sanumá becomes ill as a result of the action of evil spirits, ghosts, the spirits of dead animals offended by the breaking of taboos, or human enemies using supernatural means of attack. One of these means of attack is the type of shamanism in which certain *hekula* can be sent to cause sickness in enemy villages. Supernatural attack also includes that of night raiders (*õka dibi*) using magical preparations and techniques. This kind of attack is not responded to with shamanism, and so does not relate to my topic in this paper.

In most cases of illness, where the cause is spirit action, the *hekula* used in shamanism are, if powerful enough in a given case, able to cure the victim by killing or scaring away the offending spirit and by extracting or ejecting the illness (which may involve a pathogenic object) from the patient's body. This shamanism for the purpose of curing is, in fact, a fairly constant occurrence. It was by far the most common type of shamanism observed during the fieldwork.

Curing shamanism is, however, only one of several kinds of shamanism used. These all follow the same basic procedure of calling the *hekula* for assistance, and turning the matter over to them for their action.

PROTECTION FROM EVIL SPIRITS OR ENEMY HEKULA When there is reason to believe that *sai dibi* (evil spirits) are in the vicinity of the village (typically, if not invariably, with the purpose of causing sickness), shamanism is used to scare these spirits away, or at least to divert their attention to some other village. On one occasion when a neighbor had spent most of the night shamanizing, he said it had been because his *hekula* had awakened him to warn him that the *sai de* which causes malaria had been on its way to the village. He was able to persuade it not to harm anyone at his community (Auaris) and had sent it off to the north, to a village of Sanumá who rarely if ever have any contact with the Auaris people.

In certain circumstances *sai dibi* reveal their presence to humans. Once when a young man returning from evening hunting heard what sounded like a baby crying in an empty fieldhouse, it was realized that it must have been the *meeni dibi* (one type of evil spirit) on their way to cause harm at Auaris. To prevent this an older man shamanized that night. When a shaman's *hekula* warn him that enemy-sent *hekula* are approaching, he will shamanize to ward off their attack (see below).

FESTIVAL HUNTING SHAMANISM We also observed numerous times the use of shamanism in preparation for the ritual hunt which is always a part of a "Festival for the Dead." Shamanism of this kind is always a group performance, during the day, and always with the use of snuff.[4] A supply of snuff is usually prepared especially for the purpose. It was only in performances of this kind of shamanism that we ever saw men who are not shamans (or novices) taking the snuff. Festival hunting shamanism is primarily to call on appropriate *hekula* to help ensure success in the hunt. Many of these *hekula* are of species which in their living (*salo*) phase do in fact kill the animal which is desired by the hunters. *Hekula* of this kind are called in connection with a long list of animals and birds which it is hoped may be caught during the hunt. For example: the *kokoimane* ('buzzard') *hekula* can help the hunters catch the *paluli* (Portuguese *mutum* 'bush turkey'), the largest and most prized game bird in the area; and the *kitanani* ('cougar') *hekula* can help in the hunting of deer.

Other *hekula* called are those able to protect the hunters from dangers

---

[4] Three varieties of snuff are used in the Auaris area. These are: *sagona sai*, made from the inner bark of a tree; *palalo*, from the seeds of a tree; and *koali nagi*, from the leaves of a small shrub. The generic term *"sagona"* is applied to all three. It is thus evidently the equivalent of the generic term *"ebene"* used by the Yanomam subgroup (see Chagnon et al. 1971).

such as snakebite and the attack of evil spirits. For example, the *uli dili dibi* (one type of evil spirit) can be called, just as if they were *hekula*, and asked to refrain from their usual practice of blowing magic dust at hunters moving through thick undergrowth. Also called are spirits which can influence the weather for the duration of the hunt. For example, the *sano* ('thunder', Sky People) *hekula* can be called and asked not to make rain during the hunt. Again using appropriate *hekula*, the shamans will rid each other, and any non-shamans (especially young men) who are also going on the hunt, of "bad aim." This is considered a supernaturally caused condition (one possible cause is the non-observation of certain food prohibitions by the hunter's wife). It can be dealt with, by *hekula*, in what is in effect a minor "curing" interlude in the hunting shamanism session.

OTHER HUNTING SHAMANISM   Shamanism can also be used for everyday hunting, calling the *hekula* which can ensure one's intercepting a particular kind of animal, or successfully killing a bird or animal if encountered. This is not a common practice, at least while the hunter is at home in the village. It is, however, made more use of when a family (or larger group) is on a hunting trip and staying at a forest camp.

SHAMANISM TO ATTACK ENEMIES   The people of Auaris have *hekula* sent to attack them, especially by the Samatali (possibly a Yanomami subgroup) to the southwest. They usually send the *waduba ausi* ('vulture', Sky People), *modogi* ('sun', Sky People), and *sanuna* ('supernatural jaguar') *hekula*. To fight off these *hekula*, one young Auaris shaman told me he would use the *soinan dibi* ('bee', Sky People) *hekula* and the *pasoliuwi* ('spider monkey' — not clear if of animal or mythico-ancestral type) *hekula*. A number of other *hekula* would also be called to encourage them. This same young shaman said that he himself did not know how to do this sending of *hekula* to attack other people, but that the Kadimani village headman's father, who died a few years ago, had been especially good at it, and that his own father, an old man and a very important shaman in his day, and another senior man at his father's village could both perform that kind of shamanism.

The Acquisition of Hekula

The initial transfer of *hekula* to the novice is typically done by a senior agnate, preferably the father or father's father, or else a classificatory father.[5] When the *hekula* donor is an elder brother, or classificatory brother, he should evidently be in the "middle-aged adult" population segment, or older.

Shamanism for this purpose is done at night, and snuff is used by all involved. There is often more than one experienced shaman present, and more than one of these may give *hekula* to the novice. There can also be more than one novice at such a session. The donor shaman calls his *hekula* in the usual way and then, by the novice also performing the chant(s), *hekula* are transferred or "cross over" to the novice. When the time comes for the transfer of the novice's first *hekula*, he is expected already to know the necessary chants. This is so in spite of the fact that, no matter how many sessions of shamanism he may have attended and at which he may have participated in the taking of the snuff, he will not have been given any opportunity for formal practice of these many and lengthy chants.

Once a shaman has received an initial set of *hekula*, and if he goes on to become an active and effective shaman, he can then call new *hekula* to himself. This is done without necessarily using snuff. In some cases *hekula* will come to a shaman and offer him their services. *Hekula* are sometimes given, or exchanged, between experienced shamans as an act of friendship. Certain *hekula* (e.g. Sky People and evil spirits, when used as *hekula*) are considered particularly powerful and dangerous and will only be taken by an older shaman.

The Performance of Shamanism

The one invariable feature of Sanumá shamanism, of whatever type, is the chanting by which the shaman calls the *hekula* to his aid. This chanting (with interludes, as described below) is the main feature of the performance, whether this is done by day or at night, either accompanied by the appropriate dances or totally without the use of these, and with or without the use of the hallucinogenic snuff. The snuff is taken either by oneself sniffing pinches of the powder, or by having someone else blow a dose of snuff through a short tube into one's nostrils, each in turn. This snuff is much enjoyed, by both men and *hekula*. When the snuff is taken by the shaman, his *hekula* also enjoy its effects, become intoxicated, dance, sing, and are always more than willing to attempt whatever the shaman has in mind. In general, the snuff is only used in the daytime, in which case the participating shaman(s) usually do the dances of the *hekula* they are chanting to summon.

[5] See Ramos 1972 for analysis of Sanumá social structure and kinship terminology.

Shamanism at night (when the chest-dwelling *hekula* are in any case already awake and active) is usually done without any need of snuff. Sessions for the transfer of a novice's first *hekula*, however, are held at night and the snuff is used. Conversely, if curing shamanism, or shamanism to ward off evil spirits, is urgently needed during the day, at a time when there happens to be no snuff available, this can be done, thanks to the cooperative goodwill of the *hekula*. This, in fact, I did observe several times. Apart from the occasions of transferring *hekula* to a novice, when several experienced shamans may take part, shamanism at night, for whatever purpose, is typically a solo performance.

When the snuff has been prepared for a session of daytime shamanism, this is invariably a group session, with any visiting shamans invited to take part. This, of course, they always do, not only because the snuff is considered highly enjoyable, but also because an experienced and active shaman always welcomes any opportunity to chant to his *hekula*. No matter how many shamans may be chanting and/or dancing at one time (I have often seen sessions with four to six shamans taking part and two or three actually dancing at any one time), this is never done in unison. Each shaman proceeds with his own series of chants and his dances are quite unsynchronized with those of the other shamans.

The sessions of group hunting shamanism, which are an integral part of any "Festival for the Dead," are always performed by day, using snuff. Individual hunting shamanism, on the other hand, is likely to be a solo night-time performance, without the use of snuff.

On two occasions we also witnessed sessions of group shamanism by day, using snuff. It was insisted that these sessions were for no specific purpose, but simply for the pleasure of it. Both times, at the Kadimani village, this was the project of older shamans from the Mamugula village some distance to the south. They brought with them a supply of the *palalo* type of snuff, which is not available in the vicinity of Kadimani. These sessions were referred to by the term *polemo* ('to make like a jaguar') rather than by the common generic term *õkamo* used for the usual types of shamanism for specific purposes. Regular afternoon snuff-taking, with shamanism and/or chest-pounding duels, as Barker (1953: 453), Zerries (1964) and Chagnon (1968:90-91) have described for the Yanomami subgroup, is not practiced by the Sanumá of the upper Auaris. This may be related to differences in the supply of the snuff. Not all known varieties are locally available, and in this area there is no domesticated or semi-domesticated source of snuff, such as Chagnon et al. (1971) have described for at least some of the Yanomami villages (cf. Biocca 1971:146-148).

I have only limited information as to the content of the shamanism chants. The language used is not that of everyday speech, but a distinct, possibly archaic, form reserved for this use. What is definite is that for each *hekula* called, the same tune is sung many times over, and each time it is what might be considered a different "verse" of the total chant. It seems to be the case that, depending on the nature of the *hekula* in question, the content of the chant is either an account of the events surrounding the death of the animal or person involved, or a recounting of the myth, or a myth, associated with the being whose *hekula* is being called.

In curing shamanism, soon after he has begun his performance, the shaman may go through a sometimes lengthy and elaborate period of "diagnosis." This may or may not involve questioning the patient as to his signs and symptoms, and often entails the recognition by the shaman — intoxicated by the snuff, and receiving information from the *hekula* — of the precise procedures, movements, approach and departure routes of the spirit responsible for the illness. In curing, the interludes between the "verses" of the chants involve the vigorous massaging or rubbing of the patient's body, typically from the head downwards, ending with a clap of the hands and a throwing movement. This is all part of ejecting the illness and is accompanied by loud growling, gargling noises, and rapid-fire recitative-like speech, as distinct from the chanting proper. Certain illnesses, when duly diagnosed, require the sucking out of pathogenic objects inserted in the patient's body by ghosts (*ni pole bi dibi*) or evil spirits (*sai dibi*), to cause the illness. This is best done by a *lala de* ('anaconda') shaman, whose dangerous and rare anaconda *hekula* is expert at this task. Other shamans who are not *lala de* shamans say that they can also do this, using other spirits, but not well.

In general it seems that shamans are duty-bound to perform cures and to ward off evil, without receiving any kind of payment or remuneration, in material goods, for these services. In terms of social status and prestige, on the other hand, they do receive considerable advantage from their shamanism. When people are visiting in another village, the shamans among them will very commonly be asked by their hosts to take part in any group curing sessions which may become necessary. Important shamans may be asked to go to another village to try to cure a very sick individual. A sick person who is able to travel will, on occasion, make a special visit to another village to ask an important shaman to perform for his or her benefit.

Types of Hekula

The *hekula* used in shamanism are of the following different kinds:
(1) animal,
(2) human,
(3) mythico-ancestral (to animal species),
(4) mythico-ancestral (to human kin groups),
(5) Sky People (humanoid, animaloid, and celestial phenomena),
(6) *sai dibi* 'evil spirits',
(7) plants, and
(8) artifacts.

The most important and constantly used *hekula* are those of the first five categories. Only a very few plants and artifacts have *hekula*. These seem to be items acquired (or known about) as a result of culture contact with other Indian groups, or with whites. Regardless of the nature of the object, being, or spirit in question, its appearance as a *hekula* is always humanoid. *Hekula* look like miniature men, from ten inches to three feet or so in height.

ANIMAL HEKULA   When a shaman takes an animal *heukla* (almost invariably he takes a pair of brothers), they go to live inside his chest until he either dies or passes them on to a novice or friend. During the day they sleep in their hammocks inside his chest. At night (which is daytime for them) they are awake and alert for any approaching supernatural danger. If evil spirits or enemy-sent *hekula* do approach, they strum on the strings of the shaman's hammock to waken him so that he will shamanize to avert the danger.

HUMAN HEKULA   The spirits of dead people are already humanoid in form, but they do somewhat correspond to the *uku dubi* phase of an animal's existence in being also disposed to harm living people. Such spirits are known as *ni pole bi dibi* 'ghosts'. The ghosts typically do harm to their own surviving relatives, usually in revenge for some offense committed during their lifetimes, though it is often many years after their death before they find an opportunity to take this revenge. Ghosts can also attack their killers if ritual seclusion after the killing is not correctly observed. Disposal of the dead is normally by cremation. If the body of a dead person is incompletely cremated, his ghost can be especially dangerous: *ni pole bi dibi* are said to live in a home far off to the south in what is nowadays unoccupied territory (De Barandiaran 1965:2–3).[6] They

---

[6]   Note that this does not agree with Chagnon (1968:48), who reports for the Yanomami that the *ni pole bi dibi* go up to *hidi hendua*, the level-above-earth of the universe.

can be called from there to become a shaman's *hekula* and also to live in his chest.

MYTHICO-ANCESTRAL HEKULA The mythical ancestors of both animal species and human kin groups, after turning into animals and humans, as recorded in the myths, evidently continue to exist in spirit form and can also be used as *hekula*. They live in the forest, far to the south, where the events described in the myths are believed to have taken place.

SKY PEOPLE HEKULA The *hudomosi liuwi dibi* (Sky People) live on the level-above earth (*hidi hendua*) of the universe.[7] This level-above-earth has as its lower surface the visible sky.

Certain of the Sky People have humanoid bodies, e.g. *Omawi*, the creator twin and *Salagazoma*, his wife; some are celestial phenomena, e.g. sun, moon, sky, stars; others are animaloid, e.g. the white vulture, the (celestial) buzzard, the *koliomoni* (a large crane-like bird). These celestial birds appear from time to time on earth. I have myself seen celestial buzzards, and once a *koliomoni*, and heard hunters speak of a dead tapir that a white vulture was feeding on.

All Sky People, whatever kind of bodies they may have, have humanoid "souls," which can be called by shamans to act as *hekula*.

SAI DIBI (EVIL SPIRITS) HEKULA Some, possibly all, of the *sai dibi*, which live on this level of the universe and exist to do harm to human beings can, nevertheless, be used as *hekula* in shamanism. Young shamans are afraid to do this, but an experienced shaman has always at least a few such *sai dibi* that he can control in his shamanism and make to operate on his behalf as *hekula*.

The Relationship between the Shaman and His Assistant Spirits

It is clearly the case that the shaman-faunal *hekula* relationship benefits the shaman and his people. The *hekula* protect, and cure the sicknesses of, his friends and, in the case of certain types of *hekula*, obligingly kill his enemies. The human beings derive considerable benefit from and, in fact, are in several ways entirely dependent on the help of the *hekula*. It seems reasonable, then, to ask what benefit the *hekula* derive from the arrangement.

[7] Cf. Chagnon (1968:44–45), but note that while, for the Yanomami, the scheme of four layers of the universe is identical, the inhabitants of these layers are not entirely the same as for the Sanumá.

Sanumá informants do indicate that the *hekula* enjoy and approve of the relationship, specifying two aspects of this approval. They say that *hekula* like the house inside the shaman's chest and also that they much enjoy the hallucinogenic snuff (*sagona*) which they have ready access to when this is taken, in part on their behalf, by the shaman. Several authors speak of the use of the snuff as indispensable for the shaman's establishment of contact with the *hekula* (e.g. Chagnon 1968:24, 52; 1971:2; Goetz 1969:41; Biocca 1971:45). Among the Sanumá, at least, this is by no means the case. I have personally observed numerous sessions of curing shamanism — both at night and by day — in which no snuff was used, but a long list of *hekula* were called to assist the shaman. What does seem to be the case, however, is that the *hekula* which are thus willing to operate without snuff are those which live in the shaman's chest. These include, of course, the faunal *hekula* I am discussing.

Chagnon goes so far as to speak of a symbiosis between shaman and *hekula*, "For man cannot destroy the souls of his enemies without the aid of the *hekura*, but the *hekura* cannot devour the souls without the direction of men" (1971:3).[8] Unfortunately, he does not specify to which category or categories of *hekula* this applies. He later mentions one particular *hekula*, *hedumisiriwä*, which is used "to destroy the souls of the [enemy] babies with fire." The name of this *hekula* is cognate with the Sanumá *hudomosi liuwi*, which means both the *hekula* of the sky, and also the inclusive category of "Sky People" *hekula* (see above). The specific *hekula* mentioned in my data as used by the Sanumá, or against the Sanumá, in enemy-killing shamanism are:

(1)   the *hekula* of the sun;
(2)   the *hekula* of the white vulture (considered a supernatural being which lives in *hidi hendua* (the "level-above-earth"); and
(3)   the *hekula* of the *sanuna* jaguar.

The first two of these are Sky People; and the third, while from our point of view probably only an exceptionally large jaguar, is for the Sanumá not a game animal (*salo a*), but an inedible and dangerous being. None of the three, then, is a faunal *hekula*. It should also be noted, however, that all of these three enemy-killing *hekula* are also regularly used in curing shamanism.[9] They do not specialize exclusively in the killing of enemies. Thus, the particular symbiosis (or aspect of a symbiosis) which is mentioned by Chagnon — in which the *hekula* benefit by being

[8]   I am much indebted to N. A. Chagnon for kindly providing me with a transcription of his film *Magical Death*.
[9]   Cf. De Barandiaran (1965), where of a list of forty-one *hekula* used in curing, eight are Sky People *hekula*. Of these, one is the *hekula* of the sun and one that of the white vulture.

enabled to devour human souls — does not seem to apply in the case of the faunal *hekula* category. But, as I have pointed out, these are the *hekula* which are particularly cooperative in their relationship with human society.

THE NATURE OF THE MYTHOLOGICAL BEINGS

In mythological times, those beings which were eventually to be the ancestors of present-day fauna had the appearance of human beings. In the myths they are described as behaving just as do the present-day Sanumá. For example, the myths tell of them hunting animals, chopping wood, going on visits, dancing and singing, etc. They looked and acted like human beings and, also like human beings, they had solid bodies and immaterial, humanoid spirits. Like the other beings of mythological times, they were potentially immortal. At this stage of existence they were not distinguished from other mythological beings, including the ancestors of present-day human beings. They were simply human like all of their contemporaries and lived in harmony with the other (human) beings of that time.

In fact, they were ancestral beings and destined to become the first animals. Instead, then, of continuing in existence unchanged (and able to enjoy their immortality) something went wrong and they were transformed (*išwanižo*) into the fauna of the present day.

The other beings of mythological times still exist today, some of them quite unchanged, though they now no longer live in human territory. Many of them live on the level-above-earth of the cosmos, the *hidi hendua*; these are the Sky People discussed above.

The characteristics common to all mythological beings are, then,
(1) humanity,
(2) corporeality,
(3) indestructibility.

THE TRANSFORMATION OF THE ANCESTORS

When the animal ancestors were transformed into the original animals of the normal present-day type, their humanoid "soul" components separated to continue an immortal spirit existence. These spirits form one of the eight categories of *hekula* available for use in shamanism. Thus when certain Yanoama myths speak of the origin of *hekula*, it is *hekula* of this particular type that they refer to.[10] The corporeal component of the ancestral being was transformed into the animal. All present-day animals have mortal animal bodies and potentially destructible animaloid spirits.

The transformation of animal ancestors is always referred to by use of the verb *išwanižo*.[11] *Išwanižo* also occurs in a different but related context. In the case of certain of the faunal food prohibitions (see Taylor 1971a, 1972), the penalty for non-observance of the prohibitions involves the attack of the animal's ghost or animaloid spirit (*uku dubi*) in a particular sense. This is when the *uku dubi* makes the victim (in some cases the eater of the meat; in others, his or her child) become, to a greater or lesser extent, in some way like the animal in question. For example, a pubescent may become "piebald" like the markings of the eaten *amotha* (paca, or labba), or one's child may get a twisted wrist like that of the eaten *šimi* or *saulemi* (the two species of sloth in the Sanumá area). Such penalties are referred to as cases of *išwanižo*.

There is reason to suppose that the *išwanižo* transformation is not just a matter of "turning into" an animal, but rather one of an undesirable loss of a preferred condition. This is suggested by the nature of the situations which, in the relevant myths, precipitate the transformation. The number of adequately elaborate versions of animal-origin myths available to me is still quite limited (a total of only sixteen myths,[12] which tell of the origin of forty-one faunal categories[13]).

Nevertheless, I feel that there are strong indications in the common structure of these myths (and of certain other myths which tell of explicitly undesirable happenings of other kinds) that the *išwanižo* transformation to animality occurs as a consequence of behavior which would be judged incorrect by present-day standards. This, of course, is also true of the food prohibition penalty usage of *išwanižo*, where it is explicitly the non-observance of the prohibition which leads to the *išwanižo* ex-

---

[10]   For example, in the Yanomami myth as recounted in the film *The Myth of Naro* (Asch and Chagnon 1971), where the origin of *hekula* is referred to without distinguishing the particular category of *hekula* involved.

[11]   On one occasion when a very old man went somewhat berserk and developed the habit of wandering off alone into the darkness of the night (extremely abnormal behavior by Sanumá standards), this was also spoken of as *išwanižo*. One other application of the term is in the case of cotton thread or threaded beads becoming snarled up. I am indebted to Mr. Donald M. Borgman, missionary at Auaris, for first pointing out this usage to me, and for his comments on the meaning of *išwanižo*.

[12]   The sources of these myths are: Borgman (n.d.) for the majority, with corroborating versions in my own field data and other authors; Chagnon (1968); De Barandiaran (1968); Wilbert (1963); and Becher (1959).

[13]   Some of these are species, but several appear to be higher level categories, e.g. that of all macaws, parrots and parakeets (*ala bi*).

perience. In one of the myths this is also expressed quite explicitly: "Because a woman was forcibly led out [to dance] while she was menstruating, the [mythical ancestors] said, 'We're becoming dehumanized'" (Borgman n.d.: "The Waikas who go underwater"). In fourteen of the sixteen myths there are instances of such "incorrect behavior" explicitly or implicitly precipitating the transformation of mythical ancestors into animals.[14]

The mythological *iswanižo* transformation does not, then, occur as an arbitrary, inexplicable development. In most, perhaps (with more complete versions of the myths) all, cases it is directly preceded by behavior which would, nowadays, be considered at the least improper, if not in fact prohibited. In the myth of the origin of man's access to fire, for example, as discussed by De Barandiaran (1968), the alligator-man from whom the fire is stolen is, thereupon, transformed into animal form, becoming the first alligator. This alligator-man had been keeping the fire for his own exclusive use, guarding it in his mouth. A party was thrown with the purpose of making him laugh, so that the fire in his mouth could be stolen. With some difficulty, this was eventually done and the fire was carried to the top of a tree of the type which is used by Sanumá in making fire by the fire-drill technique.

De Barandiaran does not discuss those elements of the myth which represent what I am calling "incorrect behavior." These are possibly three. First, the alligator-man is stingy[15] in his keeping the fire exclusively for his own use. Second, when he is eventually made to laugh and thus to open his mouth, the fire is stolen (rather than requested in trade) from him. Quite apart from the fact that these two offenses appear somewhat to cancel each other out, they are less dramatically incorrect than the third. This has to do with the way in which the alligator-man is finally made to laugh — by the *hasimo* bird-man exploding a discharge of feces in his face. By present-day standards this is truly inconceivable behavior. While it is true that the Sanumá are extremely casual about where they urinate, defecation is always an extremely private and concealed act,[16] and it is considered most objectionable to have to see someone else's feces. Thus the *hasimo*-man's behavior was outrageous and the alligator-man's ex-

[14] Compare, for example, Wilbert (1970) where in thirteen of fourteen Warao animal origin myths (those in his index under "Punishment: transformation into animal" and "Creation of animal life") the transformation occurs following incorrect behavior. See also Lévi-Strauss (1970), where twenty-five of twenty-seven animal origin myths follow the same pattern.

[15] See Chagnon (1968:48) *re* the undesirable afterlife to be expected by someone who is stingy. In trading situations, Sanumá are afraid to be stingy as a disappointed visitor can be expected to retaliate by using magic to attack his stingy host.

[16] Cf. Goetz (1969:108).

perience was deeply shaming. In fact, the version of the myth presented by De Barandiaran does say, without specifying why, that the alligator-man, *avergonzado* 'shamed', went to live in the water and become animal.

A particularly elaborate animal-origin myth is the one Borgman (n.d.) has called "The Fall of the Possum."[17] In this myth the transformation into animals of some fifteen faunal categories (see Note 13) and, in the process their acquisition of distinctive anatomical features of taxonomic significance, is described. I have elsewhere discussed how this and other similar myths present an explanation of faunal "taxonomic features" (Taylor 1972:178–183) and shall here concentrate on the question of the "incorrect behavior" precipitant of the *išwanižo* transformations described.

The myth tells of how the possum-man, the mythological ancestor of one or possibly both of the two species of possum (*pumodomɨ* and *pumodomɨ tanama*)[18] known in the upper Auaris region, kills a bee-girl (*samonama* species — *yamonama* in the Yanomamɨ dialect) who has offended him, precipitating the origin of the *samonama* bees. The possum-man is then chased into hiding at the top of a tree (a mountain in the Yanomamɨ version). After much effort, a large gathering of animal-ancestors manage to chop down the tree (mountain) and the possum-man falls to his death.

At this point, appropriate behavior — by present-day standards — would involve the cremation of the body by the dead person's relatives and ritual seclusion (*kanenemo*) by the killers. In the myth, however, the killers and others with them proceed to desecrate the dead body by using its blood, brains (and feces in the Yanomamɨ version) to paint their bodies as if for a festival. They immediately *išwanižo* into animals, with colored plumage, hair, etc., in accordance with the body-painting selected by their respective ancestors.

The instances of "incorrect behavior" are as follows: three cases of taboo-breaking by a menstruating woman; two cases of personal insults; one of stingy behavior; one of throwing away food in a fit of temper; one of deceiving a mother-in-law by giving blood instead of honey (cf.

---

[17]   I refer to six different versions of this myth: three recorded at Auaris, and kindly made available to me, by Don Borgman; another I recorded myself at Auaris (all from different informants); one I recorded at Kadimani; and the Yanomamɨ version shown in the film *The Myth of Naro* (Asch and Chagnon 1971). I am much indebted to N. A. Chagnon for kindly providing me with a transcription of the soundtrack of the film.

[18]   Chagnon was so kind as to show me *The Myth of Naro* in New York, November 1971, at which time we discussed the similarities and differences between this Yanomamɨ version and the Sanumá versions. Chagnon has since confirmed that *naro* is indeed the Yanomamɨ word for one species of possum, the other being *daraima* (personal communication).

Goetz 1969:30 *re* horror of rare or bloody food); one of disobedience to a father-in-law; one of wife-stealing; one of making a nursing infant go hungry; one of non-observance of visitors' etiquette; and one of general disorderly conduct leading to expulsion from the village.

THE PRESENT-DAY CYCLE OF ANIMAL EXISTENCE

For the Sanumá, all normal present-day fauna pass through a series of possibly three phases of existence.
These are:
(1)   *salo bi* 'edible fauna',
(2)   *uku dubi* 'animaloid spirits', and
(3)   *hekula dibi* 'humanoid spirits'.

SALO BI 'EDIBLE FAUNA'   The living fauna are hunted, fished for, or collected to be eaten as food. Once an animal is killed and carried home to village or camp it will, if large enough to warrant eventual distribution and consumption beyond the hunter's immediate household, be butchered in a set manner by someone other than the hunter himself, typically by an older brother. Once butchered, the portions of the animal are distributed around the village according to set procedures. Overlying this system of distributing meat as food is the food prohibition system which requires the avoidance of this food by the members of specified sub-sets of society.

UKU DUBI 'ANIMALOID SPIRITS'   All animals, birds, snakes, fish, etc., and also all human beings have inside them, while alive, an *uku dubi* spirit. This is a miniature of, and has exactly the appearance of, the living being. At death this is released from the body and is free to move and act as a fully sentient and autonomous being. It is thus rather similar to our Western concept of "ghost." Unlike all other spirits of the Sanumá belief system, the *uku dubi* of animals can be destroyed. It should be noted that all other corporeal beings have humanoid spirits, even the corporeally animaloid Sky People (celestial buzzard, etc.), and that these spirits are in all cases indestructible. The destruction of an *uku dubi* spirit will, however, only occur as the end result of the chain of events which begins with the breaking of a food prohibition by a human being.

As I have described in detail elsewhere (Taylor 1971a, 1972) all locally edible animals are prohibited to the members of one or more of the ten "population segments" of Sanumá society. Young children, for example, should not eat kinkajou meat or they will become lazy; pubescents should avoid jaguar meat for fear of getting a sore back; the parents of a nursing infant should not eat capibara meat or the child may be drowned; middle-aged people will get pains in the rectum if they eat the meat of toads. In each case, the undesirable result or "penalty" is produced by an attack by the *uku dubi* spirit of the animal in question.

When such a situation develops, i.e. when someone does break a food prohibition and, as a result, the animal's *uku dubi* does attack and harm the offender (or his or her child), one's recourse is to shamanism. A shaman will be asked to arrange for some of his *hekula* to dispose of the *uku dubi* in question and also to remove the signs and symptoms of the patient's condition. The *uku dubi* being animaloid and the *hekula* human-oid, those *hekula* which can dispose of the particular *uku dubi* involved in any given case are always those equipped with weapons and/or skills appropriate for the purpose of hunting and killing, on the model of the hunting procedures of living human beings. For example, when the prohibition on anteater meat is broken and the *uku dubi* of the dead anteater inflicts the "stroke" penalty on the offender, the *uku dubi* has to be (1) tracked, (2) chased into ambush, and then (3) killed. The *hekula* of a *honama* (a grouse-like bird which feeds on the ground and can run very quickly) searches for the tracks, hunts, and then chases the anteater *uku dubi*. The *hekula* of a *kulemi* bird (long-legged and a fast runner), of an *amu una* (a fast-flying species of bee), and of an *uemigigi* (a fast-moving snake) all chase the anteater *uku dubi* into an ambush where the *hekula* of the *maitaliwi* (arrow-head bamboo) and *managaitili* (mythical ancestors of a specified distant group of Yanoama) are waiting to kill it with bow and arrow. If necessary, a *paso* (spider monkey) *hekula* can then deliver the coup-de-grâce with its quarter-staff.

When someone is bitten by a poisonous snake and the snake has been killed, shamanism is used to cure the snakebite. The snake *uku dubi* is first (1) found, then (2) killed. Following this, (3) the venom is removed from the patient, and (4) the patient's pain is gotten rid of. The *hekula* of certain small song-birds locate the snake *uku dubi*, which is then killed, with their staffs, by *paso* (spider monkey) *hekula*. Otter, capibara, egret, and cormorant *hekula* then wash away the snake's venom with the river water they carry in their mouths, and a *kobali* (a large hawk-like bird) *hekula* gets rid of the pain by massaging the patient with its smooth down-like feather arm-bands, held in its hands for the purpose.

When killed in this way, the *uku dubi* are considered to fall to the level-below-earth (*hidi kuoma*) of the universe, where they are eaten by the *oinan dibi* dwarfs. Thus twice-over hunted, killed, and eaten, they are totally destroyed.

HEKULA DIBI 'HUMANOID SPIRITS' If all prohibitions are correctly observed, the *uku dubi* will then (without in any way molesting human beings and thus avoiding the risk of its own total destruction) leave the forest and "go home" to the house of the humanoid *hekula dibi* spirits of its species for that particular hunting territory.

These *hekula* houses are typically in mountains, waterfalls, rivers, but not simply "in the forest." On arrival, the *uku dubi* will metamorphose into a *hekula*, a spirit with the appearance of a miniature human being. It is then available to be taken as one of his assistant spirits by some Yanoama shaman, necessarily someone living a considerable distance away in a totally different part of Yanoama territory. On its metamorphosis to humanoid form, the animal spirit acquires a miniature weapon or weapons (*lasiwi gigi*), similar to those used by human beings. These are the metamorphoses of distinctive body parts of the living animal. Using these spirit-weapons, faunal *hekula* can attack and kill or chase off the supernatural beings which cause illness and death.

The worst that can happen to a *hekula*[19] is that, if it is sent to attack a human being, other *hekula* may defend its human victim by attacking and chasing it away. The extreme form of such an attack involves actual dismemberment of the *hekula's* body. But this is only a way of establishing dominance and does not destroy the dismembered *hekula*, which will put itself back together again and withdraw.

On undergoing metamorphosis from its *uku dubi* to its *hekula* phase, the being in question has regained a state of indestructibility.

THE REGAINING OF THE MYTHOLOGICAL CONDITION

The sequence of phases of mythological and post-mythological faunal existence, and the corresponding changes in the incidence of the three basic mythological characteristics, can be shown as in Table 1.

When the mythological ancestors were transformed into animals, they lost both humanity and indestructibility, retaining only one of their three

[19] On the model of human birth and the relation between ghosts (*ni pole bi dibi*) and the living, it may be the case that these *hekula* are also available for reincarnation in newly born animals. I do not have information on this point, but will be able to check it out in the field in the near future. The particular relevance of this possibility is that it would mean that the *hekula* in question would thus revert to *uku dubi* status and be re-exposed to the risk of annihilation.

Table 1.   Phases of faunal existence

	mythological ancestor	animal	uku dubi	hekula	incorporated hekula
humanity	+	−	−	+	+
corporeality	+	+	−	−	(+)
indestructibility	+	−	−	+	+

characteristics, that of corporeality. When an animal dies or is killed (as when hunted by humans), even this corporeality is lost and its *uku dubi* (animaloid) spirit does not have any of the mythological characteristics. When it then metamorphoses into a *hekula*, the being in question regains indestructibility and humanoid appearance. But it is still only an immaterial spirit, living apart from human beings and with no direct relationship with them, as yet.

When a faunal *hekula* becomes one of the assistant spirits of a shaman — going to live in his chest, to be incorporated into his body — it then also achieves a substitute for the corporeality of its long-lost mythological condition. It is also reintegrated into the life and interactions of human beings. Its corporeality is, by all means, only a pseudo-corporeality, since the body in question belongs to the human shaman and not really to the *hekula*, but at this stage in the game it is the best available possibility. At this point the faunal being has regained, in the most complete way that post-mythological circumstances permit, all three of the characteristics of its mythological ancestor. It is at a possible end point in the series of transformations, metamorphoses, etc. of its existence. Closing the circle in this way, it has, in a sense, returned to its starting point. With luck, it will be able to remain in this state indefinitely, but this depends on its future as a chest-dwelling assistant spirit.

To begin with, there is the possible lifetime of the shaman in question. In addition there is always the possibility of being passed on to another shaman as an act of friendship on the part of the first shaman involved. Beyond this, there is the possibility of being transferred to a young novice as one of the set of first *hekula* which he has to receive from the stock of *hekula* of an experienced, older shaman. In this way the pseudo-corporeality of a given animal *hekula* may continue for a long time.

The desirability of this pseudo-corporeality is explicit in the fact that there are always some of a given shaman's *hekula* which he neither received as a novice nor called to himself once established as a shaman. These other *hekula* simply appear and offer themselves to the shaman, saying that they much admire the "*hekula*-house" inside his chest and would like to come and live there. Not only does the shaman at times have need of the particular skills of these *hekula,* but these are among the category of chest-dwelling *hekula* which will help him handle an emergency, even when there is no hallucinogenic snuff available. The *hekula,* on the other hand, are entirely dependent on the shaman for their pseudo-corporeality in what is, in this way, indeed a symbiotic relationship.

The harmony of mythological times, when all beings were human, was lost when the ancestors were transformed into animals, etc. The subsequent phase is one of hostility between animals, and their animaloid spirits, and human beings. This is resolved, and harmony is restored, when the humanoid *hekula* are incorporated into the body of a shaman, becoming assistant spirits, i.e. collaborators, in his shamanism for the benefit of his kinsmen, neighbors, and allies.

REFERENCES

ASCH, TIMOTHY, N. A. CHAGNON
 1971   *The Myth of Naro.* Film distributed by Documentary Educational Resources. Somerville, Massachusetts.
BARKER, JAMES
 1953   Memoria sobre la cultura Guaika. *Boletin Indigenista Venezolano* 1:433–489.
BECHER, HANS
 1959   Algumas notas sobre a religião e a mitologia dos Surara. *Revista do Museu Paulista* n.s. 11:99–107.
BIOCCA, ETTORE
 1971   *Yanoáma.* New York: Dutton.
BORGMAN, DONALD M.
 n.d.   "Collections of Sanumá myths. Transcriptions and translations." Unpublished manuscript.
CHAGNON, N. A.
 1968   *Yanomamö: the fierce people.* New York: Holt, Rinehart and Winston.
 1971   *Magical Death.* Film distributed by Center for Documentary Anthropology, Brandeis University.
CHAGNON, N. A., P. LE QUESNE, J. M. COOK
 1971   Yanomamö hallucinogens: anthropological, botanical and chemical findings. *Current Anthropology* 7(1):3–32.
DE BARANDIARAN, DANIEL
 1965   Mundo espiritual y shamanismo Saneva. *Antropológica* 15:1–28.
 1968   El fuego entre los indios Sanema-Yanoama. *Antropológica* 22:1–64.
GOETZ, I. S.
 1969   *Uriji jami!* Caracas: Asociacion Cultural Humboldt.
LÉVI-STRAUSS, CLAUDE
 1970   *The raw and the cooked.* New York: Harper Torchbooks.

MIGLIAZZA, ERNESTO
1972   "Yanomama languages, culture and intelligibility." Unpublished Ph. D. dissertation, University of Michigan.
RAMOS, A. R.
n.d.   "How the Sanumá acquire their names." Unpublished manuscript.
1972   "The social system of the Sanumá of northern Brazil." Unpublished Ph. D. dissertation, University of Wisconsin, Madison.
TAYLOR, K. I.
1971a   "Sanumá (Yanoama) implicit classification and derived classification." Revised text of paper presented at the Annual Meetings of the American Anthropological Association, San Diego, 1970.
1971b   "Sanumá (Yanoama) shamanism and the classification of fauna." Paper presented at the Annual Meetings of the American Anthropological Associaion, New York, 1971.
1972   "Sanumá (Yanoama) food prohibitions: the multiple classification of society and fauna." Unpublished Ph. D. dissertation, University of Wisconsin, Madison.
WILBERT, JOHANNES
1963   *Indios de la región Orinoco-Ventuari.* Caracas: Fundación La Salle de Ciencias Naturales.
1970   *Folk literature of the Warao Indians.* Los Angeles: University of California, Latin American Center.
ZERRIES, OTTO
1955   Some aspects of Waica culture. *Proceedings of the International Congress of Americanists,* 73–88.
1964   *Waika.* Munich: Klaus Renner.

Coca and Popular Medicine in Peru: An Historical Analysis of Attitudes

JOSEPH A. GAGLIANO

The cultivation and consumption of coca in Peru have aroused controversy since almost the very beginnings of the Spanish conquest. Many of the earliest coca opponents urged its destruction because they claimed that its prevalent use in Inca religious practices impeded the Christianization of the Indians. Over the centuries, subsequent critics often asserted that coca contributed to Indian crime and racial degeneration. Others affirmed that coca chewing has militated against the assimilation of the Indian into the Hispanicized culture of coastal Peru. More recent adversaries have focused their attention on the possible narcotic effects of the coca habit. Despite their polemics, these opponents historically have failed in their efforts to eradicate the shrub from the Andes because of their inability to refute the prevalent opinion that coca is a beneficial stimulant and an invaluable medicinal plant which has been essential in preserving the well-being of the highland Indians.

Preceding the Spanish conquest of Peru by at least a generation, the earliest observations relating the medicinal use of coca among the natives of the New World were those of colonists on the Caribbean Islands. Ramón Pané, a missionary on the island of Hispaniola during the closing decade of the fifteenth century, was the first to comment on the shrub and the curative virtues of its leaves (Pané 1932: II, 61). He wrote that the Indians on the island "ate" a leaf resembling Mediterranean basil, which they referred to as *guayo*. They employed large quantities of this basil-like leaf not only in their elaborate funeral rites but as a common medicinal herb to treat assorted minor ailments.[1]

[1] There are several early-sixteenth-century descriptions of the general use of

The substantial commentary regarding coca which followed the Spanish conquest of Peru initially ignored its significance as a medicinal plant among the Andean natives. Giving the coca folklore, which has grown over the centuries, a European dimension, the first observers either described its seemingly miraculous stimulative virtues or expounded its value as a barter item. In his 1539 letter to the Spanish Crown, Vicente Valverde, the Bishop of Cuzco, claimed that the natives, sustained only by this refreshing leaf, could walk and labor all day in the sun without ever feeling its heat (Valverde 1864–1884: III, 98). Pedro de Cieza de León, one of the soldier-chroniclers of the Spanish conquest, emphasized both the stimulative and anoretic properties of coca in his mid-sixteenth-century narrative (de Cieza de León 1959: 259–260). The Indians informed him that they chewed coca because it provided them with vigor and strength while repressing their hunger. Scornful of what he termed a disgusting habit fit only for the Indians, he nevertheless believed that it aided them in performing their hard work. Similarly, Agustín de Zárate, the Royal Accountant, who was assigned to Peru during the initial years of Spanish colonization, related that the natives learned from experience "that he who holds this leaf in his mouth feels neither hunger nor thirst" (Zárate 1555: 15). He appeared far more impressed, however, when witnessing their eagerness to exchange gold and silver for coca leaves. Expressing astonishment, he indicated that the Indians not only bartered precious metals to obtain leaves from the Spaniards but volunteered to work in the mines if provided with coca rations.

Detailed descriptions of the common use of coca as a medicinal plant among the Sierra and Altiplano Indians began appearing in historical literature during the second half of the sixteenth century as the shrub became the subject of controversy in Peru. Appalled by the enormous number of Indian lives lost in the cultivation of the shrub in the disease-infested montaña region east of Cuzco and convinced that the availability of the leaf (which had been frequently employed in Inca religious rites) obstructed the Christianization of the natives, for it constantly reminded them of their pagan past, many missionaries petitioned the Spanish Crown to direct the destruction of the coca plantations. These prohibitionist demands were challenged by other missionaries and viceregal officials who contended that coca served the undernourished Indians as a beneficial stimulant and nutritive supplement. Recommending protective labor legislation to reduce the death

coca in the Caribbean region. Of these, see especially de Las Casas (1951: II, 514); D'Anghera (1912: II, 369); Vespucci (1825–37: III, 252–253).

toll among plantation workers, the defenders of the leaf usually emphasized its economic significance, informing the crown that the Indians would refuse to work in the mines unless given daily coca rations.[2]

As the coca controversy became more heated, apologists for the coca habit focused increasing attention on the reputed miraculous healing powers of the leaf. Juan de Matienzo, a judge in the Audiencia of Charcas and perhaps the most articulate spokesman for the coca interests during the sixteenth century, asserted that acceding to the demands of the prohibitionists would lead to the extinction of the Andean Indians. Among the many arguments supporting the coca habit that he presented to Philip II was that it served to preserve the teeth of the Indians. If they were deprived of the leaf they would quickly lose their teeth and, unable to chew and eat their food, they would all starve (de Matienzo 1910: 89–90).

Other coca defenders catalogued its prevalence as a remedy in various illnesses among the highland Indians. The most common mixture consisted of coca leaves and quinoa ashes, which the Sierra Indians regarded as a panacea for a host of minor sicknesses. Applications of steamed seeds were used frequently to arrest such hemorrhages as nosebleeds. Cooked leaves, combined with several Sierra herbs and honey, were prescribed to alleviate stomach disorders and nausea. Mixed with egg whites and salt, ground leaves were applied in a plaster to hasten the knitting of fractured bones. This same concoction, prepared in a poultice, was administered to dry and heal skin ulcerations.[3] Perhaps ironically, contemporary references do not indicate whether this common Sierra remedy was used on the coca plantations to treat the disfiguring skin ulcerations caused by the fatal *mal de los Andes* (leishmaniasis). Presumably, only the common mercury chloride preparation known as *solimán* was used (de Toledo 1921–1926: VIII, 29–30).

Confronted with the conflicting polemics of the prohibitionists and defenders, Philip II chose to accept the claim that coca was in fact a necessary stimulant which afforded the Indians "a mitigation" for their hard work. While sanctioning official tolerance of the coca habit among the Andean Indians in a law dated October 18, 1569, Philip

---

[2] For a discussion and summary of conflicting colonial opinions regarding coca and the laws which were established to protect the coca workers, see Gagliano (1963: 43–63).
[3] Many sixteenth- and seventeenth-century chronicles describe the medical applications of coca among the Sierra Indians. Of these, see especially Cobo (1890–1895: I, 351, 476–477); Valera (1945: 131–132); de Acosta (1894: I, 381).

II addressed himself to the prohibitionist charge that the presence of coca impeded the Christianization of the natives. He urged the churchmen of the viceroyalty to maintain "a constant vigilance" to prevent its use in superstitious practices and witchcraft *(Recopilación* 1943: II, 306).

The prohibitionists regarded the crown's admonition as a justification for continuing their efforts to discredit the use of coca. Antonio Zúñiga, a missionary who had spent eighteen years among the Andean Indians, informed the crown in 1579 that the shamans employed coca more often than not for evil purposes and that the shrub was assuredly the creation of the devil, who used it to ensnare Indian souls (Zúñiga 1842–1895: XXVI, 90, 93, 94). His assertions reflected the claim among many prohibitionists that no actual distinction existed between the use of coca as a remedy in the popular medicine of the highland Indians and its employment as a fetish in their *costumbre* rituals. Likewise, these critics insisted that no distinction existed between the highland *curandero* [medicaster] and the *brujo* [sorcerer]. They chose to identify the shaman who used coca in treating the sick as a practitioner of black magic, pointing out that his ministrations were preceded by elaborate superstitious rituals.[4] Adding to the contention that the healing virtues of coca represented a diabolical illusion, an account circulating in Peru near the mid-seventeenth century described what was termed "a very subtle idolatry" which had emerged among the Christianized Indians. *Curanderos,* who were in reality secret pagan shamans, often informed the persons they were summoned to treat that their illness arose from their collaboration with the Spaniards and their submission to Christianity. The shamans then made a traditional offering of coca leaves to propitiate the gods for the ideological sins of these patients (de Vega Bazán 1655: 2–3).

Blas Valera, the Jesuit missionary and chronicler of the late sixteenth century from whom Garcilaso de la Vega, *El Inca,* borrowed generously in preparing his *Royal commentaries,* criticized the prohibitionists who denied the curative virtues of coca and clamored for its eradication because it was associated with idolatry. He indicated that long before the arrival of the Spaniards, the Andean Indians had known the efficacy of coca in treating illness. The Spaniards became aware of its obvious benefits when they observed that the natives who habitually chewed coca were stronger and better disposed to strenuous labor than those who abstained from the leaves. This was to be ex-

---

4   Emphatic sixteenth-century statements expressing this sentiment are seen in de Atienza (1583: Chapter 42) and de Vega (1600: Folios 126, 147).

pected, he concluded, for if coca had proved so beneficial as an external application in curing, its powers as a tonic were even greater when its juices were taken internally. Questioning the affirmations of the prohibitionists, he argued that if coca were the only Andean plant used by the shamans in their secret rites, its extirpation would be justified. It was, however, one among the many things of nature which the Indians idolized. The task of the missionary, he admonished, was to teach the neophytes to use coca in a Christian manner, with moderation and only for good purposes (Valera 1945: 131).

Writing in the seventeenth century, Bernabé Cobo, another Jesuit chronicler, whose understanding of the Indian mentality surpassed that of his contemporaries, demonstrated greater restraint than Blas Valera in analyzing the imprecise powers attributed to coca. From his own observations and personal experience, he realized that the shrub was a valuable medicinal plant. He concluded, however, that the Indians never completely separated its curative virtues from its avowed preternatural powers. When summoned to treat a sick person, the shaman might employ the coca he carried either as a remedy or as a fetish. If he diagnosed the affliction as arising from a neglect of worship, he instructed the person to mollify the angry deities with various offerings, including coca leaves. While the shaman watched, his patient blew some leaves toward the sun, imploring the offended gods to restore his health (Cobo 1890–1895: IV, 139; for similar observations, see de Acosta 1894: I, 381).

The growing distinction between the medical applications of coca and its role in *costumbre* practices was evident in the witchcraft cases brought before the Inquisition Tribunal in Lima during the seventeenth century. Those accused of sorcery were invariably asked whether they used coca solely in curing or also for evil purposes, such as the conjuring of the devil.[5] This distinction was also suggested in a manual prepared to guide missionaries in the highlands and published in 1631. Although admonishing the priests to remain vigilant in preventing the superstitious use of such commodities as chili peppers and *chicha* (a beer made from fermented maize) in healing, it made no mention of coca (Pérez Bocanegra 1631: *item* 43). By the eighteenth

[5] An investigation of Inquisition cases in the Archbishop's Archives of Lima demonstrates that the question appeared in virtually every witchcraft trial of the seventeenth century. For examples see Causa de idolatría . . . del pueblo de S. Juan de Macahaca (1657: Folios 4, 5, 10, 22); Información dada por . . . María de la Cruz (1681); Causas criminales contra María de la Cruz y Augustín González (1689: Folios 52, 148). The question was also asked in eighteenth-century cases. See Causa criminal contra Juan de Rojas (1723: Folios 6, 10).

century, the leaf had come to be generally regarded as an essential herb in the paraphernalia of the highland *curandero*. Acknowledging its acceptance in popular medicine, an *información* [report] submitted to the Inquisition in Lima in 1739 told of an aged shaman in Vilcabamba, known as Juan Alonso, who used a seashell filled with coca leaves both in divination and in treating the sick (Información de Brujo 1739: Folio 7). According to the report, the clergy in Vilcabamba made no serious effort to dissuade Juan Alonso from such practices because they regarded him primarily as a *curandero* rather than as a sorcerer.

In describing the prevalent use of coca in highland folk medicine, Ricardo Palma, the nineteenth-century Peruvian litterateur who wrote extensively on Indian customs, affirmed that the creoles became tolerant of the *curandero*'s practices once he incorporated Christian traditions into his diagnostic rituals (Palma 1937: 68). The *curandero* added to his chant, which had probably been sung since before the time of the Incas, an invocation of Christ and various saints. After scattering coca leaves over a poncho or shirt of his patient and again soliciting the aid of the Christian saints, he blew vigorously on the leaves. He determined the cause of illness according to the direction in which most of the leaves accumulated.

Ricardo Palma's analysis, which reflects his interest in the quaint in the process of acculturation in Andean society, ignored creole tolerance which was based on the increased acceptance of coca as a medicament among Peru's white population. Initially the creoles were reluctant to experiment with the leaf because the prohibitionists insisted that it was a satanic creation and its healing powers were actually a diabolical illusion (de Atienza 1583: chapter 16). In addition, many prominent sixteenth-century Spanish commentators shared de Cieza de León's contempt for coca, regarding its use as being appropriate only for the Indians. Nicolás Monardes, the respected Seville physician, was scornful and suspicious in describing the shrub in his 1574 treatise on the medicinal plants and stones of the New World (Monardes 1574: 115). Although including coca among the important medicinal plants of Peru, he particularly emphasized its possible euphoric effects and suggested its apparent use for ritualistic intoxication. When the Indians wished to become intoxicated or "to be out of their senses," he wrote, they chewed a mixture of coca and tobacco leaves. Monardes related that this combination caused the chewers to fall into a drunken stupor which filled them with great contentment.

The persuasive arguments of the coca apologists such as Blas Valera and Bernabé Cobo encouraged the creoles to begin using the leaf as a medicament. By the end of the sixteenth century, white colonists in the Sierra and Altiplano settlements had adopted a host of native coca remedies, including its use in the treatment of skin ulcerations and the common cold.[6] Relating his own experience, Bernabé Cobo indicated that coca had come to be regarded as an effective cure for toothaches among the white population of the highlands (Cobo 1890–1895: I, 476). He asked a barber to extract a painful molar. Advising against its removal because the tooth appeared healthy, the barber suggested that he chew large quantities of coca leaves for several days to relieve the pain. This remedy proved even more successful than Cobo had hoped, for the pain not only disappeared, never to recur, but the tooth was soon as strong and sound as the rest.

The esteem for coca as a valuable medicinal plant became evident even in Lima, the hub of Hispanic culture in Peru. While those creoles who became habituated to coca were often disowned by their disgraced families (Mantegazza 1859: 477),[7] the Limeños employed it without question in the medications their physicians prescribed. Coca preparations were recommended to treat maladies as disparate as upset stomach and rheumatism. The Limeño physicians attempted to duplicate the elaborate coca poultice, which they were informed the Sierra *curandero* administered successfully in treating patients suffering rheumatic pain.[8] In simple remedies, the leaves were usually taken as infusions in a tea. This preparation was frequently prescribed as a placebo for hypochondriacs and dyspeptics (Unanue 1821: III, 398). Ordinarily, the coca tea was taken with varying quantities of sugar to make it more palatable to white tastes. In addition, reflecting their disdain for coca chewing, the creoles believed that only those identified with Indian culture could tolerate using the limestone alkaloid or quinoa ashes the natives employed to form their plugs (Unanue 1914: II, 110; von Tschudi 1849: 315).

[6] For descriptions of the prevalent medicinal use of coca among white colonists in the highland communities, see Valera (1945: 131, 132); Garcilaso de la Vega, *El Inca* (1941–1946: III, 56–57); Cobo (1890–1895: I, 476); Unanue (1914: II, 114); Julián (1787: 31).
[7] For other comments demonstrating the social stigma attached to coca habituation among non-Indians, see especially Garcilaso de la Vega, *El Inca* (1941–1946: III, 59), Haënke (1901: 108, von Tschudi (1849: 315–316), and von Poeppig (1835–1836: II, 252).
[8] Unanue (1914: II, 97, 114). A Spanish witness testifying before the Inquisition Tribunal in Lima in 1681 informed the judges that the Indians throughout Peru employed coca leaves mixed with *aguardiente* as a remedy for several pains. Even the Spaniards in Lima, he claimed, used the concoction for medicinal purposes. See Causa criminal ... testigo ... Juan Deochoa Arada (1681: Folio 3).

The only significant exception to the widespread use of coca among Andean medical practitioners was in the presidency of Quito, whose jurisdiction encompassed much of modern-day Ecuador. Intense prohibitionist sentiment, as well as the production of a food supply more adequate than elsewhere in the viceroyalty of Peru, contributed to the virtual disappearance of coca cultivation and consumption in the region by the beginning of the eighteenth century (León 1952: 23; Unanue 1914: II, 107). Several prominent Quitans protested the complete exclusion of coca from the presidency near the end of the seventeenth century. Praising its remarkable curative virtues, which they indicated were recognized throughout the viceroyalty, they petitioned the civil officials and the Bishop of Quito for permission to introduce coca into the presidency solely for use in medicinal preparations. Their appeal was denied. Although acknowledging its medicinal value and wide applications elsewhere, the church spokemen asserted that even a limited relaxation of the coca ban to serve the worthy purpose of curing the sick represented a danger to the Christian neophytes, for the secret shamans would seize upon such an opportunity to acquire leaves for their pagan rites. The Quitan clergy regarded violation of the coca prohibition as so serious that offenders were subject to excommunication, even though they claimed to have obtained the leaves only for medicinal purposes (de la Peña Montenegro 1754: 570–571).

Increased attention was given to the importance of coca as a medicinal plant beginning in the eighteenth century with the development of significant botanical studies in Europe. Many European naturalists, who were attracted to the Andean region during the 1700's, commented on the extensive use of coca as a panacea among all classes of Peruvian society. Few of these observers, however, suggested that the shrub might serve as an equally beneficial medicament if introduced into Europe. Joseph de Jussieu, the French botanist responsible for introducing the first coca plants into Europe, and an original participant in the scientific expedition of Charles de Condamine to the viceroyalty of Peru in the 1730's, seemed far more impressed with the medicinal properties of quinine than with those of coca, having seen both used as remedies among Indians in the Andean region (de la Condamine 1751: 75, 186, 217–218). Jorge Juan y Santacilla and Antonio de Ulloa, the Spanish naturalists dispatched to the New World to survey conditions for the crown in the 1740's, made only passing references to the use of coca in their *Noticias secretas*. They did not even include it with the other medicinal plants which they listed as among the important riches and valuable crops of Peru.[9] Hipólito Ruíz, whose *Relación* was intended not only to inform Europeans concerning the flora of the New World but also to identify economic plants for the Spanish Crown, noted the prevalent use of coca in Andean folk medicine (Ruíz 1931: 294) and even sent two shrubs to Spain in 1786. He observed that the Sierra Indians used various coca preparations to treat disorders ranging from headaches to gout. Hot coca infusions served as an effective diuretic. Despite the obvious medical siginificance of coca in Peru, Ruíz did not recommend that Spain attempt to develop a European market for it as a medicinal plant.

Eighteenth-century Andean naturalists demonstrated far more enthusiasm than their European counterparts in expounding the medicinal value of coca and speculating on its potential as a major Peruvian export. One of the foremost propagandists was Hipólito Unanue, whose 1793 "Dissertation on coca" was intended in part to promote its use in Europe and North America as a stimulant and a medication. His descriptions demonstrated that no stigma was attached to its medical applications, for even in Lima it was commonly regarded as a panacea. Attempting to arouse greater European curiosity concerning its virtues, he stated that since the time of the Incas, the Indians had employed coca as an incomparable tonic for the aged. He suggested that it might prove effective in geriatrics, serving to rejuvenate the aged in Europe as it had prolonged the lives of the Andean Indians (Unanue 1914: II, 97). Although less prccise than Unanue in his analysis of coca's medicinal properties, Antonio Julián, a former Jesuit who served the Spanish Crown following the suppression of his order, was equally enthusiastic. During his long residence in New Granada, he became aware of the vigor and robust health of the Guagiro Indians who were inveterate coca chewers. Advising Charles III to consider coca as an important economic plant, as well as an invaluable medicament, he urged its exploitation so that Spain might profit, while providing European workers with a tonic which would improve their health and even prolong their lives (Julián 1787: 24–25, 31–33).

Laudatory world opinion regarding the stimulative and curative virtues of coca grew rapidly during the nineteenth century when numerous foreign travelers wrote of their experiences in the newly independent Andean nations. While these visitors suffered from the de-

---

[9] Juan y Santicilla and de Ulloa (1918: II, Part 2, Chapter 9). Although not recommending its medicinal use in Europe, they observed in their joint work that the Sierra Indians regarded coca as a panacea. See Juan Santicilla and de Ulloa (1748: I, 469).

bilitating effects of climatic aggression when they ventured into the highlands, the undernourished, coca-chewing Indian porters and guides whom they engaged performed prodigious feats of strength and endurance. In their often exaggerated narratives, these observers seemed awed by the healing powers of coca, which some viewed as almost miraculous (Gagliano 1965: 167–169). Recounting its wide use in popular medicine as a remedy for ailments ranging from stomach disorders to colds, several nineteenth-century coca commentators called particular attention to its employment as a cure and preventive for venereal diseases among the Sierra Indians (Enock 1908: 205; Fuentes 1866: 13; Freud 1884: 505). In their treatment of syphilis, the highland *curanderos* applied a poultice similar to that used in the healing of skin ulcerations.

Unquestionably Paolo Mantegazza, an Italian physician who had practiced medicine in Peru for several years, was the most exuberant coca propagandist of the nineteenth century. After returning to Italy, he wrote a lengthy article in 1859 urging European scientists to investigate the medical potentialities of Peruvian coca. Referring to the shrub as the true treasure of the New World, he extolled its efficacy in various remedies. For example, he recommended that European dentists adopt it in their practice, for it was an excellent dentrifice and tooth preservative widely used among all elements of Peruvian society (Mantagazza 1859: 497). He further claimed that the Sierra Indians had long been successful in treating hysteria with coca preparations. Suggesting that European physicians might consider experimentation with coca in cases involving mental disorders, he speculated that it would prove more effective and far less dangerous than opium, the prevailing drug used in the treatment of melancholia (1859: 498, 501). To emphasize how harmless coca was, he told of its efficacy in ending caffeine addiction. Persons in Peru and Argentina who wished to cure themselves of the caffeine habit added coca infusions to their beverage. Without indicating whether the caffeine habit was replaced by a craving for coca, Mantagazza asserted that within a short time, those following this regimen lost their desire for coffee. Terming it the "stimulant par excellence," he advised European physicians to have their patients replace their coffee and tea with coca decoctions (1859: 498–499). Much like the earlier efforts of Unanue to enhance interest in this potent Andean shrub, his works stressed its possible applications in geriatrics. Since the time of the Incas, he wrote, the Sierra Indians had known of coca's rejuvenating and aphrodisiac virtues (1859: 503).

Despite the plaudits of Mantegazza and other propagandists, some adverse commentaries appeared, questioning the value of coca as a medicinal plant. Among the nineteenth-century travelers, Eduard von Poeppig, the German naturalist who visited Peru shortly after its achievement of independence and frequently observed the ubiquitous coca chewers, was the most critical of the habit. Writing in 1836, he warned against the medical application of coca in Europe, regarding it as not only dangerous but also capable of producing effects similar to opium addiction (von Poeppig 1835–1836: II, 252, 257). Several subsequent observers, including Mantegazza, recommended cautious and exhaustive experimentation to determine whether it might have harmful effects as a medicament. Although cocaine was employed successfully as a local anesthetic after its isolation from coca in 1860, misgivings concerning its wider medical applications spread rapidly through Europe and the United States following Sigmund Freud's unsuccessful experiments with the drug in treating opium and morphine addicts.[10]

New apologists for the shrub attempted to refute the warnings that coca and cocaine were potentially dangerous. W. Golden Mortimer, a United States physician and surgeon, tried to enhance confidence in the therapeutic values of cocaine among his colleagues. Writing an encyclopedic defense of the shrub in 1901, he referred to coca as the "Divine Plant of the Incas." He emphasized that medical practitioners among the Andean Indians had used its leaves effectively since long before the time of the Incas. Often assuming a polemical tone in his attempts to reassure his colleagues, Mortimer insisted that cocaine was "not only harmless, but usually phenomenally beneficial when properly administered" (Mortimer 1901: xiii).

While controversy regarding the possible harmful effects of cocaine was evident in Europe and the United States, many prominent nineteenth-century Peruvian scientists appeared convinced that the coca shrub indigenous to their nation was perhaps the most beneficial medicinal plant known to man. Although aware of the possible hazards of cocaine, they generally denied that coca could produce drug addiction among the Indian chewers. Alfredo Bignón, a chemist, concluded from his experiments that the Indians ingested too small a quantity of cocaine to make their habit harmful. He furthermore speculated that because the Indians began chewing coca when still boys, they gradually developed a tolerance for the cocaine they ingested and

---

[10] The nineteenth-century scientific controversy concerning the possible harmful effects of coca and cocaine is analyzed in Gagliano (1965: 171–174).

could not possibly become addicted (Bignón 1885: 245–246; for similar observations written earlier in the nineteenth century, see Raimondi 1868: 125). In the 1880's, the Peruvian Government appointed a scientific commission, under the leadership of José Casimiro Ulloa, the dean of Peruvian physicians, to recommend new uses for coca which would increase its export. The commission's report, published in 1889, emphasized that coca should be promoted as an unparalleled stimulant which, if utilized in Europe and the United States, would enable miners, farmers and factory workers to derive the same invigorating benefits as the Andean Indians gained from the leaf (Ulloa, Colunga, and de los Ríos 1889: 29, 31).

The growth of the Indianist Movement in twentieth-century Peru, which concerned itself with social reform and the assimilation of the hinterland Indians into the Hispanicized culture of the coast, as well as increasing international concern that coca chewing represented a form of narcotic addiction, led to renewed criticism of the shrub's medicinal value. Hermilio Valdizán (1885–1929), a psychiatrist who became intensely active in Indianist reform projects, contended in his polemics that the use of coca was the gravest sociomedical problem of the Andes. The coca habit not only enhanced the cultural isolation of the highland Indians, preventing their assimilation into national life, but also led to racial degeneration, he insisted. He urged governmental action as rapidly as possible to prohibit the cultivation and consumption of coca (Valdizán 1913: 264, 267, 274–275).[11]

Supporting most of these affirmations, subsequent colleagues in the medical profession, who shared Valdizán's concern for Indianist reforms, proposed legislation to curtail the coca habit. In general, they recommended the establishment of a governmental monopoly that would restrict the cultivation and distribution of coca leaves, as well as the production of crude cocaine, to those levels needed for solely medical purposes (Ricketts 1936: 7, 9–14, 33–35, passim; Paz Soldán 1929: 598–599, 601; Paz Soldán 1939: 19; Luís Sáenz 1938: 220–221, passim). The efforts of these modern coca critics, which contributed to Peru's increased cooperation with the Economic and Social Council of the United Nations in seeking methods to control the manufacture of crude cocaine, culminated in the creation of a national coca monopoly in 1949 (*El Peruano* 1949: 1; United Nations 1950: 79). An agency of the Ministry of Finance, the monopoly had among its

---

[11] For early criticism of the Valdizán contention that coca chewing caused degeneration among the Indians, see especially Graña y Reyes (1940: 31); Sáenz (1933: 165).

major objectives the elimination of coca cultivation within twenty-five years.
The gradual commitment of Peru to restrict and eventually end coca cultivation and consumption in the twentieth century aroused both skepticism and controversy in scientific circles. Many sociologists and anthropologists theorized that the use of coca had become so institutionalized in the amenities, *costumbre* practices, and popular medicine of the highland Indians that its eradication or even reduced consumption seemed unlikely. Even Valdizán had conceded its prevalent medical application among the highland Indians in a joint study on Peruvian folk medicine (Valdizán and Maldonado 1922: I, 79, 99, 129, 167–169, 178–179; II, 219; passim). Writing in the 1930's, Estanislao López Gutiérrez, a noted sociologist, questioned the wisdom of attempting to curb the use of the leaf, whose healing and stimulative virtues were traditionally esteemed in the Sierra. He speculated that creating the governmental control agency which the Indianist reformers demanded might lead to the sort of gangsterism and bootlegging that attended the Volstead Act in the United States (López Gutiérrez 1938: 139, 141; a similar pessimism expressed earlier, albeit less imaginatively, is found in Castro Pozo 1924: 204–206). In his 1950 study of the role of coca in Andean folklore, Sergio Quijada Jara catalogued the extensive modern use of the leaf by the highland *curanderos*. Although speculating that an intensive and prolonged educational program of social hygiene might diminish coca chewing, he doubted whether the Sierra Indians would ever alter their opinion regarding the leaf's curative powers (Quijada 1950: 59–60, 73). In addition, proponents of the "Andean Man theory" (which affirms that the dwellers in the high Andes represent a different biological type), with their insistence that coca chewing contributes to the environmental adaptation of the Sierra Indians have stimulated an outpouring of polemics (Monge 1946: 31–315; Gutiérrez-Noriega 1948: 100–123; Domínguez 1930: 3–16). These recent and continuing controversies demonstrate the persistent divided opinion concerning the use of coca as a stimulant and a medicament which has been evident in Andean literature since the sixteenth century.

REFERENCES

BIGNÓN, ALFREDO
1885   Propiedades de la coca y de la cocaína. *El Monitor Médico* 1: 245–246.

CASTRO POZO, HILDEBRANDO
1924   *Nuestra comunidad indígena*. Lima.

COBO, BERNABÉ
1890–1895   *Historia del nuevo mundo*..., four volumes. Edited by Marcos Jiménez de la Espada. Madrid.

D'ANGHERA, PETER MARTYR
1912   *De orbe novo, the eight decades*..., two volumes. Edited and translated by Francis Augustus MacNutt. New York and London.

DE ACOSTA, JOSEPH
1894   *Historia natural y moral de las Indias*, two volumes. Madrid.

DE ATIENZA, LOPE
1583   "Compendio historial del estado de los indios del Perú, con muchos doctrinas i cosas notables de ritos costumbres e inclinaciones que tienen." Transcript from the original manuscript in Madrid made for E. G. Squier. Rich Collection, Division of Manuscripts, New York Public Library.

DE CIEZA DE LEÓN, PEDRO
1959   *The Incas of Pedro de Cieza de León*. Translated by Harriet de Onis. Edited by Victor Wolfgang von Hagen. Norman, Oklahoma.

DE LA CONDAMINE, M.
1751   *Journal du voyage fait par ordre du Roi ... servant d'un introduction historique a la mesure de trois première degrés du méridien*. Paris.

DE LA PEÑA MONTENEGRO, DON ALONSO
1754   *Itinerarios para parochos de indios, en que se tratan les materias más particulares tocantes a ellos para su buena administración* (new edition). Amberes.

DE LAS CASAS, BARTOLOMÉ
1951   *Historia de las Indias*, three volumes. Edited by Augustín Millares and with a preliminary study by Lewis Hanke. Mexico City.

DE MATIENZO, JUAN
1910   *Gobierno del Perú, obra escrita en el siglo XVI*. Buenos Aires.

DE TOLEDO, FRANCISCO
1921–1926   "Ordenanzas ... relativos al cultivo de la coca, tabajo de los indios en él y obligaciones de los encomenderos; enfermedades de indios ... Cuzco, 3 de octubre de 1572," in *Gobernantes del Perú: Cartas y papeles, siglo XVI, documentos del Archivo de Indias*, volume eight. Edited by Roberto Levillier, 14–33. Madrid.

DE VEGA, ANTONIO
1600   "Historia ... de las cosas succedidas en este colegio del Cuzco ... de estos reynos del Perú, desde su fundación hasta hoy ... año de 1600." Division of Manuscripts Library of Congress. Washington, D.C.

DE VEGA BAZÁN, ESTANISLAO
1655   *Testimonio auténtica de una idolatría muy sutil que el demonio avia introducido entre los indios ... hizo por comisión y particulares instrucciones que le dió Pedro de Villagomes, Arzobispo de Lima, 19 de octubre de 1655*. Lima.

DOMÍNGUEZ, JUAN A.
1930 La coca como factor dinamogénico de uso habitual en el altiplano argentino-chileno-boliviano. *Trabajo del Instituto de Botánica y Farmacología* 47:3–16.

El Peruano
1949 Establecase el Estanco de la Coca, Decreto Ley 11046. *El Peruano: Diario Oficial* (July 22).

ENOCK, C. REGINALD
1908 *Peru: its former and present civilization, history and existing conditions.* New York.

FREUD, S.
1884 Coca. (Translated by S. Pollak.) *The Saint Louis Medical and Surgical Journal* 47:502–505.

FUENTES, MANUEL A.
1866 *Mémoire sur la coca du Pérou* .... Paris.

GAGLIANO, JOSEPH A.
1963 The coca debate in colonial Peru. *The Americas* 20:43–63.
1965 The popularization of Peruvian coca. *Revista de Historia de América* 59:164–179.

GARCILASO DE LA VEGA, EL INCA
1941–1946 *Los comentarios reales de los Incas,* six volumes (second edition). Edited by Horacio H. Urteaga. Lima.

GRAÑA Y REYES, FRANCISCO
1940 *La población del Perú a través de la historia* (third edition). Lima.

GUTIÉRREZ-NORIEGA, CARLOS
1948 Errores sobre la interpretación del cocaísmo en las grandes alturas. *Revista de Farmacología y Medicina Experimental* 1:100–123.

HAËNKE, TADEO
1901 *Descripción del Perú.* Lima.

JUAN Y SANTACILLA, JORGE, ANTONIO DE ULLOA
1748 *Relación histórica del viaje a la América meridonial hecha de ordenes de S. Mag ...,* four volumes. Madrid.
1918 *Noticias secretas de América ...,* two volumes. Madrid.

JULIÁN, ANTONIO
1787 *La perla de la América, observada y expuesta en discursos históricos.* Madrid.

LEÓN, LUIS A.
1952 The disappearance of cocaism in Ecuador. *Bulletin on Narcotics* 4:21–25.

LÓPEZ GUTIÉRREZ, ESTANISLAO
1938 *El alma de la comunidad, bosquejo sobre la génesis y el desenvolvimiento de los aborígenes peruanos.* Lima.

MANTEGAZZA, PAOLO
1859 Sulle virtù igieniche e medicinali della coca e sugli alimenti nervosi in generale. *Annali Universali de Medicina* 167:449–519.

MONARDES, NICOLÁS
1574 *Primera, segunda y tercera partes de a historia medicinal de las*

cosas que se traen de nuestras Indias Occidentales que sirven en medicina. Seville.

MONGE, CARLOS
1946   El problema de la coca en el Perú. *Anales de la Facultad de Medicina* 29:311–315.

MORTIMER, W. GOLDEN
1901   *Peru: a history of coca, the "Divine Plant" of the Incas* . . . . New York.

PALMA, RICARDO
1937   *Anales de la Inquisición de Lima.* Buenos Aires.

PANÉ, RAMÓN
1932   "Relación . . . acerca de las antiguedades de los indios por mandato del Almirante," in *Historia del Almirante Don Cristóbal Colón por su hijo,* volume two. Edited by Hernando Colón, 35–99. Madrid.

PAZ SOLDÁN, CARLOS
1929   El problema médico-social de la coca en el Perú. *Mercurio Peruano: Revista Mensual de Ciencias Sociales y Letras* 19:584–603.
1939   Luchemos contra la esclavitud del cocaísmo indígena: sugestiones para una acción nacional. *La Reforma Médica* 25:19, 21, 24.

PÉREZ BOCANEGRA, JUAN
1631   *Ritual formulario e institución de curas para administrar a los naturales en este reyno los santos sacramentos . . . con advertenvias muy necesarias.* Lima.

QUIJADA JARA, SERGIO
1950   *La coca en las costumbres indígenas.* Huancayo, Peru.

RAIMONDI, ANTONIO
1868   Elementos de botánica applicada a la medicina e industria. *Gaceta Médica de Lima* 12:125–128.

Recopilación
1943   *Recopilación de leyes de los reunos de las Indias,* three volumes (revised edition). Madrid.

RICKETTS, CARLOS A.
1936   *Ensayos de legislación pro-indígena. Arequipa,* Peru.

RUÍZ, HIPÓLITO
1931   *Relación del viaje hecho a los reynos del Perú y Chile por los botánicos . . . extractado de los diarios por el orden que llevó en estos su autor.* Madrid.

SÁENZ, LUÍS N.
1938   *La coca: estudio médico-social de la gran toxicomanía peruana.* Lima.

SÁENZ, MOISES
1933   *Sobre el indio peruano y su incorporación al medio nacional.* Mexico City.

ULLOA, JOSÉ CASIMIRO, MIGUEL F. COLUNGA, JOSÉ A. DE LOS RÍOS
1889   Informe sobre la coca. *La Crónica Médica* 6: 27–31.

UNANUE, J. HIPÓLITO
1821   Abstract from a communication . . . to Samuel L. Mitchell, dated

at Lima, first February, 1821. *The American Journal of Sciences and Arts* 3:397–399.

1914 "Disertación sobre el cultivo, comercio y las virtudes de la famosa planta del Peru nombrada coca," in *Obras científicas y literarias*, volume two, 90–125. Barcelona.

UNITED NATIONS ECONOMIC AND SOCIAL COUNCIL
1950 *Report of the Commission of Enquiry on the Coca Leaf.* Lake Sucess, New York.

VALDIZÁN, HERMILIO
1913 El cocaínismo y la raza indígena. *La Crónica Médica* 30:263–275.

VALDIZÁN, HERMILIO, ÁNGEL MALDONADO
1922 *La medicina popular peruana, contribución al "folk-lore" médico del Perú*, three volumes. Lima.

VALERA, BLAS
1945 *Las costumbres antiguas del Perú y la historia de los Incas.* Edited by Francisco A. Loayza. Lima.

VALVERDE, VICENTE
1864–1884 "Carta del Obispo del Cuzco al Emperador sobre asuntos de su iglesia y otros de la gobernación de aquel país, Cuzo, 20 de marzo de 1539," in *Colección de documentos inéditos relativos al . . . antiguas posesiones españoles de América*, volume three (first series). Edited by J. F. Pacheco, 92–136. Madrid.

VESPUCCI, AMERIGO
1825–1837 "Las cuatro navigaciones . . . Carta al Ilustrismo Renato, Rey de Jerusalen y de Sicilia . . . [1504]," in *Colección de los viajes y descubrimientos que hicierón por mar los españoles desde fines del siglo xv, con varios documentos inéditos*, volume three. Edited by Martín de Fernández de Navarrete, 191–290. Madrid.

VON POEPPIG, EDUARD
1835–1836 *Reise in Chile, Peru und auf dem Amazonenströme, während der jahre 1827–1832*, two volumes. Leipzig.

VON TSCHUDI, J. J.
1849 *Travels in Peru during the years 1838–1842. . . .* Translated by Thomasina Ross. New York.

ZÁRATE, AGUSTÍN
1555 *Historia del descubrimiento y conquista del Perú.* Antwerp.

ZÚÑIGA, FRAY ANTONIO
1842–1895 "Carta . . . al Rey Don Felipe II, Peru, 15 de julio de 1579," in *Colección de documentos inéditos para la historia de España*, volume twenty-six. Edited by Martín Fernández de Navarrete, et al., 87–121. Madrid.

Information Concerning Court Cases

Causa criminal, 1681. Testigo . . . Juan Deochoa Aranda. . . . Archivo Arzobispal de Lima. Sección Idolatrías y Hechicerías, Expedientes. Siglos XVII–XVIII, Años 1604–1697, Legajo 2.
Causa criminal contra Juan de Rojas, su mujer y otros indios, 1723. Ar-

chivo Arzobispal de Lima. Sección Idolatrías y Hechicerías, Expedientes. Siglos XVII–XVIII–XIX, Años 1660–1850, Legajo 3.
Causa de idolatría, 1657. Los indios y indias hechiceros . . . del pueblo de S. Juan de Macachaca. . . . Archivo Arzobispal de Lima. Sección Idolatrías y Hechicerías, Expedientes. Siglos XVII–XVIII, Años 1606–1700, Legajo 4.
Causas criminales contra María de la Cruz y Augustín González, 1689. Archivo Arzobispal de Lima. Sección Idolatrías y Hechicerías, Expedientes. Siglos XVII–XVIII, Años 1660–1700, Legajo 1.
Información dada por . . . María de la Cruz . . . en la causa criminal, 1681. Archivo Arzobispal de Lima. Sección Idolatrías y Hechicerías, Expedientes. Siglos XVII–XVIII, Años 1604–1697, Abril de 1681, Legajo 2.
Información de brujo, 1739. Pueblo de Vilcabamba. Archivo Arzobispal de Lima. Sección Idolatrías y Hechicerías, Expedientes. Siglos XVII–XVIII–XIX, Años 1660–1850, Legajo 3.

Social Basis of Illness: A Search for Therapeutic Meaning

A. B. CHILIVUMBO

OVERVIEW

Most of the social investigators who have written about African society agree that belief systems as part of the structural components are causally related to illnesses (Gluckman 1966: 81–108; Evans-Pritchard 1937; Marwick 1965). It is pointed out by these writers, especially social anthropologists, that these beliefs are widespread. But in the interpretation of these beliefs and the way they cause illnesses the writers are not clear. Instead of analyzing belief systems in their broader structural context they have tended to concentrate on the structural patterns of accusations and the social functions of witchcraft belief in the societies in which they occur (Marwick 1952).

The present study focuses on the critical characteristics of the Malawi traditional societies and, therefore, the close link between the society and the individuals. One of the distinctive features of Malawi traditional societies lies in the qualities of the human relationships. They provide an encapsulation for the individual, making him live in an untenable world in which he is powerless to cope with insoluble conflicts. This leads to imaginative distortions of symbolism of reality and world view, i.e. his inside view, the ways in which the individual typically sees himself in relationship to his social map which determines the categories he uses in his perception of the familiar and strange, the healthy state and the unhealthy state, and the way in which he chooses among the alternatives before him.

This paper is based on research which was supported by the University of Malawi Research Committee. I wish to thank this organization.

In the course of growing up, the individual acquires a social map: structural orientation, which he internalizes and which provides him with alternative social routes, norms, taboos, rules, and sanctions. It provides for alternative modes of interpersonal relationships, a degree of predictability, his social contact point, and social predefinitions governing behavior. Revealed in this is the extreme importance of the link of the social-structural relationship to the healthy state of an individual and the importance of the ability to use the lines of communication to other people which are provided by the social structure which in the minds of the members is seen as all-encompassing. Ailments are seen as resulting from a person's inability for some reason to define his social-structural relationships as normal and his failure to find his social contact point.

A seemingly widespread syndrome or a cluster of ailments commonly experienced is the condition which one might call "magical fright" and "mental poisoning." Both often result in abnormal conditions of body and mind. In general they are manifested in an individual by temporary ego collapse, i.e. a state of being ill.

This article proposes to outline and examine the tenet that most of the ailments in Malawi traditional society are causally linked to a set of relationships in the social structure and that the cure is mysterious, carried out with the main objective, as understood by the patient and the *ng'anga* 'traditional doctor,' of effecting the reorientation of the patient to bring him back to his social contact point, his integration in the social fabric.

SOURCE OF DATA

Data used in this paper were gathered during a twelve-month period of research in various parts of Malawi in widely varying situations by several research assistants and through personal observations of sessions of treatment between some *ng'anga* and their patients. Material was derived from a non-random sample of patients, *ng'anga*, and others, collected through participant-observation, informal and intensive interviews covering over 200 subjects.[1] Informal interviews in the form of conversations were conducted by research assistants, most of whom were sociology students at Chancellor College. Intensive interviews with selected *ng'anga* and patients guided by question schedules probing specific

---

[1]   Most of the interviewees were illiterate and a few had no more than four years of formal education.

aspects of illness, diagnosis, methods of treatment, decision making, etc. were conducted by the author wherever appropriate during the course of research. Survey interviews were conducted largely around the districts of Blantyre, Mulanje, Zomba, and Lilongwe. Lack of funds and time precluded extending the survey to other areas. Interviews were initiated by an explanation to the respondent of the purpose of the research. To ensure cooperation, the names of most respondents were not asked. Interviews were conducted in Chichewa or English, whichever was appropriate for a particular respondent. Response was generally favorable from both patients and *ng'anga*.

CHOICES AND ALTERNATIVES OF THERAPY

Illness, a common and widespread phenomenon, is not only a highly personal affair, it arouses a wide variety of feelings in the sick person and in those close to him as they engage in a search for treatment, which becomes an immediate problem. Choices and alternatives are considered within the framework of existing knowledge and experience. Past experience of similar illnesses dictates the initial definition and diagnosis, and hence the initial treatment. People normally keep some medicine in their houses for common illnesses such as colds, fever, abdominal pains, etc. These may be roots, herbs, drugs, or tablets bought from shops. These are tried first.

A lack of response necessitates a search for more information on the illness from close friends, relatives, and neighbors who discuss and offer alternatives and suggestions regarding treatment. Subsequent failures lead to an intensive discussion of choices and a search for expert treatment from specialized parties. The choices of therapy are determined by several factors, especially the availability of a hospital and of the *ng'anga*. To many, clinics and hospitals are non-existent; they are too far away. Thus the choice is among several *ng'anga* — African medicine men. In the course of treatment several *ng'anga* may be tried consecutively or simultaneously. Where a patient is sent to a hospital, complementary treatment may still be received from *ng'anga* without the knowledge of the hospital officials.

The process is complex. For simple and easily cured ailments natural causes are imputed. But for more complex, serious, and prolonged illnesses both natural and non-natural causes are evoked. Thus one cannot easily suggest a neat division of illnesses into natural and non-natural. Instead, it becomes useful to regard illness as a complex phenomenon, one which derives its definition from the patient himself and those around him. In this postulated dimension illness is basically subjectively defined; the *ng'anga* in his diagnosis incorporates the patient's subjective definition of illness, which always involves the social structural set of the social fabric. Thus the patient, the kinsmen, and the *ng'anga* hold within the cultural framework certain perceptions of what might constitute an illness. Based on these perceptions and definitions subsequent curative steps logically follow. The value of these definitions lies in their power to dictate the direction of events.

In an attempt to assess the accuracy of these perceptions, a question of relevancy has to be decided upon. What is important from an actional viewpoint is not the objective cause or the "real" cause but rather what is DEFINED to be the cause. The cure which is meaningful to the patient is the one which sets his mind at rest. For example, a person may be somatically fit, but if he is psychologically convinced that he is not, it is the latter not the former state which is relevant. In this lies the relevance of the social structural framework of meanings. In other words, it is how the people perceive reality (in this case illness) rather than an objective assessment (of the cause of illness) which is pertinent. Thus diagnosis and therapeutic measures acquire meaning through subjective perceptions and a definite world view in which apparent irrationalities assume meaning and sense.

This is not to say that people in a traditional society suffer only from nonsomatic ailments. But, from the participants' viewpoint, each encounter with a serious ailment elicits aspects of mysticism which enter into the definition and patterns of cure.

Learning the Skill and Art of Healing

Ng'anga means a healer. Many people often know a few herbs as medicine for common simple ailments such as headache, etc. These are not *ng'anga*. The term is reserved and applied to more specialized medicine men who claim some degree of expertise. Many of the *ng'anga* interviewed were intitially patients, who after being cured learned the therapy from their *ng'anga* after paying a certain sum of money. The other category of *ng'anga* are trained herbalists, holders of certificates from herbalists' associations of either Rhodesia or South Africa. Their place of practice is in the markets in cities, towns, or district headquarters, and they tend to be commercially oriented and are often quite literate. The last category of *ng'anga* are those who claim to have attained skills through dreams or visions. Very frequently these are the *ng'anga* most sought after as their claim to cure has more mystical aura and is more in line with general expectations. Among them are a few who claim to have died and to have been resurrected. In the process they picked up therapeutic skills. Accounts from a few *ng'anga* will illustrate the process of the mysterious learning of therapeutic skills.

Dickson Mwamadi is a well-known *ng'anga* in the suburb of Blantyre City. He became a *ng'anga* after several dreams in which an old woman or several aged people one at a time came in turns to take him to the bush, showing him various medicinal plants and explaining to him the type of illness each plant could cure. Mwamadi used to tell the dreams to his parents, who would help him identify his dream visitors. By the description of their physical appearance, physique, the mode of dress, speech, and complexion the parents were able to identify the persons and informed Mwamadi of their names and their relationship to him. The process was reassuring and encouraging. The dreams carried specific instructions requesting him to cure certain people who were sick and this he did with amazing success. In the treatment he followed fastidiously the instructions supplied to him in the dream. Often, if the instructions were followed properly by the patient the illness would respond to treatment. After a period of apprenticeship Mwamadi gained ample experience and confidence to enable him to cure the patients without dreams.

Robson Likango is another well-known *ng'anga*. He also learned the skill in dreams. In his dreams he was visited by his ancestors. The visitors, who came singly, used to stand upright in front of him and would show a tree and explain the type of illness the plant could cure. The men in the dream explained in detail how to diagnose such an illness by showing him its signs, symptoms, etc. The demonstration session helped Likango to recognize the illness and the plants. The following morning Likango would write down in note form his night's experience. These instructions were given to him although there was no one who had that particular illness. He used the information later in curing illnesses when some people were ill. Success depended on the correct following of the instructions given to him, and when the patient followed these correctly he would be cured. After a period Likango gained confidence in his diagnosis and treatment of various illnesses and the dreams stopped. Now he practices without dreaming.

Bwanali is another well-known *ng'anga*. Accounts of how he learned his skills resemble those of the other two described above. He saw in a dream mysterious people who he claims gave him the skills to cure people. The visitors gave him instructions on how to treat several illnesses. Bwanali reinforces these by going to the hill-caves, where day and night for a couple of days a week he fasts, prays, and meditates. Through the meditations, treatments of mysterious illnesses are revealed to him. As a result Bwanali is a well-known *ng'anga* in the southern region of Malawi.

The *ng'anga* practice without licences. Their claim to heal is based on their success. Those who are more successful have more patients. The more successful the *ng'anga*, the more famous he becomes. Only a few have in-patients, the majority being out-patients.

A fee is often charged. The first fee, which is nominal, of about 10t is called *chipondamthengo* — payment for the trouble of getting the medicine in the bush.[2] The final fee, a more substantial sum, is paid when the patient is cured. Those who claim that their power to cure came from dreams or visions do not accept direct payment. However, they are not reluctant to receive payment in kind. The herbalists, holders of certificates from herbalists' associations, are more commercial. Patients are charged in relation to the frequency of their visits.

Diagnosis and Cure

There are no clear, well-patterned methods of diagnosis. Many *ng'anga* are guided by the information derived from the patient and the patient's escorts, and on the basis of these accounts they are able from long experience to come to some tentative decision on the type of illness and therapy. For example, the *ng'anga* asks the patient to describe how he feels. In the course of the description the *ng'anga* can ask leading questions on the symptoms and signs of the illness with which the patient agrees and this creates confidence in the patient. This process, which is dexterously done, is used often as a tactical means of gaining the patient's confidence. In the course of the discussions, the *ng'anga* will throw in hints of causes, vaguely suggesting certain individuals who might bear the patient ill will. This is skillfully done by the *ng'anga*, who throws vague hints leaving the patient himself to give substance to the hints. As the patient specifies what could be the causes the *ng'anga* nods in approval.

A commonly used method of diagnosis is divination. Several implements are employed in the process of divinition (*kuombeza maula*). Some medicine is put in the *supa*, a gourd-like container. When a patient arrives, before he tells the *ng'anga* his illness the latter looks into the *supa*;

---

[2]   Malawi uses *Kwahca* (K) and *tambala* (t). 1K is equivalent to 50 British pence and 1t is equivalent to ½ British pence.

contemplating a few minutes, he announces that he can see the one who caused the illness. For example, he may say: "I see you passing along a certain path and you urinate. Soon after your departure a certain man, youngish in outlook, who was following you but hid under the bush as you were urinating, picks up the wet soil from where you passed water and when he arrives at his home he mixes this with medicine to wish you harm." The *ng'anga* may ask, "Don't you remember this day when you passed water near a tall tree?" As people rarely use toilets, the patient can easily believe and vaguely recall some such incident.

Illness is believed to be caused by a myriad of factors. An individual can become sick if an enemy picks up sand from the mark of his foot, i.e. if you pass by, a person may pick up sand and use it for bewitching you, or a person may pick up dust from your shadow, or if he knows the name you were given when you were born he can use that as a catalyst for bewitching you. These mysterious ways of causing illnesses — juju or voodoo — are believed to cause most illnesses.

Since most illnesses carry aspects of mysticism, most of the diagnoses are equally mystical. A few accounts of diagnoses throw light on the issue. Y is a *ng'anga* who said of his diagnosis methods: "I look at the patient and with the use of medicine I hypnotize him. In this way he tells me the symptoms in a clear, detailed way. Without this the patient is not able to state exactly what his problem is." T, another *ng'anga,* had this to say: "I treat straightforward illnesses so I do not have to diagnose. What is more, I have powers of knowing, intuitively, the basis of the patient's ailment." X said: "It is difficult to diagnose illness. However, when the patient tells me signs and symptoms of his illness I am able to make out what he is suffering from." Z told us: "As for many illnesses which come to me I have a fair knowledge of their symptoms due to long experience. But I sometimes consult my magical gourd (*nsupa*), to help me." K said: "What I do all the time is to take my gourd, a special gourd with a long neck adorned with beads and filled with castor oil, and I ask it to tell me what is troubling the patient. It gives me answers which I can read and see clearly printed inside the gourd. No one else can read, see, or hear these answers." W said: "I have no problems in diagnosis. When the patient comes I have an inspiration which tells me what the real problem is and how to cure it. The inspiration comes after the patient has given me a full account of his illness." B said: "I first find out whether the patient suffers from natural or unnatural illness and I proceed to give him treatment accordingly." A told us: "I have chizimba 'detector of illness'. My father made eight tattoo marks on my left arm, but did not rub any medicine on them. Instead he got hold of lightning and transmitted it through the eight tattoo marks into me. This lightning now gives me unnatural powers, enabling me to diagnose illness easily. When the patient comes to me I hold some medicine in his hand, and the pains which he experiences are transmitted into my body and I am able to diagnose the illness, hence able to treat him." These are only a few examples of the practiced methods of diagnosis.

The treatment procedures are equally varied. Most of the procedures aim at curing both the natural and the unnatural aspects of illness. The treatment may consist of exorcism, dancing, tying pieces of roots around the neck, waist, arms, or legs, soaking roots in water and drinking the water or using the water to prepare porridge which is eaten, applying powdered medicine to tattoos or adding the powder to water or porridge.

X, for instance, told us how he cures *mauka*, an illness of the abdomen. "I take certain leaves, pound them in a mortar, and put them in warm water for the patient to wash in. After washing, the patient drains the container by pushing it with his buttocks." Another *ng'anga* said: "Depending on the illness, I either give medicine to drink like tea or I cut tattoos and rub in medicine."

Z told us of *likango* 'pile'. She believes this can be caused by either natural or unnatural causes. Its effects on a female are that as it grows inside it affects the reproductive system and leads to miscarriages. Where there is a live birth, the child dies in infancy. In girls this disease interferes with breast growth and the girl has tiny breasts or none at all. As the organism sucks blood the person is weak and loses appetite. Z treats it initially by cutting it and applying medicine to it so that the wound dries up. If this fails, the patient is given medicine in the form of roots which must be soaked in water to be taken like tea or used for porridge.

She charges her patients a nominal initial fee of a few *tambala*. When she gives the patients medicine there is a proper way of receiving it. First the receiver holds the roots, and before the *ng'anga* releases them, she makes a slight jerk of the arms and then the roots are released. At the end of the treatment there is a ritual called *kutsirika* — a process which ensures that the illness will not attack the patient again. All the roots which the patient was using are preserved and on this final day the patient carries the roots blindfolded, walking backwards or crawling to a junction of paths, i.e. where two paths cross each other, and here the roots are dropped. The *ng'anga* buries the roots in the ground. The patient is told not to eat any legs of chicken, not to touch certain plants, and not to climb on top of an anthill. Z then charges a final fee which is often 10K.

Another example is that of K, who treats patients suffering from *mizimu* 'spirits'. His cure is largely exorcism. The patient is given medicine and requested to give a feast-like sacrifice to his ancestors *(sadaka)*. Various foods are prepared and people are invited to eat. But sometimes his treatment consists of the following. The patient is covered with a cloth of any color, and a clay pot containing smoldering roots and hot water is set before him. The *ng'anga,* who sits next to the patient, tells him to inhale the steam while the *ng'anga* implores the spirit to leave the patient alone. These sessions last a few hours and are repeated until the patient recovers.

There are some *ng'anga* who treat alcoholics. The following case is a report of an observed cure of an alcoholic.

Q, a high-ranking Government official, became an alcoholic during training abroad. Modern psychiatric and medical care failed. On his return home, having of course failed to complete the course successfully, the high-ranking official was the epitome of shaking palsy. Only a bottle of Malawi gin could keep him "normal." The *ng'anga* treating him gave him a cupful of hot water mixed with one teaspoonful of ground medicine. When drinking it while holding the breasts of his wife, he repeated the following words after the *ng'anga*: "If I did not stop sucking my mother's breasts, then I should not stop drinking; if I stopped, then I must stop drinking." Many months have now passed by without his taking any liquor and there have been so far no psychosomatic side effects. The high-ranking official appears normal. The *ng'anga* demanded no remuneration.

Many other cases can be cited but some final cases of interest come from a well-known African medicine man, Mr. Bwanali of Mwanza district on the border of Malawi with Mozambique. He cures many types of illnesses. In our visit to Bwanali, we found most complaints of his patients to consist of vague bodily pains. Many complained of chest pain, of abdominal pain, of leg pains, and some complained of having suffered from pains for the past nine years. Almost all of them have tried hospitals without getting satisfactory results. Their ailments were vague, amorphous, and obscure. Some verbal reports from live discussions with the patients may throw light on the nature of these ailments.

Patient A

Questioner: How are you?
Patient: A little better.
Q.:   What are you suffering from?
P.:   I was employed at some place and while working there, some

of my fellow workers practiced magic with a view to getting me out of work. So one day as I was going home I met a strange figure on the way and I passed by it. When I reached home, I began to suffer from various illnesses.

Q.:   How do you feel now?
P.:   There is a little improvement.

Patient B

Questioner: What are you suffering from, madam?
Patient: I feel piercing pains here and there in the whole body.
Q.:   When did you come here?
P.:   Three weeks ago.
Q.:   So how do you feel now? How do you think you got the disease — do you perhaps think it's from some bad people?
P.:   I don't know whether it's from God or not.
Q.:   Is your home near?
P.:   My home is in Mulanje [100 miles from Mwanza].
Q.:   How did you come here?
P.:   I came by bus.

Patient C

Questioner: How are you, madam?
Patient: Not so well.
Q.:   Where do you come from?
P.:   I come from Zomba [100 miles from Mwanza].
Q.:   When did you come here?
P.:   I came on Wednesday.
Q.:   What is wrong with you?
P.:   I have heart troubles.
Q.:   How does it trouble you?
P.:   I feel burning pains in the chest which make me not feel well.
Q.:   For how long have you had this trouble?
P.:   This is the ninth year.

The reported illnesses carry mystical aspects. In the patient's mind, the illnesses are more than somatic and Bwanali represents a mysterious healer, a healer with extraordinary talents who reinforces his knowledge, as already stated, by habitual praying in one of the caves in the nearby hills. Through the prayers, cases which do not respond to treatment may be solved by discovering an appropriate cure or even new medicine.

In his cure medicinal potency is shrouded in the mystical influence. It operates on two levels: the biochemical process and the psyche. The method is both curative and preventive. It aims at physical cure, puts at ease the patient's anxieties, reinstates in the patient the will to live, frees him from fear, and restores him to normal functioning within social fabric. The patient gains the will to live, feels cured, redefines his reality, and gains proper perspective in his cosmos.

DISCUSSION AND CONCLUSION

The society being discussed is cohesive; the social structure provides the individual with modes of reintegration into the social fabric. It rallies about him giving him a sense of belonging and of being alive. Thus the social structure can either contract and leave the person to develop a sense of loss of orientation or give him a sense of life. Man in a traditional society lives closer to nature; his cosmos is entangled with mysticism and bewilderment. The level of technology and the development of the intellectual faculty are relatively low, with the result that individuals lack the ability to grasp their environment on an intricate level. The world around is shrouded in mysteries; unknowns and mythology lie at the heart of the explanation of daily events. Individuals are engulfed in intimate face-to-face social relationships and intense meaningful social interaction. The psychosomatic euphoria of individuals is inextricably tied to the smooth social fabric. Consequently, irregularities or disorders in the social fabric, whether actual or imagined, are unhealthy to both the society and individuals: they evoke fear of the unknown, cause anxieties and trauma affecting the individual's social orientation and his redefinition of his state of health.

Behavior contrary to predefinitions is conceived of as unhealthy. Supportive cases include ailments arising from a complex of causes. In these societies unfaithfulness is a source of illness. Sexual relations outside wedlock are deadly, causing a cluster of illnesses. Belief has it that if the husband of an expectant wife has an illicit sexual relationship, the foetus will die when he enters his house. Should the expectant mother have intercourse out of wedlock, labor will be difficult, and may even result in the death of both the mother and the baby. After sexual intercourse a woman becomes taboo. Any baby she touches contracts illness and may die. If she adds salt to relish or cooks any food, those who eat it contract *mdulo*, a blood-vomiting illness.

Other examples can be drawn from observed cases of mental poisoning. A high proportion of our respondents talked of "dangerous men" possessing dangerous powers over life or death. If they say, "You will not see the sunset," the addressee instantly contracts illness and may even die before sunset. This mental poisoning is explainable in terms of the undifferentiated cosmos of the "rural man." Not everyone can be a "dangerous man" but there were those who were suspected of witch-craft and feared in society. The words of such men possess an arsenal of power affecting the issue of life and death. Respondents talked in fear of oral threats from such people which result in illness or death. If such a person says, "Before dawn you will be sick or die," it was said that often a person may become sick or even die within the stated period. The validity of such accounts finds support in the concept of mental poisoning, in that the threat has a psychosomatic effect on the addressee by disorienting his total reality, disrupting his social map and social orientation; he becomes drugged and mesmerized; he loses the will to live.

To a technologist there is no logic in such an imputation of cause and effect. However, the logic does not lie in the scientific verification; rather it is found in the cosmos of the undifferentiated character of the thought system in which illness is conceived of as one aspect of a life in which the various aspects are intimately knitted together subsumed under one causal fabric of man, nature, and social relationships. Any breach of social predefinitions sets off a whole chain of processes; the psyche is disturbed and subsequently, in a mysterious manner, leads to a physiological maladaptive response engulfing the totality of man. Thus the causality exists in the nature of things.

Other societal disorders which were constantly encountered derived from the societal strains of changing environments. Many of these strains relate to economic changes. An individual who is richer than the rest is a target of suspicion; people start asking why he alone of all people should become rich. Any illness in the village or among his neighbors is conceived of as being linked to his wealth.

An example can be cited of a rich man's niece in Zomba, the capital of Malawi. Richness in the rural man's cosmos is seen as a social disorder and is associated with kinsmen's death. The case of M of Zomba is illustrative. M's uncle wants to buy a car and a lorry. M meanwhile contracts illness of depression (*majini*) (Chilivumbo 1972). She is very sick, has lost a lot of weight but refuses to go to the hospital though it is within walking distance of her home. She prefers to go to an African medicine man because in her mind her illness has been caused by the uncle who wishes to use parts of her body for *chizimba* as a catalyst for his wealth. She seeks a cure which consists of medicine intended to cure her psychologically, put her mind at peace, and neutralize her uncle's evil desires.

As stated earlier, so many of the illnesses are seen as derived from societal strains, and social disorders, especially in social relationships, are linked to various illnesses. Thus many people in these societies are easily susceptible to esoteric disorders which carry perilous infirmities. Bwanali's statements, along with others, give firm support to this proposition. A lot of the logic in the link between illness and the traditional society in Malawi remains unknown and requires careful study. The extent of our lack of knowledge in this aspect of Malawi life is perhaps a great source of concern and warrants more attention than it has received.

In conclusion, therefore, I wish to stress the obvious fact that illness among the Malawi traditional people is often linked to social relationships. The social structure has clear predefinitions governing behavior, and deviation from the prescribed rules is seen as a source of bad luck. Thus beliefs in taboos and witchcraft all point to the same idea, i.e. when certain predefinitions are not followed, the individuals who believe in mystical powers start a search for meanings; social disorders create loss of a contact point for individuals in their social map. The cure is intended to bring the sick person back to his contact point and to put his mind at ease.

Finally, therefore, it should be stressed that here we are making an attempt to draw attention to the relationship between illness and social structures. In the context of the discussion it appears that there is ample data to indicate that the link exists, that the mode of the link is varied, and that its specification is a matter requiring more research in specific situations.

REFERENCES

CHILIVUMBO, A. B.
  1972   Vimbuza or Mashawe: a mystic therapy. *African Music: Journal of the African Music Society* 5(2):6–9.
EVANS-PRITCHARD, E. E.
  1937   *Witchcraft, oracles and magic among the Azande of the Anglo-Egyptian Sudan.* Oxford: Clarendon Press.
GLUCKMAN, M.
  1966   *Custom and conflict in Africa.* Oxford: Basil Blackwell.
MARWICK, M.
  1950   Another anti-witchcraft movement in East Central Africa. *Africa* 20:100–112.
  1952   The social context of Ceira witch beliefs. *Africa* 22:120–135.
  1965   *Sorcery in its social setting: a study of the Northern Rhodesian Cewa.* Manchester: Manchester University Press.

Snakebite Cure among the
Rama Indians of Nicaragua

FRANKLIN O. LOVELAND

1. This paper has its origins in Evans-Pritchard's remark, "The purely ritual character of most Zande treatments is evident at a glance" (Evans-Pritchard 1937: 492–493). This remark leads us in two directions. On the one hand, we can examine curing from the perspective of "mystical" causes such as sorcery and witchcraft which in turn relate to the social situation. On the other hand, these "mystical" causes operate in concert with natural causes, which are also important to the Zande as the causes of disease. The question remains, however, for us as anthropologists, how we can meaningfully approach the study of "mystical" causes and "ritual" treatments in contrast to natural causes and natural treatments. It is this question which is central to medical anthropology.

In a recent paper (1971), F. B. Welbourn indicated that, "Zande medical practice thus asserts that in the aetiology of every disease there is in principle, both a "natural' and a 'social' factor; and this dual causation is recognized also in contemporary western social medicine, which tends to use endo-psychic instead of exo-psychic symbols." Turner, in discussing Ndembu medicine likewise sees this dual aspect of medicine. Certain Ndembu cures are private and involve only herbalists while other diseases involve "mystical" causes and "therapy becomes a mat-

This paper is based on fieldwork done at Rama Cay, Nicaragua, during the summer of 1969 and February–October, 1970. The research was supported by grants from the Duke University Graduate School, a National Institute of Mental Health Training Grant, Public Health Service Grant No. PHS # 5SO5 FRO 7070-04, and by the Wenner-Gren Foundation. I would like to thank my Rama informants, Cornelio Omier, Willie Macre, and Felix Williams. Also I would like to thank Dr. Weston La Barre and Dr. Christopher Crocker who encouraged me and my wife, Christine Loveland, whose cogent counsel made a final draft of this paper possible.

ter of sealing up the branches in social relationships simultaneously with ridding the patient (*muyeji*) of his pathological symptoms" (Turner 1970: 360).

Finally, a discussion of Glick's illuminating model for the analysis of evidence, process, and cause in medical diagnostic systems and negatively and positively directed therapeutic systems seems appropriate (Glick 1967: 35–38). In this model, evidence is equated with symptoms, process with pathological processes, and causes with instrumental, efficient, and ultimate causes (Glick 1967: 35–37). Negatively directed therapies remove or neutralize "malevolent sources of power" while positive systems of therapy try to restore the power of the victim himself (Glick 1967: 37). It will be seen that each of these concepts is important in analyzing medical systems but that certain cures such as those for snakebite focus on immediate processes rather than on causes *per se*. However, the "positively directed" therapy associated with snakebite cure makes conceptual statements about the ultimate causes and effects of snakebite, and it is in this context that this type of medical system may be fully understood.

The theoretical background of this paper is one of emphasis on social and cultural correlates of medical practices. This paper will deal with the snakebite cure of the Rama Indians of eastern Nicaragua. In a recent paper which analyzes the origin myth of this cure, I have shown that the snakebite represents exchanges at the highest level of Rama conceptual order and further justifies the processual model of Rama society and culture (F. Loveland n.d.: 1). These exchanges occur on several different levels of Rama society; in same sex and cross-sex groups, between siblings and brothers-in-law, and in the context of domestic groups (F. Loveland n.d.: 5). They also refer to two types of sexuality. One is associated with reproduction, the domestic group, and hence may be termed "restricted" sexuality; the other is associated with unfulfillable sexual desire (incestuous and phallic libidinal pleasure) in the context of potential sexual partners outside the domestic group, and may be termed "unrestricted sexuality" (F. Loveland n.d.: 7, 11).

Both the cure and the myth manipulate these conceptual categories, at several levels of the social structure, by integrating or isolating the patient so as to achieve a cure. At the same time, the myth and the cure represent a basic non-elaborated cuisine and a return to cultural basics, such as lack of condiments in food, the elimination of sexually hot foods, and elimination of foods that are hunted, i.e. meat. All of this points toward the idea that Rama snakebite cure must first be anchored in this conceptual framework to be understood. Our purpose here is to focus on the ethnographic data of Rama snakebite cure and then to analyze it in the context of certain crucial social-cultural factors which relate to exo-psychic as well as endo-psychic factors. This paper may be conveniently divided into three parts. Section 2 will briefly introduce the reader to Rama culture ethnographically and discuss the Rama view of snakes generally. Section 3 will present the ethnographic data on Rama snakebite while Section 4 will analyze it.

2. The Rama Indians are members of the Chibchan language family and presently reside in four major settlements in the lowland tropical rainforest of the Atlantic coast of Nicaragua. Census data indicate that the present population numbers some 450 individuals. The largest settlement of Rama is located in the southern portion of Bluefields Lagoon on the island of Rama Cay. It is this community upon which this research is based.

The Rama[1] practice slash-and-burn agriculture at plots on nearby rivers. Agriculture is supplemented by hunting, fishing, and gathering activities. These activities correspond to seasonal variations in the rainfall and in turn to the constant changes of faunal environment created by the corresponding changes in salinity levels of Bluefields Lagoon. The Rama live in a liminal environment, that of the estuary lagoon, which seasonally alternates between the saltwater of the ocean and the freshwater of nearby rivers, corresponding to the dry and wet seasons respectively.

The basic social group for the Rama is the *kwimah* or *kwinbalut,* the household unit or extended family. Some married children may live adjacent to the household, but generally the household consists of three or four generations. The household is built around the household head, *nu abing* 'houseowner', a middle-aged man or woman. Also the household unit provides a kinship network through which partners in economic or subsistence activities are chosen. In fact, marriage itself is seen as an economic partnership which involves a number of affinal obligations beyond the economic obligations of the spouses to one another. Ideally residence is neolocal, but with the shortage of land on Rama

---

[1] Hereafter, Rama refers to the Northern Rama of Rama Cay, Nicaragua. This ethnographic description of the Rama is meant to serve as an introduction to their culture. Virtually no major ethnographic work on the Rama in English has appeared in modern times. However, the situation is changing and two articles will soon be available. Bernard and Judy Nietschmann's "Change and continuity: the Rama Indians of Nicaragua" will soon be published in *America Indigena*. Also Christine Loveland's "Rural-urban dynamics: the Miskito Coast of Nicaragua" was just published.

Cay it is not always possible. At the death of a household head, a struggle over inheritance ensues between the brothers-in-law and the children of the household head.

Local level political processes among the Rama take the form of opposition of factions, headed by *nakiknah ma* 'big men'. In 1969–1970, there were two factions on Rama Cay: one controlled by the Christian group which advocated a more traditional viewpoint, and the other faction headed by a young *ladino*-ized Rama who advocated change and more involvement with Bluefields, a nearby city. This second faction's leader eventually lost power because he had an affair with a stepdaughter of the leader of the other faction.

The traditional religion of the Rama was built around *turmali* or seers. *Turmali* apprenticed by seeking visions through fasting in the bush. *Turmali* also cured illnesses. In 1859, the Moravian Mission established a mission at Rama Cay and attempted to change the religion. However, the Rama belief system remains intact in spite of Moravian efforts to change their beliefs and the strong influence of Western culture in recent years.

The general term for snakes in Rama is *albut*. Modern-day usage indicates the term is now used to refer almost exclusively to harmful snakes of the water moccasin and boa constrictor groups, although in the past it referred to the *fer de lance* group. The Rama also utilize the term *tamigar* to refer to harmful or poisonous snakes generally, and particularly those of the *fer de lance* group.

The Rama distinguish between eleven different types of snakes. Several different species of *fer de lance* are recognized, also the coral snake and water moccasin, boa, and several species of harmless snakes. The flexibility of usage of taxonomic names among the Rama requires further investigation. In general, though, we may conclude that as only two of eleven taxonomic names of snakes in Rama refer to harmless snakes, the Rama are much more concerned with poisonous and harmful snakes.

In general, the Rama believe that snakes are similar to men, as they were like men in creation times and have homes like men today. As noted previously, the Rama believe most snakes are harmful or dangerous. They do not eat snakes because that would make you sick. Also snakes, unlike most other land animals, are considered to have cold blood by the Rama. Their bite causes great heat to accumulate in the victim's body and the snakebite cure attempts to "cool down" the patient by removing sexually dangerous individuals from him and by isolating him socially and culturally. Let us turn to the snakebite cure itself.

3. At the time of our fieldwork there were two practicing snakebite curers on Rama Cay. One of these was in the process of completing an apprenticeship under a third snakedoctor who had given up his practice shortly before our arrival on Rama Cay because of the death of two of his patients. The other snakedoctor had apprenticed under a Sumu man in the Punta Gorda River area of Nicaragua. He had been curing snakebite since he was fifteen years old. His practice at Rama Cay did not begin until many years later when he migrated to the Rama Cay area. The retired snakedoctor had been an apprentice under a Black Carib Indian from Orinoco, Nicaragua, a man by the name of Isedroe Zenone, the great grandson of John Sambole, the founder of Orinoco.[2] This apprenticeship took place some seventeen years before the time of our study. Much of this retired snakedoctor's knowledge follows the Black Carib method for curing snakebite (Damon n.d.: 1). Interestingly enough there has been some diffusion of snakebite cures from the Rama to the Black Carib during this apprenticeship as well as diffusion of Miskito and Black Carib herbal and cosmological knowledge to the Rama. It is for this reason that any consideration of Rama snakebite curing techniques also involves a consideration of Miskito, Carib, and Sumu medical knowledge and associated beliefs concerning the cause and cure of snakebite.[3]

According to Lehmann, Rama snakedoctors, *albut ain kauling* 'snake his people', are "Besondere Männer die mit Giftschlangen geschickt umgehen und im Rufe stehen, übernatürliche Kräfte zu besitzen" (Lehmann 1914: 24). Certainly, Rama snakedoctors are skillful in removing snake poison as evidenced by the high recovery rate (see Table 2), but the question may be raised whether modern-day Rama snakedoctors rely on supernatural powers in curing snakebite victims. In

[2] Solien de González noted that, "A few Carib individuals, some with their families, have moved to other regions . . ." (Solien de González 1969: 24). John Sambole was one of these individuals whose family migrated to Nicaragua five or six generations ago. John Sembole married a Miskito woman and it is this marriage which is cited as proof of kinship with neighboring Miskito villages. This is an adaptation to a new environment which proved successful for the Caribs. However, the situation is changing today. See Solien de González (1969: 25, 27–29) for a discussion of this problem.

[3] It could be argued that the Rama do not have an indigenous form of snakebite cure because their present-day snakedoctors apprenticed under Black Carib and Sumu snakedoctors. Missionary records and autobiographical statements indicate clearly that the Rama have been curing snakebite using their own *materia medica* from the precontact period to the present. In recent times, the Rama have relied more on the herbal knowledge of neighboring peoples following the Miskito pattern of purchasing herbal remedies for snakebite (Peck 1968: 84). Also the Rama rely on a Miskito prophet for curing certain classes of supernatural illnesses. For an account of a Miskito prophet see Peck (1968: 82–84).

all accounts of snakebite cures given to me by informants, including snakedoctors, there was no mention of the use of supernatural power to attain the cure. Prophets do have supernatural power to see or foretell the future, and this power might be employed in curing. To resolve this conflict it is hypothesized that in the postcontact period the importance of supernatural power declined, especially in the last fifty years when the *turmali* decreased in numbers. It is also plausible that after contact with the Miskito, the Rama snakedoctors relied more heavily on herbal knowledge than supernatural power. For the Miskito, the role of supernatural power is minimal, as Peck notes:

Snakebites are not treated by the *sukya*. Bush snakebite medicine is fairly widely known. In fact the knowledge can be purchased from people who know the specific herbs to use for specific kinds of snakes (Peck 1968: 84).

Some associated beliefs concerning the relationship between people, animals, and snakes and the cause and cure of illness complete our understanding of Rama beliefs concerning snakedoctors and their role in Rama society. The Rama believe that certain people can transform themselves into animals (*aisukya*) and that certain diseases (*yakuki*) are brought on by seeing certain animals. These illnesses are cured by the *turmali*, using supernatural power to cure them. It is not clear whether the *turmali* transform themselves into animals in order to achieve the cure and whether or not the illnesses are brought on by seeing people who have transformed themselves into animals or just by seeing certain animals or both. In the myth presented in a previous paper, it was shown that the snakes were transformed into people in the land of the snakes in creation times (F. Loveland n.d.: 3). It is conceivable that this inverse relationship on the mythic level sets apart the class of illnesses related to snakebite and justifies it. Although there is no direct evidence, one informant noted that snakedoctors are "close to snakes." Another informant, Cornelio Omier, a snakedoctor himself, mentioned that a snakedoctor cannot kill a snake or he would surely die. He told a story to make this point. One day, he was returning from weeding some bananas at Western Hill across from Rama Cay. When he returned to his dorry (*ut*), he found a large snake of a poisonous variety under his dorry. In spite of all his efforts to get it out from under the dorry without killing it, he could not. (At this point in telling the story the informant's expression changed, revealing a real fear of the snake, possibly because he believed that it was not an ordinary snake.) He walked up and down and as night drew closer he became anxious. Finally, he managed to get the snake out from under the dorry and quickly paddled toward Rama Cay. The snake, to his amazement, followed him and then he knew it was not an ordinary snake and he could not kill it. He said he did not feel well for several days thereafter. We cannot be sure what the relationship is between the snakedoctors and snakes, but it is possible that in mythic time as well as linear time, they participated in a unique relationship — that of *aisukya* — in which snakes can be transformed people and people transformed snakes.

Rama snakedoctors are recruited through several channels. First, a snakedoctor usually has been bitten and cured, and this serves as a prerequisite for his apprenticeship. Second, kinship ties and status affect the recruitment of snakedoctors. In one case, a man taught his wife's sister's son how to cure snakebite. This same man was quite important in the Rama Cay community, and it is said that he learned how to cure snakebite because some years before he had been bitten by a *samut* in the Corn River area and had survived because of anti-venom shots administered by a prospector. Also his wife's father's brother had cured him of a snakebite in the Tswani River area. All of these factors may have affected his decision to apprentice. The other snakedoctor on Rama Cay did not have any close relatives who were snakedoctors. However, he was a well-respected man in the Punta Gorda area, especially since he spoke Spanish and successfully made the transition to the *ladino* world there. As a career possibility, then, snakedoctoring usually enhances the individual's status, which usually is already higher than that of the average individual in Rama society. Notice also that in at least one case, most of the important kinship relationships in snakedoctor apprenticeship are affinal relationships that are operationalized as the basis of a career in snakedoctoring.

The apprenticeship usually involves a period of sexual abstinence and a number of trips to the bush to learn the names and uses of various medicinal plants. It could not be determined whether the initiate underwent a period of fasting to obtain supernatural power as is the case with the *turmali*. Informants concentrated more on detailing the knowledge of herbal medicine and did not indicate whether one had to seek supernatural power. It is presumed that the fact that one had survived snakebite and sought out a snakedoctor under which to apprentice made one a "snakeperson" and therefore a good candidate for snakedoctoring. Exactly how much time was involved in becoming an apprentice and learning snakebite cure is not clear. The first patient an apprentice treated usually was a friend or relative. In two recorded cases, one snakedoctor treated a cousin as his first patient, the other treated a member of his own or wife's family. In all cases, the first cure was a success, and the snakedoctor's reputation was built from that cure.

The cure of snakebite wounds is accomplished through the use of leaves, roots, and the powder of the head of a snake (*tamigar*). Table 1 presents a list of the most common leaves and roots used in snakebite cure on the Miskito Coast. Such material has been touched upon by Heath (1950) and also in an unpublished manuscript (Heath n.d.). This list represents a compilation of those sources, Hodge and Taylor (1957), Conzemius (1932), and unpublished fieldnotes of Fred Damon for the Black Carib and of myself for the Rama. The leaves and roots are prepared in a variety of ways and utilized in compresses, decoctions, poultices, teas, or even chewed raw. These *materia medica* are gathered by the snakedoctors alone. They are the only ones to know all the names and functions of plants used in snake medicine. Individuals do learn something about certain important first aid snakebite remedies, but the body of systematic knowledge about herbal remedies for snakebite cure is encompassed in the knowledge of the snakedoctor. He is the only one who knows all the plant names and who can classify and utilize them in curing snakebite. Some doctors will gather the plants only at night. Others will gather them during the day but they must be sure no one sees them or they will lose their power to cure snakebite. One snakedoctor made a small garden near his house where he kept the plants to be ready if needed. Most of the plants are non-domesticated plants and must be gathered in the tropical rain forest surrounding the homes and agricultural plots of the Ramas. Informants did not disclose how long it took to gather the necessary plants and roots. They did say that they dried the medicine and kept it in a special place ready to be used in the event someone was bitten. The doctor who cured by using plants from his small herbal garden did not have these difficulties because he could use the plants from his garden as they were needed.

The basis of the snakebite cure of the Rama is a powder made of the leaves and/or roots of thirteen to thirty different plants (see Table 1). As noted above, the leaves or roots are roasted or smoked over the cooking fire in order to prepare them to be ground up as a powder. Also added to this powder of various leaves and roots is the powder of a smoked snakehead (*tamigar*) which is prepared in a way similar to the leaves. The snake is one which has bitten someone and has subsequently been killed and prepared by the snakedoctor for use in snake medicine. The Black Carib say the head must come from a female snake with no eggs and that it must have both fangs present (Damon n.d.: 1). As with the roots and leaves, the head of the snake is placed above the fire where eventually the smoke from the cooking fire dries it out. It is then put in a small paper sack where it is kept until it is needed. The dried snakehead is ground up into a powder and added to the herbal teas and infusions which are given to the patient during the cure. The Ramas are aware of the danger the poison presents especially if the snakehead is that of a *tamigar*. At all stages of the preparation of the medicine, the utmost caution is exercised to make sure that none of the snakehead powder gets into a cut or sore. In spite of the powder's poisonous effects, the Rama say that the medicine would not help the patient if it did not include the snakehead powder and therefore it is utilized. It is hypothesized that the snakehead probably contains less venom than normally would be expected, especially if it comes from a snake which had recently bitten someone. However, this contradiction in their belief system which, on the one hand, says the medicinal value of the dried snake head is significant and, on the other hand, that the snakehead can kill someone if the poison gets into a cut or sore, does not create confusion for the Rama. For when the special status of the snakebite victim is considered, i.e. being hot in relation to the cooler condition of other people, it is clear that the poisonous snakehead operates on a principle of analogy, hot with hot. It is also possible that the Rama believe the ashes of a snake who is hostile will somehow counteract the snake who is presently overwhelming the victim. In turn, this corresponds with their belief that in spite of destruction even to the state of ashes the essence of life forms remains.[4]

After a person has been bitten, the first thing that must be done is to kill the snake that has bitten the snakebite victim. Although the snake itself is not used in the cure, it must be killed or the patient cannot be cured. If a person is alone, it is his responsibility to kill it immediately. Under no circumstances must the snake be shot with a gun or the patient could not be cured (La Barre 1969: 195, Note 2). If the snakebite vic-

---

[4] Although this statement might seem to be mere conjecture, it is based on several ethnographic facts. First, the Rama associate ashes with the Milky Way where the souls of the dead go. According to Lehmann, someone spreads hot ashes over the path where the souls of the dead must go (Lehmann 1914: 65). According to an informant, in the old days ashes and leaves were placed on the heart of a dead person to preserve the body for four days while the members of his family kept watch. Second, besides the equation ashes+ = death–, we have a myth "The Jaguar and His Drum" which tells how a jaguar is outwitted by a sandcrab. The sandcrab is inside the jaguar's drum and makes music so the people can dance. The jaguar becomes angry and destroys the drum trying to stop the music of the sandcrab. In a series of acts which include chopping up the drum and burning it, the drum is reduced to ashes yet the sound issues forth from the ashes. The jaguar throws the ashes in the river and the music continues. It is for this reason that the jaguar walks along the river; he is looking for his drum.

Two ideas emerge from these data: (1) that ashes are associated with death; (2) that the essence of life remains in the ashes or residue after death. Unfortunately, I could not learn if the Rama made the association between the ashes of the snakehead and the possibility of cure in the context of these ideas.

Table 1. A list of common plants used by Rama, Carib and Miskito Indians in snakebite cure (after Conzemius 1932; Damon n.d.; Heath 1950, n.d.; Hodge and Taylor 1957)

Native name*	Common name	Scientific name	Used by*	Preparation and other uses
kangbala-M	(Buttonweed)	Borreria ocymoides or B. laevis	C, M, R	Root boiled for tea. Decoction and poultice.
maksixsa-C	maksixsa	unknown	C, R	Roasted and boiled for tea. Used with campasia.
campasia	campasia	unknown	C, M, R	Root boiled for tea.
lalbaiwra-M	guaco	Aristolochia guaco	C, M, R	Boiled and decoction.
kuntribo-M	contribo	Aristolochia tribolata	C, M, R	Poultice and decoction with rum. Also for tea.
sirsaika-M	Bitterbroom Weed	Scoparia dulcis	C, M, R	Poultice and decoction.
yukwaika-M	Soft Broom	Scoparia sp.	M, R	Leaves used in tea.
quassia	quassia or Bitterwood, Bitterbush (ash)	Picramnia sp. or Quassia sp.	C, M, R	Decoction.
—	Swelling Bush	unknown	C, R	Poultice, used with hot bush.
—	Hot Bush	Campyloneuron sp.	C, R	Poultice.
—	Trumphet	Cercopia peltata	C, M, R	Boiled to syrup which is drunk alone to remove headache from fever.
Cercasee	Monkey's Ladder	unknown	R	Decoction of vine.
tmaring-M	Jamaican Calaica	Aristolochia sp.	R, M	Infusion for pain or fever.
—	Annatto (achiote)	Bixa orellana	R	Seeds for tea.
—	White Lily	Pancratium sp.	C, R	Leaves and roots boiled for tea to cure bites of water snakes (Agkistrodon).
—	White Lily, Lettuce	Nymphoides humboltianum	C, R	Leaves and roots boiled for tea to cure Agkistrodon bites.
mukula-M	Antidote Bean	Fevillea cordifolia	C, M, R	Poultice.
—	Bellyful Bush	unknown	C, R	Roasted and boiled for tea.
riruk-M	Wild Plantain	unknown	M, R	Roots boiled and eaten as wobol.
—	Sour or Wild Cane	Gynerium saggitatum	C, R	Boiled in water for tea and drunk for pain and sleeping sickness.
limi dusa-M	Tiger Bush (Tree Fern)	Acrostichum sp.	C, M, R	Boiled and used for bathing.
—	Running Bush	unknown	C, R	Roasted and boiled for tea.

Name	Common Name	Scientific Name	*	Use
borbor	Stuco Bush	*Caesalpinia crista*	C, R	Decoction with rum.
—	Beach Morning Glory (Potato Wit)	*Ipomaea pes caprae*	C, R	Boiled with *contribo* for snakebite. Also used for bath.
borbor	borbor	unknown	C	Roasted with coconut.
—	Ginger or High Lily	*Hedychium coronarium*	R	Boiled for bathing.
nesca	Nesca	unknown	R	Tea.
After Heath (1950)				
basala-M	Three-cornered Vine	*Serjania inebrians*	M	Used with *guaco* and antidote bean; also with garlic and ginger.
limsi-M	Turpentine Tree	*Elapharium simaruba*	M	Bark used as poultice and chewed.
pankalkal-M	Ash	unknown	M	Decoction of bark used to stop bleeding.
pyuta dusa or *pyuta kaiora*-M	Gramanty Bark or Coby Wood	unknown, seed known as "snake okro"	M	Decoction of bark. Seed protects against snakebite.
tuburus-M	Guanacaste	*Enterolobium cylcocarpum*	M	Decoction of bark and poultice.
tuktukya-M	—	unknown	M	Seed of flower used internally and externally.
After Heath (n.d.)				
suhar kumka-M	—	unknown	M	Poultice.
yukutu-M	Pokeweed	*Phytolacca* sp.	M	Poultice and decoction or tea of leaves.
After Conzemius (1932)				
brum sirpi-M	—	*Scoparia* sp.	M	Poultice.
culmecea	China Root	unknown	M	Root is boiled and decoction is drunk to clean blood.
daka-M	—	unknown	M	Decoction.
kisauri-M	Fits Weed	*Eryngium* sp.	M	Decoction and poultice.

* C = Black Carib, M = Miskito, R = Rama.

tim is with someone else, the other person must kill the snake; if the patient were to kill the snake in someone else's presence, he might not be cured. Snakedoctors cannot kill snakes because they would have to give up their curing and might be endangered as was Cornelio when he just saw a snake. If a snakedoctor is alone and is bitten, he tries to summon someone else to kill the snake and then immediately seeks the aid of another snakedoctor (see Table 2, Juan Vanegras).

The next step is to give the victim a root to chew until he returns home. In many cases, this root will be *campasia* or perhaps the root of the white lily (*Pancratium* sp.) or even a decoction of the vines, *contribo* (*Aristolochia* sp.) and *guaco* (*Aristolochia* sp.). The time which elapses between being bitten and being treated varies. It may be from one to twenty hours before the patient is seen by a snakedoctor depending on the locale where the patient is bitten. However, the patient MUST be brought to his own home, and preferably his home on Rama Cay, where he is put in bed.[5] Members of the family and others present when he is brought in MUST HUG HIM. If they don't hug him, he will die, or so say the Rama. Also once the cure begins, people who were with him when he was bitten must stay with the patient until he is cured. Care must be taken to insure that the patient does not see any pregnant woman, especially one in his own family. Again, if the snakebite victim does see a pregnant woman, his condition will worsen and he cannot be cured. Also if a pregnant woman were to see a snakebite victim it is believed that the child would miscarry or be born without a face (see Taylor 1951: 89).

Once a snakedoctor begins a cure he must not leave the patient until the patient is well. Normal activities are suspended for the snakedoctor and members of the household who are watching over the patient. Also strangers or outsiders may not see the patient until he is well. The Black Carib say that if a stranger passes the house and "looks in" on the patient, the patient will feel pain and both the patient and the onlooker must undergo a ritual cleansing. This is especially important for pregnant women whose presence places the patient in immediate danger. Both the patient and the pregnant woman must undergo a special ritual (Damon n.d.: 2). While the Rama fear the presence of pregnant women and the harm the snakebite victim might cause the fetus, they did not mention any ritual the patient or woman must undergo.

[5] There is a problem in defining what the Rama mean by "his own home." In most cases this would be the house of his family of marriage or if he were single, the house of his family of birth. For a woman, it would mean either her husband's house or that of her natal family. In most cases, a person who was bitten upriver would be brought to Rama Cay. However, if a doctor were nearby, the victim would be brought to his upriver home.

As soon as the patient has been hugged and put to bed, he is isolated from all those who did not hug him by white sheets of mosquito netting. It is not clear whether the Rama follow the Black Carib practice of covering the snakebit patient with a white cloth (Damon n.d.: 2). However, the patient must be wrapped up with blankets (white?) to keep him warm and help him sweat. The snakedoctor and his assistants serve as go-betweens between the patient and the outside world. They also begin the infusions of herbal teas and place the poultices and plasters of tobacco and other herbal medicines on the patient's wound. As the patient perspires from the tea, fever, etc., the blankets must be changed and new doses of tea administered.

It should be noted that during the cure the patient is on a special diet, prepared in a special way. All foods and medicines must be prepared over a separate fire. This fire is not the domestic fire but a special fire built in an area apart from where the normal cooking goes on. It is understood that if the snakebite victim were to be fed food or medicine cooked on the household hearth, it would endanger his life as well as the lives of household members.[6] The Rama say that a snakebite victim should not eat meat. Also, as mentioned previously, the snakebite victim should not have salt, sugar, or plantain *wobol* with seeds or salt in it. The *wobol* must be made from roasted plantains rather than boiled ones. As with the Black Carib, who use cassava (*Manihot dulcis*) and fish, the Rama depend on a roasted staple for the basis of the snakebite victim's diet.[7]

The medical objective of the cure is to stop the patient from vomiting and urinating blood, to lower his fever and in turn, to assist him in getting rid of the poison. As the poison has less effect, the patient will hold down the tea and become cooler. The Rama believe the snake poison makes the blood boil. The cure is aimed at cooling the blood and making the patient clean, or without poison. The cooling of the blood must be accomplished gradually as the patient could die if he were given some-

[6] This belief is a derivative belief of the general prohibition against cooking a midwife's or menstruating woman's food over the household fire, especially when they are unclean. I am not sure if this prohibition applies to women who have recently given birth. Unfortunately, the Rama never gave an explanation of the significance of this prohibition although the Freudian implications are tantalizing.

[7] The Black Carib elaborate much more on the food taboos than the Rama. One who is snakebitten cannot eat *wari* or white-lipped pecarry (*Tayassu pecari* ssp.) or the fat of the *wari* because the *wari* roots. Also one cannot eat the meat of animals which are cooked with their skins on: *wari*, pig, or *paca* (*Cuniculus paca* ssp.). One cannot eat chicken or eggs, perhaps because the chicken roots or pecks. Fish may be eaten only if they are roasted. Also one may not have salt or sugar, especially sugar in coffee. Bananas are also prohibited in a snakebite victim's diet in contrast to cassava which is recommended (Damon n.d.: 1–2).

Table 2.   Record of snakebite cures by a Rama snakedoctor, Rama Cay, Nicaragua

Name of person bitten	Place bitten	Where bitten	Type of cure (leaves, bush powder, tea, etc.)	How much blood	How long to cure
Isaac Daniel	Tshwani River bank	Left hand	—	Spot of blood for two days, no heavy flow of blood	5 days
Mohrland Macre	Duckuno River	Left foot	Powder, bush parch with the snake head; tea for cooling stomach	No blood flow (his foot became inflamed and bled a little)	Was well in 8 days but was not allowed up for 10 days
Victor Macre (my brother-in-law)	In the bush of the Kukra River where he was working	On the foot	—	He spat up much blood; could not urinate or go out in the night glare	12 days
Josefa Macre	Kukra River at dusk	Left foot	(I did not find one of the bites until the next day)	Threw up blood and also urinated blood	12 days
Olevarto Macre	Duckuno River at 8 A.M.; did not receive any attention until 2:00 P.M.	On the foot	Tea; and plaster on bite	Spat blood for 3 days	14 days (it took him a long time to heal because of a lame foot)

Juan Vanegras (Other snakedoctor)	Rama Cay at 9:00 A.M.; received no treatment until noon	On his fingers	Felt better after receiving medicine 3 times	Vomited much blood for 2 nights	1 day
Lydia Álvarez	Kukra River, place named Santa Rita; was 2½ days before she received medicine	On the foot	Gave powder to drink and used powder; bathed her	Spat and urinated much blood	Died within 8 days from heart sickness
Margenno Macre	Kukra River; brought him back to island late in evening; didn't call me to bandage; other doctor made excuse, "I had no medicine"; they called me later	—	Plates tea medicine, snake head (I did all I knew how to do but nothing worked)	Did not spit up blood and was in severe pain	Lived only one day before he died

thing too cold (water that had not been boiled) or too bitter (food or drink with salt, sugar, or seeds in it). It is also important to the doctor that the patient be clean if he should die. Otherwise, the doctor's credibility suffers. Repeated administrations of the herbal tea serve this dual function, while the poultices keep infection out of the wound (snakebite victims often die from gangrene; see Ambrose 1956: 328–329). Also the patient may chew *campasia* or some other root to expunge the poison.

The symptoms of the snakebite victim include: vomiting and urinating blood, fever, pains, and inflammation of the area in which the wound occurred (most often the hand or foot).[8] As the medicine takes effect, the symptoms lessen and usually the patient begins to hold the tea. The lowering of the fever and the stoppage of loss of blood are the most significant changes in the patient's condition for the Rama, as the state of hot blood or loss of blood is thought to be one of imminent danger. Loss of blood is equated with loss of physiological and supernatural power by the Rama. Boiling blood has no antecedents in the cosmology of the Rama except perhaps the idea that it is unnatural for man to have hot blood when he is constantly losing physiological power with age. Normally, it is supernatural power which counteracts this loss of physiological power, and boiling blood introduces an element of dissonance into the system. The resolution occurs when the patient's fever goes down and he returns to the normal cool condition of his fellow human beings.[9] After two or three days, the patient may begin to feel better and his appetite returns.

The average time required for a cure is nine days, the shortest time being three days and the longest time fourteen days (see Table 2). In a sixteen-year period, one snakedoctor on Rama Cay treated eight cases of snakebite, curing six and losing two. In one case the snakedoctor did not begin treatment until twelve to twenty-four hours after the person was bitten and in the other case, the patient was an older woman who died clean but was, according to the curer, a heart attack victim. The other doctor at Rama Cay has lost one patient in some twenty-five years

---

[8]   For a discussion of medical symptoms associated with snakebite cases in Central America, see Ambrose (1956: 327).

[9]   Further discussion of the concept of hot-cold in Rama medicine is precluded by the fact that I did not research humoral medicine. The Rama use these concepts in an abstract manner in their cosmology but do not talk about these concepts when discussing curing. In their cosmology the Rama utilize hot-cold in the following ways: (1) in categorizing animals, as land animals are hot and those of the water are cold; (2) in discussing the physiological state of old people, who have cold blood according to the Rama; (3) in classifying certain foods; and (4) in connection with death, hot ashes are placed on the heart of the corpse and strewn across the path of the souls of the dead in the Milky Way.

of practice. The mortality rate from snakebite wound is very low, 1 per 2,000 per year, so we can assume that the cure is fairly effective (75–87.5 percent) and that snakebite wound is not frequent, with a rate of 2.6 bites per 1,000 per year[10] (see Table 3). Snakebite usually occurs on the hand or foot. Most patients are young or middle-aged men (75 percent) who are bitten along the river while doing chores. Some women are bitten. Snakes hide in the grass around the house, in the storage boxes under the bed, or in the rafters of the house. I have heard of only one child dying from snakebite. She was

Table 3. Deaths by snakebite, Rama Cay, Nicaragua. Taken from Moravian missionary records, 1859–1966

Date of death	Name	Remarks
10/ 1/1889	Ferming Rudolph Macre	He was bitten by a snake on the river and died four days afterwards.
7/??/1895	James Smykel	
11/24/1902	Emiline Judith Benjamin	She served in the Mission here very well. She was bitten by a snake in Kis-Kis point on November 22. The case was delayed and neglected and on the 24th she died senseless.
8/13/1905	Dimitri Daniel	1904 — He ran away with Rachel when she was with her father in his plantation in the Kukra River.
9/14/1913 a	Downs Bliard	Shortly after he committed adultery, a snake bit him.
7/ 2/1928	Delecia Hodgson	—
2/20/1930	George Martinus Macre	Dropped June 28. Fornication with Fern and Judith underage.

a Died of dysentery.

[10] The limitations of this type of statistical analysis should be noted. The lack of data on all cases of snakebite and snakebite cure among the Rama is a possible source of error. It is improbable that the population structure remained constant over a sixteen-year period.

However, it should be noted that there are comparative statistics available among the Cuna of Panama (Nordenskiold 1938: 14, 396) and from the United Fruit Company in Central America (Ambrose 1956: 324–326). The Cuna data indicate that 1.3 persons per 1,000 per four-month period were bitten at the village of Ustup or Puturgandi during the dry season of 1931 (January to May) when a majority of the bites occur. Extrapolating from this figure, we can assume the maximum number of bites during the year 1931 in this village was 3.9 per 1,000. Unfortunately, data on curing and mortality rates are not available during this year, so we cannot compare the Rama data on this point with that of the Cuna. Data presented by Ambrose (1956) show clearly that in Central America Western medical technology results in a lower mortality rate, 4.3 percent lower than that among the Rama, 12.5–25 percent (Ambrose 1956: 324).

playing by the river; a snake bit her and she died soon after. I am sure that more children are bitten but unfortunately no attempt was made to gather all cases of children being bitten by snakes in recent times. The Moravian Mission records of deaths for Rama Cay support the hypothesis that men are most frequently bitten (see Table 3). From 1889–1930, seven persons were recorded as being bitten by snakes, six of whom died of snakebite wound. While these data do not include all cases of snakebite during this period, it is significant that five of the seven were men, one was a woman and the other was a young woman.

As soon as the patient regains his appetite the final phase of the curing ritual is initiated. The doctor is able to leave his patient and the patient's isolation is replaced by reintegration into the family group. Also the house is swept out and life returns to normal. The patient now may eat salted food, meat, *wobol* with seeds in it, and drink coffee with sugar in it. Pregnant women have nothing to be afraid of, and the cured snakebite victim gains a measure of respect from other members of the community, as does his own family. Also the snakedoctor receives some reinforcement in the form of social recognition that the cure was a successful one. A doctor who is not successful in curing victims of snakebite is censured by the community. In one case, it is hypothesized that this censure to some degree influenced a snakedoctor to give up curing. It is at this point we must examine some of the social-cultural, symbolic, and psychological components of Rama belief in and practice of snakebite cure.

4.   From the presentation of the data on Rama snakebite cure, it may be concluded that Rama snakebite cure is a social as well as natural phenomenon. The cure utilizes endo-psychic and exo-psychic symbols. The social nature of the cure is reflected in the fact that the patient is integrated or isolated at several levels of the social structure during the cure. This is evidenced by the facts: (1) that the person with the snakebite victim at the time he is bitten as well as the snakedoctor must remain with him until he is cured or dies; (2) that the family must hug the patient when he is brought into the house; (3) non-kin, strangers, or outsiders are excluded from seeing the patient; (4) pregnant women are excluded from seeing the patient; while (5) older people are permitted to see the patient because their blood is cold and they can survive the heat of the snakebite victim. The important point concerning this isolation and integration of the snakebite victim is that the Rama consider these prescribed rules of social behavior ESSENTIAL to the cure's success. Potentially, the entire kinship network of an individual could participate in a cure but

it is clear that the domestic group is being emphasized here in the context both of the myth and of the ritual. It is the domestic group which stands to lose the most should an important member of the household die (such as the household owner (*nu abing*) who is usually the snakebite victim). In this sense then snakebites threaten the social order especially because of the potential disruption of the household and the ensuing fight over inheritance.

Cutting across these categories are the bonds of partnership and economic cooperation, which is the probable basis of the relationship between the patient and the individual with him at the time the patient was bitten. Also there is the prestigious snakebite doctor who is in a special category (*abut ain kauling*) which gives high status and a link to the supernatural. Finally there is the category of older people and pregnant women. Older people in general are considered special in Rama society. Their inclusion is significant because they are asexual and thought to have cold blood. Pregnant women, on the other hand, are very sexual and also carry potential heirs. The exclusion of the sexual pregnant women and the inclusion of the asexual older people make logical sense for the Rama as the cure de-emphasizes sexuality.

The cultural component of Rama snakebite cure is that associated with cooking, the dyad of hunting-homicide, and the dimension of hot-cold. The absence of meat from the diet of the snakebite victim and the necessity of killing the snake after it has bitten the victim are interrelated. The killing of the snake symbolizes revenge for potential homicide and the absence of meat represents a return to a non-hunting-based subsistence system. (Fish are gathered, not hunted.) The dimension of cooking, using only roasted or boiled foods without condiments for the patient, represents a non-elaborated cultural cuisine. The separate fire signifies the liminal status of the patient as well as the household. Finally, the hot-cold dimension elaborates the idea that the body may not be overheated or surely the patient will die.

The third level of meaning and metaphor in Rama snakebite cure is that of sexuality, both libidinal and reproductive. The Rama believe that potential sexual unions (i.e. adultery) are potential causes of snakebite.[11] Therefore, one might argue that snakebites symbolize adulterous desires and, in turn, generalize anxiety relative to unfulfilled sexual desire. At a second level the anxiety takes the form of prohibitions surrounding pregnant women. These prohibitions refer to the reproductive or restricted sexuality associated with the domestic group and child bear-

[11] The Jívaro of Ecuador believe that "after intercourse, he is particularly susceptible to being bitten by a poisonous snake" (Harner 1972: 82).

ing.[12] The prohibitions are designed to insure the continuance of an ordered social and psychological atmosphere to promote the birth of the child.
In conclusion, it is apparent that the understanding of Rama snakebite cure lies in a multifaceted approach to its myth and ritual. It is hoped
that this paper has provided a starting point for this type of analysis
in the future. As Speck noted long ago, "Ethnoherpetology indeed offers unlimited prospects for exploration into native cultures far and wide,
beginning with study in the environs of the Indian tribes in the Americas" (Speck 1946: 355).

REFERENCES

AMBROSE, MICHAEL S.
1956 "Snakebite in Central America," in *Venoms*. Edited by Eleanor
E. Buckley and Nandor Porges, 323–329. American Association
for the Advancement of Science, Publication 44. Washington D.C.
CONZEMIUS, EDUARD
1927 Die Rama Indianer von Nicaragua. *Zeitschrift für Ethnologie* 59:
291–362.
1932 *Ethnographical survey of the Miskito and Sumu Indians of Nicaragua*. Bureau of American Ethnology Bulletin 106. Washington,
D.C.
DAMON, FRED
n.d. "Snake curing in Orinoco: Isedro Zenone." Unpublished manuscript.
EVANS-PRITCHARD, E. E.
1937 *Witchcraft, oracles and magic among the Azande of the Anglo-
Egyptian Sudan*. Oxford: Clarendon Press.
GLICK, LEONARD B.
1967 Medicine as an ethnographic category: the Gimi of the New
Guinea Highlands. *Ethnology* 6:31–56.
HAMBLY, WILFRID D.
1931 *Serpent worship in Africa*. Field Museum of Natural History
Anthropological Series 21(1):3–85. Chicago.
HAMILTON, KENNETH G.
1939 *Meet Nicaragua*. Bethlehem, Pennsylvania: Comenius.
n.d. "Miskito myths and beliefs." Unpublished manuscript.

[12] There was a sterile woman on Rama Cay who found a snake under her bed.
The snake had offspring and the Rama thought this most strange, especially since
she was infertile and had a fondness for all animals. Traditional beliefs would lead
to the conclusion that the woman was an *aisukya*. Also it could be argued that the
woman was an asexual being with a reproductively sexual snake under her bed
(which ironically represents the height of human sexuality for the Rama), and it is
this contrast which creates the significance of this event for the Rama.

HARNER, MICHAEL J.
1972 *The Jívaro.* Garden City: Doubleday.

HEATH, GEORGE REINKE
1927 *Grammar of the Miskito language.* Herrnhut: F. Lindenbein.
1950 Miskito glossary, with ethnographic commentary. *International Journal of American Linguistics* 16(1):20–34.
n.d. "Salts and leaves." Unpublished manuscript.

HOCART, A. M.
1952 *The life-giving myth.* Introduction by Lord Raglan. London: Methuen.
1954 *Social origins.* London: Watts.

HODGE, W. H., DOUGLAS TAYLOR
1957 The ethnobotany of the Island Caribs of Dominica. *Webbia* 12(2):513–643.

LA BARRE, WESTON
1969 *They shall take up serpents* (paperback edition). New York: Schocken.

LEHMANN, WALTER
1914 Vokabular der Rama-Sprache. *Abhandlungen der Königlichen Bayerischen Akademie der Wissenschaften Philosophisch, Philologische und Historische Klasse* 28(2):1–124. Munich: G. Franz'-schen.
1920 *Die Sprachen Zentral Amerikas,* two volumes. Berlin: Dietrich Reimer.

LÉVI-STRAUSS, CLAUDE
1967 *Structural anthropology* (paperback edition). Garden City: Doubleday.

LOVELAND, CHRISTINE
1973 Rural-urban dynamics: the Miskito Coast of Nicaragua. *Urban Anthropology* 2(2):182–193.

LOVELAND, FRANKLIN O.
n.d. "Snakes and social order in southern Middle-America." Paper presented at the 1973 Pennsylvania Sociological Society meetings.

MALKIN, BORYS
1956 Sumu ethnozoology: herpetological knowledge. *Davidson Journal of Anthropology* 2:165–180.
n.d. "Moravian Mission records, Rama Cay." Unpublished manuscript.

NIETSCHMANN, BERNARD
1973 *Between land and water.* New York: Seminar Press.

NIETSCHMANN, BERNARD, JUDY NIETSCHMANN
i.p. Change and continuity: the Rama Indians of Nicaragua. *America Indigena.*

NORDENSKIOLD, ERLAND
1938 *An historical and ethnographical survey of the Cuna Indians.* Edited by Henry Wassén. Comparative Ethnographical Studies 10. Göteborg: Walter Kaudern.

PECK, JOHN G.
1968 "Doctor medicine and bush medicine in Kaukira, Honduras," in

Essays on medical anthropology. Edited by Thomas Weaver, 78–87. Athens, Georgia: University of Georgia Press.

RANDS, ROBERT
1954   Horned serpent stories. Journal of American Folklore 67:79–81.

SOLIEN DE GONZÁLEZ, NANCIE L.
1969   Black Carib household structure. American Ethnological Society Monographs 44. Seattle: University of Washington Press.

SPECK, FRANK G.
1946   Ethnoherpetology of the Catawba and Cherokee. Journal of the Washington Academy of the Sciences 36(10):355–360.

TAYLOR, DOUGLAS MAC RAE
1951   The Black Carib of British Honduras. Wenner-Gren Viking Fund Publications in Anthropology 17. New York.

THOMPSON, J. ERIC S.
1970   Maya history and religion. Norman, Oklahoma: University of Oklahoma Press.

TURNER, VICTOR
1970   "A Ndembu doctor in practice," in The forest of symbols, 359–393. Ithaca: Cornell University Press.

VILLA, JAIME
1962   Serpientes venenosas de Nicaragua. Managua: Novedades.

VOGEL, J. P.
1926   Indian serpent-lore. London: Probstbain.

WASSÉN, HENRY, editor
1938   Original documents from the Cuna Indians of San Blas as recorded by the Indians Guillermo Haya and Rubén Pérez Kantule. Comparative Ethnological Studies 6. Göteborg: Walter Kaudern.

WELBOURN, F. B.
1971   "Missionary stimulus and African responses," in Colonialism in Africa 1870–1960, volume three: Profiles of change: African society and colonial rule. Edited by Victor Turner, 310–345. Cambridge University Press.

WESTROPP, HODDER M., C. STANILAND WAKE
1975   Influence of the phallic idea in the religions of antiquity (second edition). New York: J. W. Bouton.

WISDOM, CHARLES
1940   The Chorti Indians of Guatemala. Chicago: University of Chicago Press.

The Traditional Folk Medicine of Taos, New Mexico

JANET S. BELCOVE

In the summer of 1972, material for a paper concerning the traditional Spanish-American medicines of Taos, New Mexico, was gathered at the Fort Burgwin Research Center near Taos. This center, a branch of Southern Methodist University, is a field school for anthropological training. The data were collected by the author, who was then a student in the field school, by conducting informal interviews in English with knowledgeable Spanish Americans. Another colleague supervised field-work at Fort Burgwin that summer. The paper reporting this research in full was published in 1973 (Belcove and Aceves 1973). Here we give a short outline of our findings.

Taos has been called "an ethnic zoo" by some because of its complex melange of ethnic groups. The population of Taos and the surrounding counties shows a majority of Spanish Americans with minority populations of Anglos and Indians. The term "Spanish American" is important. These people trace their ancestors back to the *Conquistadores* and the colonists who established such towns as Santa Fe, San Gabriel, and Santa Cruz and who founded Taos as a frontier post in the late sixteenth century. In the eighteenth and early nineteenth centuries, some settlers moved north, settling in small self-sufficient agricultural communities. Culturally they have close ties with Spain. The stress upon Spain and not Mexico as the "patria" is important; the *Taoseños* refer to Mexicans as *Mejicanos* — *Mejicanos* or *Mejicanos de Mejico.*

One of the problems facing an ethnic group in an area of diverse ethnic groups is the problem of maintaining its own cultural integrity. Language is one way of doing this; adherence to folk customs such as the traditional medical practices described in the paper is another.

It is significant that the traditional medical practices described are practiced more by the older people than by the young. The purpose of the paper is to present data without a wider analysis as to the meaning of the practices in relation to the maintenance of Spanish-American identity. It is possible, however, that the use of traditional medicine may reinforce this identity.

The primary curative agents in the pharmacopoeia of Spanish-American traditional medicine are herbs. The importance of herbal remedies in the Taos area is demonstrated by the following statement of a *curandero:* "Everything belongs to herbs and medicine if you study and know how." The paper contains a listing of herbs, how they are used, and what ailments they cure. Not only do they alleviate "scientific disorders" such as cancer, influenza, ulcers, arthritis, the common cold, high blood pressure, diabetes, etc., they are also used to alleviate "folk illnesses": illnesses not formally recognized by physicians but well known to those afflicted with them. Such folk illnesses as *mal de ojo, susto,* and *empacho* are commonplace in Taos and are also described in the paper.

Since we know of no publication about Spanish-American traditional medicine (as opposed to Mexican and South American traditional medicine about which there is a large body of literature), we feel this data will be useful to ethnologists for purposes of cross-cultural comparisons.

REFERENCES

BELCOVE, JANET S., JOSEPH B. ACEVES
  1973   Medicina tradicional en Taos, Nuevo México. *Etnica, Revista de Antropología* 5:193–208. Barcelona.

Different Approaches to Medicine among Different People

MICHIO TSUNOO

In Japan we owed the progress of modern medicine mostly to Germany until World War II; thereafter influential impact came from the U.S.A. When I visited the University of Chicago a decade ago, I had a deep impression of the modern instrumentation in the hospital and clinic. Everything seemed mechanical and there was frequently a lack of the personal touch. Although chaplains, social workers, and psychologists were working together with doctors, medical treatment was systematic and objective. In Japan, an in-patient clinic seems to have an atmosphere of a small residential community, while an out-patient clinic is usually too mechanical because of the number of patients. Each patient's consultation lasts only thirty seconds. In spite of this, the patient usually visits the clinic without an appointment. The Japanese health insurance system does not pay for the doctor except for the first consultation.

Nowadays, I do not think any difference exists in the hospitals of developed countries from a medical point of view. The spoken language, the working people, and ways of visiting patients are different in each country. However, the actual practice of medicine is almost the same. Consider for a moment the victim of a car accident who is taken to the hospital. The X-ray instrument, EEG, EKG, blood for transfusion, oxygen, etc. are all ready in the emergency room. If the EEG, spinal fluid, and X-ray show brain damage, a neurosurgeon will be called on the phone. I think all such procedures are similar in all modern hospitals. It should make no medical difference to the patient whether he is hurt in the U.S.A. or Japan. However, this may be the special occasion — emergency.

In ordinary daily life, medical practice consists of mutual reliability between patients and doctors for various reasons. One of these reasons is emotional, and many diseases are accompanied by emotional disturbances. You can see many foreign doctors' offices in Tokyo, which is now the center for the Far East — economically, culturally, commercially, and politically. Foreign people in general avoid indigenous physicians, even if there is no communication problem in terms of language. Patients choose the doctor who can best understand them.

When I worked at Billings Hospital in Chicago, the heart transplant in South Africa shocked all laboratories, and reactions from lab people were mostly concerned with the successful surgical technique and the prospects of the transplanted heart. Then, the news from Palo Alto and Houston caused a similar reaction. After I returned to Japan, one Japanese surgeon succeeded in a heart transplant. In contrast to America, that caused an ethical rather than a medical problem. A group of lawyers and the parents whose son was the heart donor sued the surgeon for his incomplete recognition of the donor's death. No surgeon followed him, and he could not try again. Where does the different response between the American and the Japanese people come from? It is hard to explain this difference. I would say a part of this comes from different spheres of medical concern. Japanese medical concern is domestic rather than social, individual rather than humanistic. Eye- and blood-banks are less developed in Japan than in America. It is also still not easy to perform an autopsy in a hospital in Japan.

Recently, acupuncture anesthesia in China attracted much attention from foreign medical professionals. While we, the Japanese, have used acupuncture for neuralgic pain for quite a long time, nobody thought of acupuncture anesthesia. This shows the medical creativity of the Chinese people. Japanese medicine, as well as Western medicine, is dependent on chemical drugs which produce various adverse reactions. Prompt induction and recovery have become successful through acupuncture anesthesia. I do not want to try to go deeply into this point. In China medicine belongs to the people, while Western medicine is concerned mostly with the disease of human beings. This difference is political.

In regard to artificial abortion and narcotics, there are differences among the U.S.A., England, and Japan. These are legal ones, although this problem includes religious and social factors. In any developed country there are many environmental and iatrogenic diseases. These are caused mostly by industry and by medical treatment. The former can be cured by a change of environment, but this is not economically easy. The latter often comes from the doctor's incomplete understanding of drugs or techniques. Japan is the country where chinoform has been withdrawn from the market because of SMON (subacute-myelo-optico-neuropathy) caused by overdoses of chinoform which were prescribed by doctors. These are artificially caused diseases, however, and are outside the area I want to discuss.

Scientifically speaking, although medicine is not a real science, the medical approach to disease should be similar everywhere. An EKG or an X-ray photo of a patient can be sent electronically to an expert far away, and adequate treatment can be prescribed by a computer. In the near future, all medical information will be stored in a data bank and will be available everywhere in the world. The medical treatment throughout the world becomes more and more equalized. This information about medical treatment is comprised for the most part of technical procedure, and technique is important to cure disease. On the other hand, can the people of the world be equalized even if the genes are well distributed among the people? The world even in the infinite future will consist of different people, who will always be influenced by their own culture and thought. Medicine is under the influence of the culture of each group of men and cannot be replaced only by technology. Medicine is an integrated science about human beings, and, as far as science must depend upon human beings, different approaches to medicine will continue to exist among different people.

Post-Partum Salt Packing and Other Medical Practices: Oman, South Arabia

HARVEY DOORENBOS

Oman is a very traditional Middle Eastern Arab society where certain parts of the interior have been minimally affected by Western society during the past several hundred years. We still see a few interesting, challenging situations in medicine, carry-overs of the prescientific era which can be seen in any society minimally affected by the scientific explosion. I would like to refer to just one specific problem. I am a surgeon and therefore have noted a large number of gynecological complications which come to our hospital as a result of post-partum packing of the vagina with ordinary table salt. This post-partum technique is prevalent only in certain areas of Oman, and when asked why they do this most of the local midwives only answer that it has always been done this way. They do not have a conscious reason for doing it that we can elicit. Of course this technique causes many complications, from minor scarring of the vagina to total obliteration of the vagina. The secondary complications can range from mild difficulty in delivery of subsequent children all the way to totally retained menses. What we have noted so often has been vaginal atresia of the moderately severe degree, which allows pregnancy but not delivery — and therefore depending upon how late the woman comes for medical attention, she may require either a cesarean section or perhaps already have a ruptured uterus requiring emergency surgery. The obstetrical staff of the maternity wing of the hospital has been teaching against this practice for many years and we are now beginning to see a decrease in its incidence, but at one time three years ago, four patients were in the hospital recovering from a ruptured uterus, and over a period of thirteen months we saw fourteen cases of a ruptured uterus. I have not totaled up the number of cases of complete vaginal atresia requiring vaginal plasty for retained menses but this of course is considerably more than the total number of ruptured uteri. Our c-section rate also is higher than normal. The indication for the great majority of the cases requiring c-section is vaginal atresia from salt packing.

A couple of other interesting social habits regarding medical practice in Oman include the practice of burning an area of the body with a hot metal rod where there is pain. This is practiced quite widely throughout Oman, and patients sometimes come to the hospital with a very large number of burns. Some cases of chronic abdominal pain may have up to several hundred individual burn scars from different courses of treatment. Occasionally this is given to newborn babies — usually four burns are applied immediately adjacent to each quadrant of the umbilicus on the assumption (stated by the families) that the crying of the newborn is because of abdominal pain. The disfigurement caused by these burn scars when on the face is sometimes rather grotesque, but at the present time in the society of Oman not considered a social handicap.

As I presume is the case in most developing countries of the world, we have here local bone-setters who are occasionally over-vigorous in applying splints to fractures of arms and legs and who cause vascular occlusion and gangrene of the limb involved. We see four to five cases per year of gangrene of arms and hands following misuse of splints for bone fractures. Perhaps this is not a very alarming incidence of complication considering the number of fractures that must occur in this society, but when such a case arrives in our hospital we naturally are somewhat horrified.

We still occasionally have a situation where a child bride, immature in development, has been taken in marriage by an older man, and attempted sexual intercourse has caused a severe perineal laceration.

One other disease that I would like to comment on is mental illness as it is seen and treated here in Oman. Quite often the person and family of a mentally disturbed person consider that the cause of the mental illness is the "Devil." There is a very strong belief in God and in the Devil, and therefore the mentally ill person may believe that he is possessed by an "Evil Spirit." Generally, to treat such a case a religious man is called in, and he reads for several hours to the person from the Holy Quran. Some people report healing of mental illnesses from this. Other people report intermittent attacks of demons' possession in their lives. Still others do not think that all mental illness is from an evil spirit, but simply think that the person is crazy and the general treatment then is to keep the person in a home. If the person is violent he may be chained. Occasionally the person is nonviolent but needs some protection from himself and from other people and some identification as someone who is crazy. Shackles will be put on the ankles of such a person and he will be allowed to walk around in the community but will sometimes be assisted back to his home at evening. My general impression is that the incidence of mental illness in this society is low.

SECTION TWO

Specific Subject Papers

Introduction

DANA RAPHAEL

In this section, we will be dealing with papers which go deeply into one specific aspect of medical anthropology.

Dr. Bela Römer's paper, "The use of argillaceous earth as medicament," is a discussion of geophagy, or clay-eating — a phenomenon that occurs in many cultures and is especially prevalent among pregnant women. The active ingredients include aluminum hydrosilicate. The most important characteristic of the clay is the caloidial structure. Dr. Römer, who is a physician, is making a nutritional analysis of the clay. And, finally, we are going to have a connection between the nutritional and cultural practices. The paper by Mary Parthun, Ph.D., is on "The incidence of mental illness among Italians in an English-Canadian city." The hypothesis that rapid acculturation causes a high incidence of mental illness is NOT confirmed here. This is very exciting because the Italian family is traditionally a well-integrated family. The reasons for this are discussed in her paper. Dr. Dana Raphael, Ph.D., has a paper entitled, "Warning: the milk in this package may be lethal for your infant." The World Health Organization suggests infant mortality rates have risen in newly developing cultures, partially due to the use of powdered milk replacing breast-feeding as women move into a new and Western economic life style. The reasons for this and the solutions to these problems are discussed. We are seeing marasmus as early as three months from birth in these infants and they are dying. We may add that these are allergic reactions to milk that are very pertinent to prob-

Raul Slovinsky, a member of the Congress Service Corps, put together the abstract of the abstracts of this part of the session. It was really a great job and we are thankful for the same.

lems here in the United States. We insist that black children, who are often particularly allergic to cow's milk, drink it in school at lunch time. They get sick. We are discussing this problem. Dr. Dale Ritter — a medical doctor — and his archeologist son, Dr. Eric Ritter, have a paper entitled "Prehistoric pictography in North America of medical significance." Petroglyphs and pictographs at these sites in the western United States may have medical significance which include magical, religious, and supernatural concepts and practices. The hypothesis is that these glyphs and graphs should be used as an ethnographic analogy. The direct historical approach and other methods are used. This is something we need to do to give medical anthropology a deeper dimension. Miss Sheila Cosminsky has done a paper on the "Cross-cultural perspectives on midwifery." This is a cross-cultural survey on the role of the midwife. Case materials from a Guatemalan community — as well as from many other communities — are given. A discussion on research goals and methods and the place of midwives in the whole structure is given. The next paper, "Cerro Sechin: medical anthropology's inauguration in Peru?" by Fr. Francis X. Grollig, S.J., Ph.D., calls attention to this site in Peru which includes various monoliths depicting a good working knowledge of anatomy that the artists had 3,500 years ago. The accompanying designs are copied from photographs by the author.

Editor's Note: On this work-session and consequently this section, Dr. Haley commented that it "was devoted to a group of papers that were individual in their own right — they didn't relate in great depth to other papers. Some of these presented some rather unique ideas."

The Incidence of Mental Illness among Italians in an English-Canadian City

MARY LASSANCE PARTHUN

The Italian immigration to Canada began in the late nineteenth century in connection with the construction of the great Canadian railways and the general exodus from Italy during the period. Prior to 1900, there were a few hundred Italian arrivals each year, rising to several thousand per year in the first decades after the turn of the century (Foerster 1968: 17). The bulk of Italian immigration to Canada followed World War II.

The Italian experience in Canada has been unique in many respects. Until recently, the Italians have not been acknowledged politically or socially. Their arrival in significant numbers came after other ethnic groups had staked a claim on higher status levels in the social system. Because Canada tends to possess a tightly stratified social system, in which ethnic background figures prominently in social status (Porter 1968), this historical factor has been and will probably continue to be a key factor in Italian-Canadian life.

The Canadian custom of referring to ethnic and cultural groups as "races" in an era when race has become a divisive factor, serves to accentuate further the differences between ethnic groups and to increase the sense of isolation from the community at large and from other ethnic groups. Isolation of immigrants whose mother culture is different from that of the new country tends to be marked geographically as well as socially. Among southern Europeans this extends even to subgroups of their own culture (Darroch and Marston 1969).

Thus, the social resources available to these groups are lessened and their social isolation is greater, should any disruption of the family group take place. The potential reference group is thus limited and the position of the individual in the larger society becomes more vulnerable. As Castellano (1959: 74) indicates, when this isolation is combined with physical or emotional estrangement from the individual's family, the alienation is profound.

Another factor in this isolation may be the sense of transiency felt by those who regard their Canadian experience as a temporary situation while they accumulate enough wealth to return to Italy and end their days there in comfort. In this situation, the motivation to become established in Canada may not be strong. However, the reality of daily living can be untenable under these circumstances, as the goal of return becomes ever more remote, often eventually becoming clearly impossible. The increasing awareness of this can, in itself, be tragic.

An Italian-born psychiatrist has described in moving terms the interplay of desire for success in Canada and longing for Italy as two core motivations among Italian immigrants, both of which, too often, are doomed to failure (Marcilio 1971: 9).

For the descending generations, the focal point of problems changes from culture conflict and culture shock to the problems of minority status. The position and status of Italians in Canada have been well documented by Porter (1968: 87). Ethnic and cultural discrimination limits the potential for social mobility, while raising problems of self-esteem and conflict about identity within individual members of the minority. The Italian-Canadians' difficulties are compounded by the association of Italians with organized crime in the minds of other Canadians, a factor tending also to enhance isolation.

Insularity which stems from a family-centered agricultural society is further accentuated by continuation of the geographic and linguistic divisions brought from Italy. This divisiveness retards group action and identity. A study of leadership among Toronto Italians, for instance, revealed rivalry among potential leaders and distrust of their motives (Jansen 1969: 41). This bears out the experience of applied fieldworkers as well (Earlscourt Project 1971).

Such a situation makes leadership and group action difficult and keeps the Italians far less powerful than their numbers would suggest. The result is that success must be achieved on a highly individualistic basis and, in a country such as Canada where power lies in the hands of a powerful ethnic and religious group, the likelihood of ultimate success is slim and can occur only if one purges oneself of all traces of one's Italian cultural heritage.

At the same time the enduring image of North America as a land of promise nurtures hopes for a better lot. Contrary to stereotypes about Italian indifference to learning and their children's academic progress, professionals engaged with working-class Italians report a strong desire for education and upward mobility for their children (Marcilio 1971: 10; Earlscourt Project 1971). The dissonance caused by living with high expectations induced by a social system which at the same time limits upward mobility is a negative mental health factor.

With a discriminated-against minority status comes lower social and economic status, a factor demonstrably associated with more severe mental disorders (Hollingshead and Redlich 1958: 194 ff.; Srole, et al. 1962: 210 ff.). In the midtown Manhattan studies, for instance, difficulties of Italian and other immigrants tended to be related to low socioeconomic status rather than to cultural factors *per se* (Srole, et al. 1962: 295). Indeed, the sheer physical burden entailed in being a member of the working poor seemed to be a factor in the illness of a group of Ontario Hospital patients who were Italian immigrants (Castellano 1959: 72–73). One finds men accepting jobs that are too heavy for them physically and woman not only managing housework and family without labor-saving devices but also working at physically strenuous jobs outside the home.

Both immigrant and native-born Italian-Canadians are rendered vulnerable to adjustment problems because of the combination of stress and isolation. Potential hazards to the mental health of immigrants and members of ethnic minorities are many. Allodi (1970: 8–11) has described a series of stages which the immigrant undergoes, any of which, given unfavorable circumstances, can lead to malevolent psychological states.

During LANDING ANXIETY, the immigrant suffers for one to two months from wakefulness and a preoccupation with physical security. This is often followed by depression, and if no security or help is forthcoming, these patterns can crystallize into pathology. Lack of language skills coupled with adversity and insecurity predispose the individual to paranoid ideas (Castellano 1959: 69).

The mass postwar immigration of Italians to Canada has heightened the need for study of the mutual accommodations of Italians and the members of the larger Canadian society in its various aspects. Among professionals, general concern has been expressed, and specific studies have been made of adjustment problems in large urban centers (Allodi 1970; Castellano 1959). The situation of those Italians who filtered out into areas of less dense population has received little attention.

In view of this, the present study was undertaken to investigate the adjustment of members of an early established Italian community in a small city in Ontario.

Readily identifiable minorities often feel Canadian social distinctions quite harshly. However, in the large urban Italian communities, the realities of the greater society are cushioned by the trappings of the old culture which surround daily life. The constant flow of immigration, the visits of members of the group back to Italy and stories brought by returnees maintain a constant fresh input of Italian culture into the community.

By contrast, the problems of minority status are accentuated among those arrivals who settled at a distance from dynamic urban centers, where status tends to remain fixed and social mobility is slow and undramatic. From the historical and social perspective of today, the situation of those first Italian migrants is poignant and provocative. Sometimes marooned in remote communities by the exigencies of railway construction, they and their descendents become small islands in the midst of the predominant culture. Lacking sufficient numbers to form a sizeable buffer within the British-dominated culture, they are faced with the alternative possibilities of either becoming insular and ingrown or being forced to assimilate in an unwilling and unwelcoming larger society. It was postulated that such a situation would have a deleterious effect on the mental health of the members of the Italian minority in this situation.

The area chosen for study is located in central Ontario, Canada. The city of Rockberg (fictitious name), with a fairly stable population of fifty-five thousand, is a service and commercial center for a large rural catchment area. It is regarded as being so typically Canadian that for twenty years it has been an official testing area for opinions and products under both government and private auspices (Williams 1968: 63).

Rockberg was founded in 1825 and was originally settled by Scottish and Irish immigrants. The first Italian settlers arrived some fifty-five years later as transient laborers on the Grand Trunk Railroad (Spada 1969: 281). An elderly Rockberg Italian reports three Italian families here when she arrived in 1904. The accident of continuing employment, first on the railway, then on a huge hydraulic lift lock, and subsequently in local fledgling industries fixed these transients in Rockberg.

With sponsorship, natural increase, and independent immigration, the total Italian population grew slowly and steadily. The Italians formed a small, separate social, if not economic, entity within the community. The British Protestants and the Irish Catholics had already begun and indeed fixed the characteristic Canadian vertical mosaic. The Italians were Catholic but the church was Irish. They were under the burden of illiteracy, which inhibited the acquisition of a flexible command of the English language. Accordingly, they did their socializing among themselves and looked to Italy for their brides.

To an Italian, it was not only the culture that was inhospitable. Situated in a damp valley, Rockberg has a treacherous, bitterly cold winter with immobilizing snow. The summer is beautiful but brief — for a short period the otherwise harsh drabness of the city is softened by trees and foliage and a glimpse of the sun. Harbingers of autumn begin in August when the evening, and often the day as well, is chilly and rain is frequent. The architecture is monotonously brick, with scant wooden trim, usually painted in one of four standard shades, making a subdued touch of color.

In such surroundings, it was customary on Sundays for the Italians to gather after the main meal to reminisce about the visual and sensual delights of Italy. One descendant, now in his seventies, after hearing one of these sessions, once asked his father impatiently why he had left Italy, and his father replied, "Italy is beautiful, my son. But, oh, the hunger."

This tough-minded acceptance of economic exile and an almost contractual loyalty to Canada is noted, while often misunderstood, by the Anglo-Canadian. The same Italian informant once asked his father whether, if the two countries should ever be at war, he should fight for Canada or Italy. He was told simply: "Kiss the hand that gives you bread."

In spite of this loyalty, the acceptance of the Italian presence by members of Rockberg's founding groups has always been marginal. In 1904, a feature story in the local paper hailed a new arrival as the "first fair-skinned Italian bride" to arrive in Rockberg. Sixty-eight years later the same paper chose to cover the international reunion of the distinguished Ronca family that was held in Rockberg by focusing on a wealthy car collector in the family and described a Mafia-like arrival of Italians in vintage Cadillacs, armed not with machine guns but with forks — for an orgy of eating. The gathering was actually a sedate multigenerational affair at which a light summer buffet was served. Feeling about the article was bitter in the Italian community, but they chose to express these feelings among themselves, and no formal complaints were directed at the newspaper.

In spite of the flashes of ugly prejudice, surface acceptance has become easier with the acquisition of language and other skills. In the meager times of the economic depressions, the Italians personified the frugality, piety, strict sexual morality, hard work, and stamina which were paramount values among the working people of the community. Members of the second generation were attending school and rapidly assimilating Anglo-Canadian values, building ties of friendship, and occasionally intermarrying. No threat was felt by the larger community from the continuing immigration which was composed of the economically serious, whose goals were modest and whose numbers were insufficiently great to constitute an economic threat.

By 1961, Italians were the fourth largest non-British ethnic group in Rockberg, numbering 980. Of these, 492 were male and 488 were female. The population is well distributed according to age, the largest numbers being concentrated among prime-age adults and pre-teen children, indicating a growing and vital population. Of the total population, 344 listed Italian as their mother tongue, all of them immigrants, although some had arrived a very long time ago. It does indicate a substantial number of foreign-born in the Italian population.

Surveys of occupational status in Canada show that Italians are generally overrepresented in low status manual occupations (Porter 1968: 87). In Rockberg, however, the general Italian occupational level is higher than in the nation as a whole (see Figure 1):

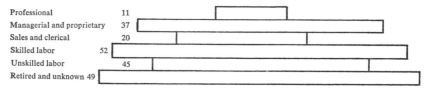

Professional   11
Managerial and proprietary   37
Sales and clerical   20
Skilled labor   52
Unskilled labor   45
Retired and unknown 49

Figure 1.   Italian occupational distribution in Rockberg for heads of families

Of the 214 heads of households for whom data are available only forty-five were employed as laborers. Representation is found at all social levels except among the secular power elite. As a correlate of this, there are no self-employed professionals, and young Rockberg Italians who have gone into these prestigious fields have chosen to settle in other areas. Interestingly, the bishop of the diocese of Rockberg is a descendant of one of the oldest Italian families. The Executive Director of the local Family Counselling Agency, a professional social worker, is Sicilian-born and came from outside the community to succeed the Irish-Catholic priest who founded the agency.

Beyond these significant isolated professionals, there is clustering in traditional "Italian" occupations such as the artisan building trades, barbering, hairdressing, and the retailing and wholesaling of produce, both on the sales and management levels. These areas open the way to independent entrepreneurships, and many stores and services in the above category are owned and operated by Italians. Success within these businesses and other small businesses is the key, to a modest degree, for enhanced social prestige and solid financial security. The older people, usually first or second generation, who achieve this kind of success, maintain the same modest working-class standard of life, reflecting their general conservatism and perhaps a fear of economic insecurity.

To date, Italian aspirations have been modest, within what seems to suggest "acceptable limits." Individuals are active in church-based groups, the Roman Catholic Parent-Teacher Association (PTA), church hockey groups, and the like, which have no real power, although they are eminently respectable. However, Italian names are missing from the rosters of school boards and municipal government, and from boards of directors of both social services and businesses. Moreover, personal slights, such as the example of thoughtless humor described previously, are reported by Italians and those married to Italians.

In the voluminous book on Rockberg County and its history, published in honor of Canada's centennial in 1967, the word Italian is not mentioned, a devastating slight that did not pass unnoticed in the Italian community. The only notice of minorities by the editors consisted of a chapter on new immigrants written by a member of the old Rockberg power elite, a chapter on the wealthy conservative Jewish community of three hundred persons, and mention of the prehistoric (but not the current) Indian population of the area.

The acceptance of Italians in Rockberg is still qualified, and as a group they tend to maintain a low profile. Officially ignored, fixed by economic factors in an essentially alien environment, the members of the Italian community of Rockberg would appear vulnerable to emotional problems. It was postulated that mental and emotional problems would be marked in such a situation. How this situation affects the incidence of psychiatric difficulty among Rockberg Italians will be examined. It was decided to determine this through a survey of the incidence of contact with psychiatric facilities among those of Italian origin and descent.

For the purposes of this study, a case survey was undertaken. The cases were obtained from the two psychiatric resources which serve the psychiatric and psychological treatment needs of the Rockberg area. These are the Mental Health Centre in Rockberg itself which provides a preventive and consultative service to the community as well as a direct treatment service for inpatients and outpatients and the receiving Ontario Hospital for the area of Queensville (fictitious name), 150 miles away. The latter serves as a treatment center for long-term and seriously incapacitating illnesses. While it is possible that a few individuals may be seeking treatment in out-of-town facilities, expense and isolation would generally rule this out.

In preparation for the case survey, a list of the Italian families in Peterborough was prepared by a university student of Italian descent, who is a lifetime resident of Rockberg and a descendant of one of the oldest families there. The list was prepared from census material and city and telephone directories.

With the aid of this master list, the records of all Italians (both immigrants and those of Italian descent) were selected from the admissions records of the Ontario Hospital and the Mental Health Centre. The period chosen for the study was that of January 1960 to July 1971. This period coincides with the establishment of an inpatient psychiatric facility in Rockberg. Moreover, use of this recent period gives insight into the current situation.

The total sample consisted of forty-six cases from both facilities (see Table 1). This total includes an age span from four years and ten months to seventy-one years and ranges from preventive work with children (usually in the area of learning disabilities) to incapacitating and largely irreversible functional and organic psychoses.

Of these cases, nine were hopitalized in the Ontario Hospital (three of these were treated at the Mental Health Centre as well).

Table 1. Number of patients in each facility by sex

		Male	Female
Ontario Hospital	9	6	3
Mental Health Centre and inpatient	6	5	1
Mental Health Centre and outpatient	31	20	11

Of the forty-six receiving special help of a psychiatric or psychological nature, seventeen, or almost one-third, were children under eighteen. Of these seventeen, nine, or over one-half, had learning disabilities; three were mentally retarded; the remaining five suffered from neurotic and behavioral disturbances (see Table 2). It is interesting to note that of these seventeen minors, only three, or less than one-sixth, were female.

Of the twenty-nine adults, the male-female ratio is less disproportionate — seventeen men, twelve women — although, as will be seen, the men

Table 2.   Patients under eighteen by sex and diagnosis

	Male	Female	Total
Learning disabilities	8	1	9
Mental retardation	2		2
Neurosis	2	2	4
Behavior disorder	2		2
Total	14	3	17

tended to suffer from more malevolent and incapacitating disorders. For instance, of the fifteen (one-half of the adult patients), who required hospitalization, only four were female. Moreover, in contrast to the women, seven incidents of personality and behavior disorders were found in the male population, all in patients under the age of twenty-six. This syndrome is, of course, quite resistant to modification.

This pattern is precisely opposite to the pattern typical for the geographic area, in which the ratio of female patients is predominantly higher. In general, two-thirds of the Mental Health Centre patients are women and one-third are men. In the Italian population the proportions are reversed. This may reflect the more sheltered status of the Italian women of the community.

Another clustering occurred among males in the next age level, with four men, aged twenty-eight to thirty-six, suffering from anxiety syndromes. Interestingly, one-half of the women (six) were in this general age group (twenty-nine to forty-five) and suffered from anxiety syndromes.

Of the sample, seven were born in Italy, ranging in age from eight years to seventy-one years. The diagnostic categories were the following: a young boy suffering from a learning disability; two women (aged thirty and thirty-two) suffering from anxiety with depressive features; two men (aged twenty-eight and thirty-two) suffering from severe psychosomatic problems, one affecting the musculo-skeletal system; and a man (aged sixty-four) and a woman (aged seventy-one), both suffering from organic psychoses.

The seven individuals in the sample who were born in Italy fit into classical types of disturbance and dysfunction described elsewhere in the literature (Allodi 1970; Castellano 1959). The school-age boy in this part of the sample, suffering from a learning disability, has probably been the victim of language and cultural difficulties.

In the total sample of forty-six, thirty-one surnames were represented. One extended family had six members who had been in contact with the psychiatric facilities during the time of this study. Twenty-three patients were the only members of their families to receive such help.

It is interesting to note as well that three highly achieving extended families had more than three members who received treatment. It is possible that higher achievement standards, along with the accompanying sensitivity to the reality of Italian minority status, are a contributing factor. "Who dares much risks much."

The overall occupational level of the remaining patients suggests that individuals of Italian descent tend to reflect their socioeconomic status rather than any cultural heritage. The adult patients would seem to corroborate other findings that marked disturbances tend to be related to low socioeconomic status. On the other hand, more sophisticated services, such as preventive and remedial services for children, tend to elicit response from better educated, achievement-oriented parents.

The occupational level of the adult sample tended to be lower and more marginal than that of the Italian community at large. The occupational level of the fathers of the children in the sample tended to be higher, a feature that is easy to explain, inasmuch as more sophisticated parents tend to become aware of learning disabilities more quickly and to take action to seek or pursue assistance for their children.

However, in spite of these trends, the overall rate of treatment for psychiatric or psychological problems was low. During the ten-year-plus period under study, only one-twentieth of the total Italian population received assistance from the facilities studied — a relatively low rate as compared with the population in general. A key factor is the financial security enjoyed by the group as a whole. Another factor is the degree to which members of the community have selected goals which are acceptable to the larger community, thus diminishing conflict and frustration.

An unknown factor is the degree to which chronic or passing disorders are handled by support from family and clergy — there is no evidence to indicate how prevalent this is. Another unknown factor is the degree to which problems and conflicts are somatized. Such a process may result in the more "respectable" physical breakdown, rather than the mental or emotional breakdown which is less approved. An investigation of the incidence of psychosomatic illness could be explored.

In general, in spite of apparent negative mental health factors following from rapid enculturation and minority status, adjustment to difficulties in the economic, religious, and psychological spheres, as measured by treatment rates, has been good. Adjustment is enhanced by economic success, modest expectations, and the high value placed on integration in the larger community.

REFERENCES

ALLODI, F.
1970 "The Italians in Toronto: mental health problems of an immigrant community." Unpublished manuscript.

CASTELLANO, V. G.
1959 "Mental illness among Italian immigrants." Unpublished master's thesis, University of Toronto.

DARROCH, A. GORDON, WILFRED G. MARSTON
1969 Ethnic differentiation: ecological aspects of a multidimensional concept. *International Migration Review* 4:71–95.

EARLSCOURT PROJECT
1971 Interview with staff of the Earlscourt Project, October 5.

FOERSTER, ROBERT F.
1968 *The Italian immigration of our times.* New York: Russell and Russell.

HOLLINGSHEAD, A. B., F. REDLICH
1958 *Social class and mental illness: a community study.* New York: John Wiley and Sons.

JANSEN, CLIFFORD
1969 Leadership in the Toronto Italian ethnic group. *International Migration Review* 4:25–43.

MARCILIO, M. P.
1971 Anguish in a new land. *The Globe Magazine* (July 3):7–10.

PORTER, JOHN
1968 *The vertical mosaic: an analysis of social class and power in Canada.* Toronto: University of Toronto Press.

SPADA, A. V.
1969 *The Italians in Canada ethnica,* volume six. Montreal: Riviera Printers.

SROLE, LEO, *et al.*
1962 *Mental health in the metropolis.* New York: McGraw-Hill.

WILLIAMS, TONI
1968 "Test Town, Canada." *Toronto Telegram,* February 24:68.

Warning: The Milk in This Package May Be Lethal for Your Infant

One estimate has it that if all the women of mainland Asia were to stop breastfeeding, an additional herd of 114 million cattle would be needed! This alone would be sufficient cause to take a hard and unsentimental look at lactation. But there is yet another critical factor. In underdeveloped and developing countries, an increasing number of children are malnourished or dying from protein deficiency, aggravated by weaning diarrhea associated with the use of artificial animal milk.

As women in developing countries move into new economic and social patterns, they incorporate many new traits, one of which is the use of artificial milk. Ironically, the move from breastfeeding to artificial feeding parallels an increase in infant mortality. This tragedy is caused by the disparity between the Western concepts that are implicit in the development and sale of the product and the misunderstanding of that product by those who buy it.

For example, imported powdered milk is improperly used, mixed with impure water and rendered bacteriologically unsafe. It is usually unrefrigerated and so becomes dangerous to the infant gut if it is not consumed within a limited safe period of time. The directions for preparing the milk are described in the terms of a chemical formula and so they are frequently ignored, not understood, or adjusted and readjusted to fit another set of cultural needs and values.

While working on this problem recently, I singled out four distinct socioeconomic, culturally unique groups of mothers — those who BREASTFEED EXCLUSIVELY and are generally living in primitive cultures or villages apart from urban centers; those BREASTFEEDERS WHO ARE BEGINNING TO USE ARTIFICIAL MILK AND BOTTLES and usually live in towns or in village areas that involve market economies; those who are EXCLUSIVELY BOTTLE FEEDERS and are always close to urban centers; and, finally, the modern urban and suburban women who, though living in a bottle-feeding culture, CHOOSE TO BREASTFEED (Raphael 1973b).

Each of these four patterns occurred in sequence in the United States over a period of sixty years (Raphael 1966). This cycle of breast-to-bottle-to-breast is now happening in a similar sequence in other cultures, though with one major change — the process is running its course within one generation rather than two or more.

It will take time to avert the mortality which accompanies this cycle. However, we can slow it down and move as quickly as possible to eventually reverse and eliminate the deleterious effects caused by such fast-paced changes. For instance, we can attempt to keep women breastfeeding for longer periods of time. And, at the same time, we can develop a non-dairy weanling food which does not require elaborate preparation and care and which, if misused, would not lead to illness or death.

But, before we try to implement such ideas, we need to know more about these women, the patterns of their lives and their motivations. Let us look first at the breastfeeding groups. The women who breast-feed exclusively still live in inaccessible areas, in places where contact with the more economically developed sections of the society are minimal, or within the lowest rungs of the economically developed countries. There are no choices for these women, no alternatives. The modern RETURN-TO-THE-BREAST GROUP, however, are women whose mothers used bottles but who do have a choice and clearly choose breastfeeding despite an all-pervasive bottle-feeding atmosphere around them.

Both these groups need a supportive system around the mother/ neonate which protects and succors the mother during the lactation phase. The physiological process of breastfeeding is extremely sensitive to the networks of personal rituals and public rites which surround the pair during this early sensitive and critical period. In order for this protective network to work, it almost always includes the presence of a mothering figure, a *doula* (Raphael 1969) who helps construct such an environment around the mother. Within these cushioned surround-ings, she has time to establish and maintain her milk supply. When such a mothering figure is absent, breastfeeding failure increases dramati-cally.

It is interesting to note that this cultural factor, the presence (or absence) of a supportive other person, sets up and permits (or inhibits) the environment which allows the ejection reflex of lactation to occur. This physiological process whereby bundles of mammary cells contract and eject the milk within them through the breast ducts and into the nipple area where it becomes available to the infant is an essential part of the function of lactation. If it works well, the mother breastfeeds. If it does not, the milk remains in the cells, the infant cannot suck it out, lactation is inhibited, and breastfeeding must be discontinued.

The supportive *doula* was found in most of the 270 cultures where lactation was investigated cross-culturally (Raphael 1966). Interestingly, there was a preponderant preference for the mother's mother or mother's kin to perform this role. In fact, the maternal kin were most often there to play out this *doula* role with women during the birth of their first live infant.[1]

The EXCLUSIVE BREASTFEEDERS have this pattern of supportiveness built into their culture. When it breaks down, when the *doulas* within those cultures are absent or their activity is minimized due to extreme economic or social stress, the mother fails to keep her infant alive. Among the Westernized, affluent group of breastfeeders, the kinship patterns have largely disappeared, and with them the *doula* figure. Also gone is the knowledge of what makes breastfeeding work. All the rituals and folklore which are part of the complex of supportiveness have also disappeared. In order to breastfeed, these women have had to invent new networks. They have had to develop interpersonal friend-friend relationships or pseudokinship arrangements in the form of an organization, e.g. La Leche League International, primarily an American phenomenon, operates at this level. Individual members of this organized group act as *doula* for each other and the organization as a whole acts as a kind of "collective *doula*," whose availability and accessibility are an essential part of the supportive network. As a result, La Leche women succeed.

Recent studies show that full lactation, that is, lactation without supplementary feeding of any sort, correlates highly with delay in ovulation (Pérez, et al. 1971). In this way the total breastfeeders in underdeveloped areas, where contraceptive devices are hard to get or expensive, have the potential of delaying the next pregnancy. This provides the immediate nursing infant that much more chance at life.

In the more affluent cultures, the infant's life is not at stake, but expectations of the mother for a fuller relationship with her child still

---

[1] Another study has demonstrated that the majority of women are at the matrilocal residence or return to their natal home for the birth of their first infant (Suzanne Wilson, unpublished material).

provide a strong motivation to breastfeed. This should be assured to her.

One way to lessen the syndrome of infant mortality is to keep women who are breastfeeding at it. This may mean strengthening the *doula*/mother pattern.

Now for those women who use artificial methods. The ELITE BOTTLE FEEDERS are an affluent class composed of professionals, semiprofessionals, and business and political leaders. Extensive Western influence on this population has resulted in the almost exclusive use of bottle feeding. Since refrigeration and precautions in preparing bottled milk prevail in this segment of the society, the use of artificial feeding does not usually result in infant mortality.

Not so with the EMERGING BOTTLE FEEDERS. They represent the vast majority of the women described here and the largest group of infants affected by the syndrome of artificial food, malnutrition, and related illnesses or death.

Cultures at this stage are in the midst of what the Jelliffes (1970) call the "urban avalanche" of Westernizing nations. They are set in towns or villages situated close to more urban centers. One of the most predictable features of groups going through this stage of change is the use of bottles and artificial milk. The bottle tends to become imbued with the mystique of Westerners and affluent urbanites, who are seen as larger in size, politically more powerful, better educated, and who seem to live in a sterilized, scientific, mechanical, and medically superior environment. Bottle feeding, among these Western megamen and megawomen, becomes part of the symbol of the future.

Attempts to persuade the EMERGING BOTTLE FEEDERS that the robustness of Western infants is not necessarily due to bottle feeding, or to dissuade them from using artificial food is looked upon as a sly and subtle attempt to reduce the population of the underprivileged by proposing the old and less successful method. The problem, then, with this group is how to encourage a more extensive period of breastfeeding even while the use of artificial milk, at some point, is inevitable.

Pleading is useless. We have documented evidence where such supplication did NOT work. In the United States, doctors became alarmed around the turn of the century over what they saw as a relationship between bottle feeding, infant diarrhea, and death. They beseeched mothers not to discontinue breastfeeding. Their pleadings fell on closed ears (Raphael 1973a). The phrase "that dangerous second summer" was coined to express the danger of feeding babies cow's milk that was delivered unrefrigerated during the summer months. In the city, milking by workers hired off the street was done in the filthy basements of breweries, where the cows could be fed cheaply from the leftover grains. Under such conditions, milk became bacteriologically dangerous in wintertime, too.[2] Despite all these warnings, mothers denied the relationship between the "modern" bottle and childhood illness. They rationalized that many bottle-fed children were bigger, healthier, and often much better off on this diet. And SOME were.

But for many, the crisis of diarrhea and infant death continued until some thirty years ago, around the time of World War II, when the widespread introduction of electric refrigeration came about and made artificial milk safe.

A similar refusal to accept the dangerous relationship is occurring among the EMERGING BOTTLE FEEDERS. Their use of contaminated water or overdiluted formula causes an appearance of marasmus as early as three months.

Many years ago Margaret Mead suggested that it would be important to find ways in industrial societies to move the nursing working-class mother to adopt the practices of the more affluent middle-class breast-feeding woman, but avoid the stage of bottle feeding in between. Now we find women moving from preindustrial cultures into market, industrial, and Western economic states with a parallel change in infant feeding methods, and we are still searching for a method to skip the bottle stage.

The American example just described and the current trends around the world do not mean that mothers are callous, that life is cheap, or that some women are ignorant. These are simplistic conclusions. My analysis leads me to more complex insights. Bottle feeding comes as part of a complete sociopolitical package of promises that all things are going to be better. Expectations are for better housing, better education, better living standards, better health, better chances for one's children. The wonderful, powerful, clean, elite bottle is part of this vision. It would be akin to entering a market economy and trying to do so without money. Bottle feeding is part of the winds of change, the whole cloth that goes with the new movement. Breastfeeding, seen as something that will hold back the future, comes to be perceived as a lesser way of loving. It is viewed as a deterrent to the child's chances for a better life.

What can we say then to women in developing nations who want to join the new world and regard breastfeeding as inhibiting? How can

---

[2] The clean milk clinics established by Mrs. W. R. Hearst, wife of the noted publisher, were a response to the lethal effects of artificial feeding.

we convince them that breastfeeding and a new lifestyle can be compatible? If they feel that independence, self-sufficiency, and new economic gains lie outside of the home, and if that is where they want to be, what rewards are realistically available that will satisfy their desire for this change and at the same time keep their infants alive?

We have mentioned that information campaigns that plead with mothers to continue breastfeeding are generally ineffective. They meet with little opposition, yet result in no effective response. The power of the Western culture's bottle-feeding tradition within the social groups mediates against it. However, it is important to continue these campaigns for the impact they have on the influential people who play a pivotal role in diffusion and change processes. The idea that breastfeeding has ecological and health advantages can make some headway among the professional and well-educated classes. Therefore, in some cases, the cost of such a program is after all worthwhile.

Equally realistic would be to have the governments of developing nations step in and subsidize mothers during their initial postpartum period. This income would permit the mother to remain at home and breastfeed, rather than rush back to work.[3] It would be a powerful demonstration of the worth of breastfeeding for governments to actually pay women to encourage them to continue. It may also help to demonstrate that breastfeeding and the new lifestyle are compatible. Here again, each additional month of breastfeeding gives the infant that much greater tolerance against weanling diseases, malnutrition, and even death.

If the EMERGING BOTTLE FEEDERS can be influenced to stay with breastfeeding, they can tap the resources of existing *doulas* within their still integrated kinship groups. If so, these *doulas* too should be rewarded for their supportive roles. In modern terms this may mean financial aid to them, as well, because the mother's mother is often also working.

[3] The financial difference between a program that subsidizes mothers for the first six months after childbirth (to prevent early marasmus, etc.) and another program that focuses on cures for the malnourished child, shows the wisdom of the former. For example, subsidization of Jamaican mothers over a six-month postpartum period would have cost $250-300 (U.S.) in 1970. On the other hand, costs for curing a child of marasmus and other related diseases and returning him home to the same semistarvation environment totaled over $800 (U.S.) (E. F. P. Jelliffe 1970). To these medical costs must be added the price of dealing with adult problems directly related to infant and childhood malnutrition (Alland 1967), such as the cost of treating, supporting, and giving extra and special education to the mentally retarded child and adult whose subnormal intelligence is a result of nutritional deprivation. Additional cost to the culture for the untold loss in man-hours of work and creative energy should also be considered.

We suggested earlier that the development of a high-protein weanling product would prevent millions of infants from being adversely affected by the misuse of artificial milk. The product would have to be a food that does not require cautious preparation nor should its misuse be lethal for human infants. Foods produced from non-dairy ingredients or from adjusted dairy products that are not susceptible to rapid spoilage do not require the use of water or cause the allergic reactions that often occur from milk. Their development is well within our technological capacities. Only the commitment to invent these foods and funds to produce them are required.

Such an innovation would have two other values. The first would be to reduce the increased use all over the world of cattle and feed and space for both, which seems to mount endlessly in our hungry world. The second would be the benefit to the "lap child." A broad-based plan for supplementary food could be used to wean the healthy breast-fed child as well. As it is now, this older period is one of the most serious ones, during which some children who were formerly well sicken, weaken, and often die.

International organizations such as the World Health Organization can serve as catalysts to get local government and industry, as well as world powers, to act. It is sad, but past history has shown that altruistic programs that lack motives of self-interest are hard to sell. Infant-feeding programs are ticklish subjects. In the past, like fertility programs, they have been laden with nationalist/racist implications that end in charges of attempts to interfere with social progress and keep the recipients "backward." Suggestions of limiting the use of powdered milk have also been seen as a threat to profits.

Resistance likewise comes on ethical grounds. In the nineteenth century, even people with feelings rationalized failure to act on the grounds that the unfortunate malnutrition and infant mortality were "nature's way," or inevitable and irreversible manifestation of the "survival of the fittest." In the same way, sick or dying babies are being ignored in the twentieth century by those who sigh the sad refrain, "That's the natural way. That's overpopulation."

This is an expression of the same confusion that exists in regard to some of the United States government-aid programs. It appears to be a comfortable American cultural pattern to dole out huge amounts of money on a crisis basis only. Infants are fed in famine or disaster zones, temporary repairs are made, and the aid withdrawn. Such programs are wasteful, harmful, and often immoral.

There are areas of common concern and mutual self-interest that can be tapped to reverse the trend in infant mortality. Take the question of overpopulation. The death of one's children is one of the major fears of most of the world's parents. It often leads to an overproduction of offspring. Only when parents are convinced that their children will survive to adulthood can they afford to limit their number. Reduced population can stem from the survival of a woman's first offspring.

In summary, we have an urgent responsibility to encourage governments to accept a direct role in the problem of infant feeding, to fund programs in support of maternal benefits and infant survival, to provide incentives for industry that would encourage companies to develop products that will keep infants alive while their mothers make a dramatic change in their way of life. There is a critical need for anthropologists to become involved in such projects and to use their insights into medicine, nutrition, processes of change, and patterns of social structure to stay this terrible waste of human life.

REFERENCES

ALLAND, A.
   1967   The anthropology of war. *Natural History* (special supplement) 76 (December).
JELLIFFE, D. B., E. F. P. JELLIFFE
   1970   The urban avalanche and child nutrition. *Journal of the American Dietetic Association* 57 (11).
JELLIFFE, E. F. P.
   1970   *Report of the Tropical Metabolism Research Unit, Jamaica, West Indies.* (Case histories of the last ten children discharged November 1, 1970.)
PÉREZ, A., P. VELA, R. POTTER, G. S. MASNICK
   1971   Timing and sequence of resuming ovulation and menstruation after childbirth. *Population Studies* 25(3):491.
RAPHAEL, DANA
   1966   "The lactation-suckling process within a matrix of supportive behavior." Unpublished doctoral dissertation, Columbia University.
   1969   Uncle Rhesus, Auntie Pachyderm, and Mom: all sorts and kinds of mothering. *Perspectives in Biology and Medicine* 12 (winter).
   1973a *The tender gift: breastfeeding.* Englewood Cliffs, New Jersey: Prentice-Hall.
   1973b The role of breastfeeding in a bottle-oriented world. *Ecology of Food and Nutrition* 2:121–126.

Prehistoric Pictography in North America of Medical Significance

DALE W. RITTER and ERIC W. RITTER

INTERPRETIVE APPROACHES

The interpretation, functional analysis, and explanation of petroglyphs and pictographs can be examined in light of two integrated methods, direct and inferential. The direct approach uses historical documentation, informant discussions, and, rarely, direct observation. The inferential approach is divided into inductive and deductive reasoning. Binford (1968: 16) has stated that "traditional methodology [in archaeology] almost universally espouses simple induction as the appropriate procedure, and the archaeological record is viewed as a body of phenomena from which one makes inductive inferences about the past." In this manner inferences regarding rock art are guided by ethnographic analogy, by our knowledge of contemporary peoples, and by certain other data or principles such as geographic distribution, classification of content, style, patination, mineralogical composition of rock used, environmental and archaeological associations, and the law of superimposition. By these processes, increasing confidence in the inferential generalization about the past is possible. Binford (1968: 17) argues that "the generation of inferences regarding the past should not be one end-product of the archaeologist's work." Furthermore, he wants to see a shift to a rigorous hypothetico-deductive method with the goal of explanation. Deductive inferences concerning the interpretation and explanation of rock art, that is, working from the general to the particular, or the testing of our hypotheses derived from induction have been

All figures and photographs are by the authors. Photographs, figures, and tables copyright © 1972 by Ritter and Son.

often neglected.

Our general proposition is that a large portion of rock art has medical significance, some of which is shamanistically derived, and we deduce that particular motifs are thus medically oriented. Here we regard the modern concept of medicine as much more restrictive than the aboriginal and prehistoric concept. Support for this deductive logic is garnered from the direct historical approach and from inductive logic based on interpretation of modern medical fact; i.e. a hand that lacks a joint is obviously an abnormality of medical significance. In this study we are interpreting and determining at an explanatory level the meaning, associations, and uses of scattered motifs from North America, believed to be products of medically oriented art. We do not mean to say that all North American rock art is medically oriented in either the modern or the aboriginal sense. The proposition that much of rock art has medical significance should not detract from the consideration that rock art was often multifunctional to either the maker, the viewer, or their groups.

What is argued here is that the generation of inferences regarding the past should not be the end product or only product of the archaeologist's work. Although an awareness of a great range of variability in sociocultural phenomena is possible and the citations of analogy to living peoples are not belittled here, a main point of our argument is that independent means of testing propositions about the past must be developed.

Because rock art and related pictography in North America are largely representative, abstract, or symbolic, classification, interpretation, and explanation are not easy. Seldom is a direct interpretation by the maker recorded in the literature. Relatively secure interpretation is available for prehistoric specimens only when a particular practice (such as making totemic records) or specific content (such as certain mythical beings) continues into historic times. Examples are the clan symbols or totems recorded by Catlin at the pipestone quarries in Minnesota (Winchell 1911: 564) and those at Willow Springs, Arizona, noted by Gilbert (Mallery 1886: 46) or the study of *Kokopelli* by Renaud (1948: 25–40; Lambert 1967: 398). The tradition of making petroglyphs and pictographs has continued in many areas of the West from prehistoric, through protohistoric and historic, into modern times — particularly in the Southwest. The Navajo, Hopi, Zuñi, Paiute, Kutenai, Blackfoot, Sioux, Stony, Northwest Coast tribes, Eskimo, and others still make them. Practicing members of the Grand Medicine Society of the Ojibwa are still active. This archaeological and ethnological continuum and its spatial and temporal modifications and projections offer a valuable opportunity for a dynamic study. A similar opportunity can be found in the circumpolar regions, Africa, and Australia.

A small number of symbols are widely recognized (e.g. handprint, cupule, spiral, circle, cross, maze, serpent, sun, or swastika). Even these may represent a certain idea or object to one person or group, but something else to another (Cartwright and Douglas 1934: 44). The problem is further compounded by the possibility that the maker of some glyphs may have intended several interpretations or functions. Likewise, some individuals of the maker's group may have viewed the work in differing interpretations or functions. A totem carving could have served as a clan or personal identification and, at the same time, as a record of a visit or a sign of ownership. A hunting scene could serve not only as a record of the event but also as sympathetic magic of the hunt, or perhaps as art alone.

It is also recognized that petroglyphs or pictographs can have recreational or incidental meaning. In Monument Valley, Arizona, in 1957, Navajo children were noted painting white pictographs during play, and in 1968 a demonstration in the techniques of making petroglyphs was witnessed at Hanalei, Kauai, Hawaii (see *Sunset Magazine* 1968: 30). There are also references in the literature in which reliable informants alleged that they were made in fun or to "while away the time" (Heizer and Baumhoff 1962: 227; Gifford 1936: 290; 1940: 154). Similarly, Keithahn (1940: 130) was advised that a Tlingit chief assigned the carving of rocks as occupational therapy for slaves, "to keep them out of mischief."

In the study of petroglyphs and pictographs in western North America, there are now enough data collected that hypotheses and ideas which can be experimentally tested must be presented — right or wrong. The collection of data alone, the detailed listing of symbols, or other near-sterile and even misleading presentations must be replaced or reformulated.

MEDICAL PERSPECTIVES

To modern men of advanced civilization, medicine is apt to mean the study, prevention, and treatment of disease or injury. To prehistoric men, however, it had a much broader meaning (see Table 1). It was a concept that included not only health and the cure or prevention of illness, but also direction of good or bad fortune, success or failure in the hunt, war, love, or revenge, the attainment of the desirable, preven-

Table 1.   Profile, province, psychodynamics, and practice of the medicine man
(proposed outline including witch doctoring and shamanism)

I.   *Attributes, assets, qualifications, modalities*
  A.   Spiritual, supernatural, magic, religious
    1.   recovery from death
      a.   resurrection
      b.   reincarnation
      c.   rebirth
    2.   recovery from illness (especially self-cure)
    3.   revival
    4.   altered or trans states *
      a.   transformation
      b.   transfiguration
      c.   possession states
      d.   transcendentalism
      e.   consecration
      f.   personification
      g.   narcosis
      h.   trance, dissociation
      i.   self-hypnosis
      j.   other (hysteria, amnesia, faint, fugue, coma, seizures, sleep, som-
           nambulism, somniloquy, etc.)
    5.   transmigration *
      a.   visitation
      b.   transcend
      c.   ascend
      d.   descend
    6.   spernatural communication and liaison *
      a.   by 1, 4, & 5
      b.   pictography
                 magic symbols
                 magic signs
                 (including rock art)
      c.   visions, portent
      d.   divination, augury
      e.   dreams, oneiromancy
      f.   hallucination
      g.   totem relationships
      h.   communion
      i.   incantation
      j.   conjure
      k.   prayer, worship
      l.   hypnosis
      m.   coitus, bestiality
      n.   omens, oracles, astrology
      o.   necromancy
      p.   other (plastromancy, scapulomancy, etc.)
    7.   supernatural skills *
      a.   exorcise
      b.   charm
      c.   hypnotize, induce

---

*   Rock art and other pictography may be instrumental or associated.

Table 1 (continued).

---

      d. sorcery, voodoo
      e. cast spells, hex
      f. other (e.g. 4i, 6b–f, 6i–p)
    8. personal spirits and spirit control *
B. Natural, real
    1. physical
      a. certain imperfections
          deformities
          epilepsy
          other
      b. recovery from illness
      c. immunity to illness
      d. dexterity, coordination
      e. stamina
      f. male (preferred)
      g. other
    2. mental, emotional
      a. motivation
      b. intelligence
      c. wisdom, sagacity
      d. insight
      e. observant *
      f. intuition
      g. creativity *
      h. artistry *
      i. drive
      j. persuasiveness
      k. compassion
      l. psychoneurosis (sometimes)
      m. psychosis (seldom)
      n. other (clairvoyance, etc.)
    3. social
      a. training, education *
          preceptorship *
          initiation *
          restitution, fee
          knowledge
          ventriloquism
          legerdemain
          other skills *
          histrionics
      b. reputation, rapport
      c. selection
          kinship
          inheritance
          circumstance, chance
          custom
      d. interrelationships
      (patient, student, group, audience, kin, to practitioner)
          credibility

Table 1 (continued).

---

                    confidence
                    conditioning
                    fear
                    faith
                    love
                    hysteria
                    awe
                    other
II. *Functions* *
     A. Maintain order (correct disorders)
         1. individuals
         2. society
         3. universe, nature
     B. Assure success
     C. Assure good luck
     D. Avert evil, bad luck (or cause them)
     E. Propitiation
     F. Spiritual guidance
     G. Absolution
     H. Prophecy, interpretation
     I. Communication, liaison
         1. supernatural
         2. dead
         3. living
         4. nature
     J. Cure and prevent illness
     K. Inspiration, leadership
     L. Training, teaching, advice
     M. Custodial care (sacred materials, beliefs)
     N. Officiate, consecrate
III. *Media, vehicles, aids*
     A. Arts *
         1. picture art, "3D" art (including rock art)
         2. drama
             a. ceremony
             b. ritual
         3. dance
         4. music
         5. architecture (kivas, etc.)
     B. Science, pseudoscience
         1. pharmacy, alchemy
         2. surgery*
         3. psychology *
         4. physical sciences
         5. natural sciences *
         6. palmistry, phrenology
         7. astrology *
         8. other (logic, philosophy, etc.)
     C. Intermediaries, mediums
         1. supernatural *

---

*   Rock art and other pictography may be instrumental or associated.
** Emphasis on personal disease (vs. societal, universal).

Table 1 (continued).

---

      2. real
- D. Accouterments *
  1. charms, talismans
  2. fetishes, idols, figurines
  3. sucking tubes, knives, needles
  4. musical instruments
     a. rattle
     b. drum
     c. flute
     d. other
  5. medicine, drugs, herbs
  6. medicine bundles
  7. baton, mace, staff
  8. weapons
  9. various paraphernalia
- E. Dress * — animal parts & disguise
      allegoric symbols
      magic adornments

IV. *Concepts of disease* **
- A. Etiology, pathology
  1. supernatural
     a. soul-less
     b. intrusion
     c. trans states
     d. spell, hex, curse *
     e. breach, sin, transgression
            taboo
            custom
            law
            moral
            principles
            other
  2. real
     a. stress
            psychic
            physical
     b. injury
     c. genetic
     d. poisoning
     e. allergy
     f. infection
     g. malnutrition
     h. other
- B. Diagnosis
  1. supernatural communication,* ESP
  2. observation, experience, logic
  3. testing, trial & error, analysis *
  4. hypnoanalysis, psychoanalysis
- C. Treatment
  1. correct etiology *
     a. recapture the soul (may use soul catcher)

Table 1 (continued).

---

      b. remove intrusive objects (sucking, legerdemain)
      c. remove curse, hex
      d. spirit control
      e. other
  2. physical therapy
      a. exercise or rest
      b. heat, cold, sweats *
      c. massage, flagellation
      d. acupuncture, tattoo * (also act as magic, psychotherapy)
  3. medicine, drugs, herbs *
      a. emetics
      b. cathartics
      c. counter-irritants
      d. hallucinogens
      e. narcotics
      f. other
  4. surgery *
  5. midwifery, obstetrics *
  6. set and splint fractures
  7. hypnotherapy, suggestion
  8. psychotherapy, sociatry *
  9. ritual and ceremony *
      a. curing
      b. maturation
      c. fertility
      d. hunting
      e. crop
      f. apotropaic
      g. mortuary
      h. other
10 magic (sympathetic, contagious) *
11. offerings, sacrifice, atonement *
12. prayer, incantation, worship *

---

* Rock art and other pictography may be instrumental or associated.

tion of the undesirable, and influence over fellow men, animals, nature, spirits, and gods. These goals were achieved more often through the use or intervention of the supernatural than through natural or scientific means. The earliest attempts to combat illness seem to have developed in two directions, magical and empirical (*M. D. Medical Newsmagazine* 1959b: 89). Often in prehistoric times the practitioner had to be not only an expert in healing, but a medicine man, shaman, sorcerer, priest, magician, hypnotist, and seer. Medicine, magic, and religion were so closely intertwined that now in retrospect it cannot be determined where one began and the other ended (Corlett 1935: V, 65; Gunn 1966: 700–706; Lommel 1967: 9; Vogel 1970: 14, 22, 26). Fox (1967: 255) reminds us that illness — both mental and physical —

though based on universal psychobiological factors, is culturally patterned in its expression. Illness in one culture may be religious fervor in another. Certain illnesses in modern North American culture would have been considered in many past cultures as a supernatural gift and even an asset leading to selection as a shaman (e.g. epilepsy). On the other hand, almost all illnesses have at least some common psychic components such as fear, anxiety, rejection, anger, and depression that transcend population and cultural boundaries. Success in healing must include relief of these and in this the prehistoric medicine man or shaman was often adept. However, at times he capitalized on these reactions to achieve credibility or personal gain.

The terms medicine man, shaman, and sorcerer will be used somewhat interchangeably because they all share the role of healer. Subtle differences are recognized such as the methods by which one is chosen, the limits or spheres of their practices, the methods by which they heal, and colloquial usage. The roles of all three are poorly defined and merge, making it difficult to know which term is most appropriate (Lommel 1967: 7–9, 242; Corlett 1935: V, 65).

SUPERNATURAL ART OF PREHISTORIC MEDICAL PRACTITIONERS

The associations of shamans or their intermediaries with the practice of medicine (both concepts) and with the use of art (including petroglyphs, pictographs, and pictography in general) have been reported by several authors.

At one time the very idea of preserving man's thoughts and deeds was considered a miracle, and very often attributed to divine inspiration. A knowledge of writing during certain periods of the world's history has been considered dangerous, for it was used in the beginning primarily as the tool of priests and magicians (Cadzow 1934: 95).

However, Okladnikov (1970: 213) describes the origin and function of secular and shamanistic art with these statements:

In actuality, like everything else of vital importance in the culture of primeval man, pictographic writing was created not by sorcerers and priests but by the people themselves, and the sorcerers only tried to use it for their own ends. The pictography which served the needs of real life was not derived from magical signs, but vice versa.

Part of the artistic heritage left by prehistoric shamans, sorcerers, and other creative aboriginal men was pictography, a precursor to writing (Blum 1970: 536; Covarrubias 1954: 79; see also Tables 2 and 3).

Table 2.   Rock art of the medicine man, with doctor or shaman (proposed characteristics)*

A. *Site selection*
   1. associations
      a. ceremonial
      b. hunting
      c. crops
      d. habitations
      e. routes
      f. spas
   2. areas of natural attributes
      a. scenic
      b. resources
            water
            food
            minerals
            pipestone
            wood
            etc.
   3. physical properties
      a. visibility
      b. vantage
      c. shelter
      d. caves
      e. facings
      f. accessibility
      g. rock type
      h. rock size
      i. surfaces, cliffs
      j. rock alignments
   4. previous site
   5. present site
B. *Site use*
   1. special function
   2. special communication
   3. secondary uses
      a. shrine (including healing)
      b. meeting place
      c. refuge
      d. ritual, ceremony
      e. burial
      f. cache
      g. other
C. *Spatial relationships*
   1. restriction
   2. condensation
   3. composition
   4. grouping
   5. incorporation of rock features
   6. incorporation of prior art
   7. directional orientation
   8. enclosures

---

* Not exclusive and may be associated with secular art.

Table 2 (continued).

---

    9. superimposition
   10. revamping
D. *Temporal relationships*
    1. superimposition
    2. reuse, revamping
    3. continuum of use
    4. evolution
    5. negation
E. *Special content*
    1. themes, topics
      a. cosmology
      b. mythology
      c. dichotomy
      d. altered, spirit, trans states
      e. supernatural communications
      f. sympathetic magic
      g. other magic
    2. motifs
      a. projections
      b. life or heart lines
      c. consanguinity lines
      d. continuity lines
      e. ground lines
      f. X ray (exposed rib)
      g. composite animals
      h. bipolar animals
      i. distorted animals
      j. labeled animals
      k. totems
      l. eye motifs
      m. genital
      n. receptive female
      o. phytomorphs
      p. sacred object
      q. weapon
      r. sun circle
      s. cross
      t. celestial
      u. combinations
      v. other
    3. miscellaneous (other artistic, graphic devices)
      a. perspective
      b. 3D
      c. motion
      d. esthetics
      e. scenes
      f. abstractions
      g. conventionalization
      h. impressionism
      i. representation
      j. pictograms

Table 2 (continued).

---

       k. ideograms
       l. rebus?
       m. other
    4. typical examples **
       a. supernatural anthropomorphs
          medicine men
          shamans
          sorcerers
          gods, kachinas
          ancestors
          spirits
       b. hunting magic (imitative)
          wounded animals
          spirit animals
          weapons
          hunt scenes
       c. healing magic
          fertility rocks
          sand paintings
          serpents
          ritual art
F. *Color significance*
    1. red
       a. used most
       b. associations with the supernatural noted
       c. associated with ceremony, ritual
    2. black — 2nd most common
    3. white — 3rd most common
    4. study is needed

** Combination of:
    a. A1a, A3b, C4, E1a, E2a, E2p, E2q, and E3g.
    b. A1b, A2b, C6, D1, E1f, E2b, E2q, E3e, and F1b.
    c. A1a, B3a, C1, D3, E1f, E1g, E2g, E2m, and E3g.

Gunn (1966: 703–706) further states that although a shaman often used medicinal and physical aids, his main field, prerogative, and forte was psychotherapy, using suggestion, fear, persuasion, illusion, and hypnosis. Individual and mass hysteria, faith of the people, and his faith in himself contributed to his success.

It does appear that the art of prehistoric or primitive medical practitioners and shamans can be linked with a series of pictures, themes, motifs, artistic devices, graphic tricks, or styles which portray mediumistic, supernatural, or shamanistic myths, concepts, or ideas (Mallery 1893: 237, 463–467; Maringer 1960: 195; Strong 1959: 120; 1969: 175; Lommel 1967: 25; Ritter 1970: 399, 409; Ritter and Ritter i.p.; see Tables 4 and 5). Lommel (1967: 25) states that visual art, especially

Table 3. Natural content of rock art (functional aspects)

A. *Identification*
1. personal (idiographs) *
2. group
   a. residency
   b. culture
   c. totem
   d. kinship
   e. nature
   f. socioeconomy
   g. politics
   h. status
   i. religion
   j. other
3. geographic
   a. territory
   b. boundary
   c. ownership
   d. natural resources
   e. trails
   f. maps
   g. graves
4. celestial
   a. stars
   b. planets
   c. sun
   d. moon
   e. constellations
   f. planetariums
   g. celestial maps
B. *Records* *
1. visits
2. events
3. exploits
4. messages (semiotica)
5. stories
6. legends
7. myths
8. tallies
9. testimonials
10. memorials
11. calendars
12. objects
13. conditions
C. *Mnemonic devices*
D. *Visual, teaching aids*
E. *Practice, experiment*
F. *Pastime*
1. doodling
2. games, puzzles

---

* Dermatoglyphics and fingerprints shown in handprints may be useful records of prehistoric illness or physical anthropology.

Table 3 (continued).

---

3. occupational therapy
4. decoration
G. *Art alone*
H. *Multifunctional*

rock paintings, is partially derived from shamanism. The shaman is above all an artistically productive man (1967: 8). In the practice of medicine he is most successful in psychotherapy (the art of medicine?) (1967: 9). Lommel further suggests that shamanism and art were derived from primitive hunting cultures, emphasizing that shamanistic regalia is an animal disguise (1967: 107, 128). The earliest example of this is probably the "Sorcerer" at Trois Frères Cave in southern France (Kilgauer 1959: 44).

Table 4.   Themes, topics

A. *Cosmology*
   1. origin
   2. creation
   3. cosmos
   4. celestial arch
   5. celestial bodies
   6. space concepts
   7. time concepts
   8. seasons
   9. world order
   10. other
B. *Mythology* (also legend)
   1. pantheon
   2. deification
   3. heroes
   4. totemism
   5. ancestors
   6. spirits
      a. beneficent, guardian
      b. evil, destructive
      c. personal
   7. medicine men, shamans, sorcerers
   8. migrations
   9. contests
   10. conquests
   11. quests
   12. roles
   13. interaction
C. *Dichotomy*
   1. evil vs. good
   2. male : female
   3. death : life
   4. heaven : hell
   5. conflict of supernaturals

Table 4 (continued).

---

    6. twin relationships
    7. natural : supernatural
    8. negation
D. *Altered, spirit, and trans states*
    1. transmigration
      a. ascendency
      b. descendency
      c. transcendency
    2. transfiguration
    3. transcendentalism
    4. transformation
    5. personification
    6. animation
    7. animism
    8. possession
    9. resurrection
    10. reincarnation
    11. consecration
    12. illness
    13. death
    14. other
E. *Supernatural communication* (also liaison, rapport)
    1. divination, portent
    2. vision portrayal
    3. dream portrayal
    4. visitation records
    5. intermediaries, messengers
    6. coitus
    7. bestiality
    8. prayer
    9. incantation
F. *Sympathetic magic* (mainly imitative) (see G, H)
    1. hunt
    2. curing
    3. crop
    4. rain
    5. fertility, increase
    6. love, sex
    7. hate, hex
    8. stealing
    9. war
    10. other
G. *Other magic*
    1. symbolism and signs
      a. good luck
      b. bad luck
      c. death
      d. life
      e. illness
      f. rain, water
      g. cupules
      h. genital

Table 4 (continued).

---

      i. coital
      j. parturition
      k. parent with young
      l. nursing
      m. magic objects
      n. sacred objects
      o. maze
      p. other
   2. spirit control and influence
   3. exorcism
   4. sorcery
   5. legerdemain
   6. contagious magic
      a. curing shrines
      b. accouterments
      c. dress
      d. other
H. *Ritual, ceremony*
   1. see F
   2. maturation
   3. apotropaic
   4. mortuary
   5. worship
   6. sacrifice
   7. offering
   8. quest
   9. supplication
   10. consecration
I. *Combined, merging, and other themes*

Table 5. Motifs

A. *Projections*
   1. extracorporeal, external
      a. cephalic
         coronal
         orbital
         oral
      b. corpus
         navel
         nipple
         back, etc.
      c. caudal
         tail
         anus
         genital
      d. pedal
      e. manual
   2. juxtaposed
   3. trajectory, protruding missiles
   4. types
      a. straight line

Table 5 (continued).

---

      b. broken line
      c. zigzag line
      d. *wakan* line
      e. spiral
      f. circle
      g. curve
      h. dots
      i. halo
      j. involute
      k. rays
      l. arrows
      m. feathers
      n. horns
      o. other
   5. significance
      a. supernatural qualities
      b. supernatural power
      c. supernatural status
      d. transfer of
          power
          information
          spirits
          disease, etc.
      e. illness, wounds
      f. exorcism
      g. other relationships
B. *Life or heart lines*
C. *Consanguinity lines*
D. *Continuity lines*
E. *Ground lines*
F. *X ray or exposed ribs*
   1. skeletal
   2. internal organs
   3. fetus
   4. involute
G. *Composite animals*
   1. part human, part animal
   2. parts of various animals
   3. pregnant
H. *Bipolar cephalic animals*
I. *Distorted animals*
   1. absent parts
   2. added parts
   3. head or mask only
   4. size distortions
   5. shape distortions
   6. common or shared parts
   7. incongruous parts
      botanical
      inanimate, etc.
   8. wounded
   9. dead

Table 5 (continued).

---

      10. split
      11. unfolded
      12. other
J. *Tagged or labeled animals*
      1. geometric
      2. symbols
      3. magic signs
      4. genital signs
      5. other
K. *Totems*
L. *Eye motifs*
      1. weeping eye
      2. open eye
      3. forked eye
      4. eye and hand
      5. eye and joint
M. *Genital*
      1. cupules
      2. vulviforms
      3. phallic
      4. ithyphallic
N. *Receptive female*
O. *Phytomorphs*
      1. medicines
      2. tree of life
      3. sacred plants
      4. corn
      5. pollen
P. *Sacred objects*
      1. drum, rattle, flute
      2. mace, club, staff
      3. prayer stick
      4. medicine bag
      5. medicine bundle
      6. feather
      7. pottery
      8. gourd
      9. shell
      10. other
Q. *Weapons*
      1. *atlatl*
      2. axes
      3. spears
      4. bow and arrow
      5. knife
      6. shield
R. *Sun circle*
S. *Cross*
T. *Celestial*
U. *Combinations of motifs*
V. *Other motifs*

In supernatural or shamanistic art, parts of several animals are combined arbitrarily into a COMPOSITE ANIMAL; e.g. a panther may have a stag's antlers or a stag may have several heads, and a part may be shared by two or more animals (Lommel 1967: 128). Examples from Russia and Siberia are known. A two-headed moose or elk petroglyph from the Angara River in Siberia is illustrated by Okladnikov (1969: Plate 15).

Crow Indian medicine bundles were considered to hold various mythical creatures and their power, including the chief of the underwater animals called the "long bug." This creature was thought to possess the body of a huge snake and to be double-headed. One of its heads resembles that of a cow with two long horns and has "eyes as large as sunflowers." The other head looks like that of a human being, with a long nose and a single eye. Protruding above the single eye is one large horn. Among the Crow Indians the snake is recognized as the chief of all "insects" and is the medicine *par excellence* used in doctoring, particularly in dangerous and severe cases (Wildschut 1960: 11–12).

A grotesque, composite Indian image or idol, part animal and part human, found along the Mississippi River is pictured in Josephy (1961: 156) being destroyed by early explorers and missionaries. It resembles some reproductions of the former *Piasa* pictograph of the Illini also found in that vicinity. Squier (1851: 110, 136, Figures 20, 24) describes a double-headed cat, jaguar, or lynx at Uxmal and an "astronomical serpent" in the Dresden codex.

Spinden (1957: 53–57) describes "two headed dragons" or serpents with clawlike or cloven feet found at various places in Central America like Copán, Palenque, Piedras Negras, and Yaxchilán. He also states (1957: 34) that parts of other creatures are often added to the body of the snake in Mayan art. Among the myths of the Iroquois pertaining to the reign of Atotarho IV (pre-Columbian), a double-headed serpent which destroyed the people of a fort (Emerson 1965: 540) is mentioned.

A two-headed, doglike animal and a serpent whose body forms a cloud symbol in the center but with a head at each end are found among the petroglyphs at San Cristobal, Santa Fe County, New Mexico (Sims 1950: 6, 8, Plates II, XI). A serpentlike, double-headed animal found among pictographs of the Northwest Coast Indians will be discussed later. Other illustrations of composite animals include: the two-headed sheep or deer petroglyphs of the Coso Range, Inyo County, California (see Figure 1); the *Piasa* pictographs formerly located near Alton, Illinois (Armstrong 1887: 2); the two-headed bear and owl fetishes of the

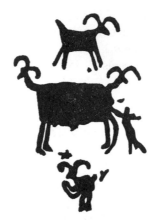

Figure 1. Big Petroglyph Canyon, Coso Range, California. Many examples of two-headed sheep or deer can be found in this region.

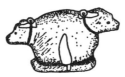

Figure 2. Zuñi fetish. Occasionally the Zuñi hunters will use a double-headed fetish for hunting luck because "it has twice the power"

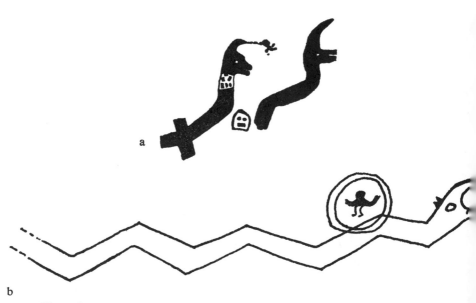

Figure 3. *Awanyu*, the horned or plumed serpent, a widespread composite animal occurring on many media, including rock art panels: (a) San Cristobal, New Mexico; (b) Pueblo Blanco, New Mexico

Zuñi (see Figure 2); the *Awanyu* of the Southwest (see Figure 3); and an occasional instance of shared parts, usually with superimposition, such as occur at Renegade (Little Petroglyph) Canyon, Inyo County, California (see Plate 1), Nine Mile Canyon, Duchesne County, Utah (see Figure 4), and Indian Creek, San Juan County, Utah (see our Plate 2; Ritter 1970: Figure 204).

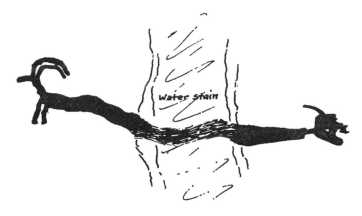

Figure 4.   Nine Mile Canyon, Utah. This interesting sheep-serpent is found pecked where it is crossed by a water seep. Speculation is aroused as to whether this is an intentional or accidental location, and if intentional, whether it relates to water supply

A second general characteristic of shamanistic art given by Lommel is the portrayal of SHAMANISTIC BATTLES in which shamans are disguised as animals. He suggests the scene at Lascaux showing a prostrate anthropomorph before a wounded aurochs as an example — only one participant has assumed the form of an animal (Lommel 1967: 128–129). This concept is difficult to accept and prove, but perhaps the bear fight scene at the McConkie Ranch, Ashley Canyon, Uintah County, Utah, or the archers' scene at Renegade (Little Petroglyph) Canyon (see Figure 5) could be interpreted similarly.

Another characteristic of supernatural art is the X-RAY STYLE commonly seen in the prehistoric and historic art of the Northwest Coast and Great Plains (see Figure 6 [Columbia River, Washington], Figure 7 [Sproat Lake, Vancouver Island, Canada], Figure 8 [Wrangell, Alaska]; see also Figure 9 [Massacre Lake, Nevada], Figure 10 [Kenton, Oklahoma], and Ritter 1961: 4). Along the Columbia River, Strong (1959: 120) identifies this common stylistic element as the EX-POSED-RIB MOTIF.

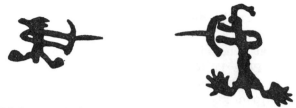

Figure 5. Little Petroglyph Canion, Coso Range, California. This pair of archers might represent Lommel's shamanistic art theme of conflicting supernaturals or might be a record of some battle or duel

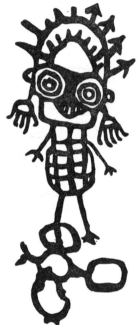

Figure 6. This anthropomorph formerly located about ten miles above The Dalles on the Columbia River has been destroyed by vandals

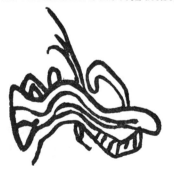
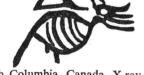

Figure 7. Sproat Lake, Vancouver Island, British Columbia, Canada. X-ray or exposed-rib style of portrayal is noted in the water monster on the left and the stylized animal on the right

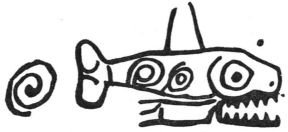

Figure 8. Wrangell, Alaska. This killer whale, identified by his large dorsal fin, has been made by the X-ray style typical of the Northwest Coast region of North America

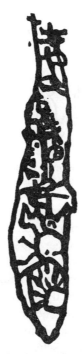

Figure 9. Massacre Lake, Nevada. Located near dry pluvial beds on the rim of the Great Basin is this magnificent five-foot petroglyph of a primitive sucker-type fish done in X-ray style. Its location also represents a peripheral extension of this style from the Columbia River plateau

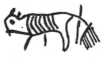

Figure 10. Kenton, Oklahoma. Ribs are shown in this bison or buffalo figure carved in a sandstone rock shelter

Lommel (1967: 57) includes the HEART-LINE MOTIF in addition to the exposed-rib motif as a form of X-ray style and gives many examples from Siberia, Lapland (109), Scandinavia (130–132), Australia, and Eskimo art (133) (see also Black 1964: 16). Cheng TeK'un (1966: Plate 24) presents an anthropomorph with the exposed-rib motif found painted on Yangshao pottery from China. This same bowl is illustrated by Covarrubias (1954: 61) and compared with pottery bowls from the Southwest (Pueblo II–III). The heart line is a common motif among the Ojibwa bark pictographs (James 1956: 181, 345), the medicine tipis of the Blackfeet (McClintock 1936: 123), the Sioux winter counts (see Figure 11), the kiva walls of the Pueblos (Dutton 1963: 74), and

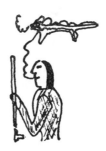

Figure 11. Sioux winter counts painted on buffalo robes occasionally show the heart line or life line. Also shown are a consanguinity line and cephalic projection

is found among petroglyphs and pictographs of a similar yet wider geographic distribution (Connor 1962: 29; Erwin 1930: 65, Plate 12; Renaud 1938: Plate 12). Maringer (1960: 195) states that the magical character of circumpolar art also is indicated by the LIFE LINE. He notes that this practice was observed among the Ojibwa as late as the 1890s; their sorcerers drew exactly the same sort of "life tine." It is also found among the rock art of the Pueblo and Navajo cultures in Arizona and New Mexico, on other rock pictures in North America, in Siberian engravings, and in Lapp art (Schaafsma 1963: 41, 60). Zoomorphs with heart lines found in a rock shelter in Harrison County, West Virginia, are described and illustrated by Mallery (1893: 475, Plate XXXI). Others are found in Ohio County, West Virginia (Swauger 1962: 34, Plate I; 1964: 6, Figure 2), in Columbiana County, Ohio (Swauger 1968: 6, Figure 2), and in central Baja (see Figure 12). It should be noted that some workers call the line from mouth to heart a life line rather than a heart line.

These lines are not to be confused with the CONSANGUINITY LINES between two animals or objects, especially between adult and young,

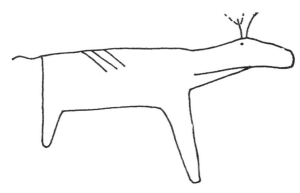

Figure 12. In the central highlands area (Sierra de Zacatecas Range) of Baja, figures such as this deer showing a heart line are frequently found

which indicate a close relationship or kinship (see Figure 13). Such a line is also seen between an anthropomorph and his totem animal, e.g. in pictographic autobiographies or the tribal rosters of the Ogalala and the census of Red Cloud's band (Mallery 1886: 165–187). This special line device therefore might serve a secular purpose, and also might be shamanistic at times.

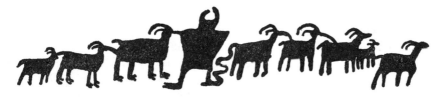

Figure 13. Minnie Maud Canyon, Utah. This diagram, taken from a larger panel showing a hunting scene, illustrates the consanguinity (affinity, relationship, kinship) line

Animals shown with the heart line were considered supernatural by the Ojibwa and Zuñi. Among the Ojibwa and Dakota, spirals indicated *wakan* [spirit] and animals shown with these are also intended to be supernatural. Ojibwa animals connected with certain sacred ceremonies are represented as encircled (Mallery 1893: 773–774). *Gitche-a-nah-mi-e-be-zhew* or *A-nah-me-be-zhe, ne-kau-naw* [the underground wildcat], who derives his power from medicinal roots and herbs, is shown encircled by his tail or with a spiraled tail. Mallery (1893: 495, Figure 698) also mentions spiral *wakan* lines in some pictographs of the Dakota which indicate the act and power of a medicine man or shaman to "shoot" objects into a victim and cause injury, disease, or death. He also illustrates the Dakota symbols for medicine man or shaman which include wavy or zigzag lines (1893: 463, 464, 467). Such lines among the Ojibwa meant magic influence (1893: 237, Plate XVIII).

Medicine Hunts

Pictography in western North America associated with medicine hunting or sympathetic magic of the hunt is sometimes made or controlled by a hunt shaman, medicine man, or the hunter himself. Some of the animal figures involved show three of Lommel's characteristics of shamanistic art (i.e. parts combined arbitrarily, X-ray style and the heart line). Some animal figures may represent spirit animals or souls of animals and some are thought to be capable of remote control, even reincarnation (James 1956: 164, 181, 341; Ritter 1970: 397; Schoolcraft 1851: 382–388). The content of pictography associated with sympathetic magic of the hunt includes prestige animals, wounded animals, successful hunting scenes, animal parts, spoor, prints, traps, weapons, fertility signs and scenes, even special anthropomorphs thought to be gods of the hunt, "keeper of the animals," the hunt shaman, or his spiritual counterpart and assistant. Certain petroglyphic hunting scenes with *Kokopelli* and kiva wall paintings of *Paiyatuma* are good examples of the latter (see Plate 3) (Wellman 1970: 1681; Ritter 1970: 397, 399; Dutton 1963: 75, Figure 88; Stevenson 1904: Plate XLI). The fact that a majority (87 percent) of field-studied petroglyph and pictograph locations with hunting content are found in or near present, historic, and prehistoric hunting areas (game trails, hunting blinds, box canyons, water holes, buffalo jumps, etc.) supports the postulate that they were used as hunting medicine or magic (Ritter 1970: 397; Schaafsma 1965: 7, 9; Heizer and Baumhoff 1959: 904–905; 1962: 239–240). The occasional graphic tricks of placing an animal facing the sun, a trap, an obstacle, or a maze, of making his tracks face in the opposite direction from the way he is facing, or of placing him in association with signs which may stand for supernatural or magic powers, confusion, or peril (e.g. the snake, heart line, maze, or spiral) also imply hunting medicine or magic (Ritter 1970: 399; Dutton 1963: 74). The possibility that some are hunting records also must be recognized.

In a study of the Zuñi, Stevenson (1904: 439) documents the relationship of pictographs to hunting medicine: "There is a good drawing in blue-gray of a deer on the face of a mesa 30 miles southwest of Zuni, which is shot at by all the hunters who pass that way, and success is inevitable for the one whose arrow strikes the mark." Judging from the techniques of manufacture and artistic merit, an ordinary hunter or artist could have made most of the petroglyphs and pictographs found in western North America. Because of his special rapport with the spiritual or supernatural, the shaman or medicine man probably would have been preferred in the manufacture of these art forms, however.

Heizer and Baumhoff (1962: 242, 281) suggest that shamans of the Great Basin may have made petroglyphs as part of a hunting ritual. These authors do not suggest a relationship to medicine, except perhaps the relationship between successful hunting and good nutrition, or between sympathetic magic (of the hunt) and "medicine" in its more comprehensive sense. In the San Joaquin Valley and the neighboring Sierra Nevada, some pictographs are said by native Yokuts to have been made by shamans (Steward 1929: 135, 227; Heizer and Baumhoff 1962: 226). Grant (1965: 65) states that the main function of the California shaman was to cure disease. These shamans were reported to be able to turn themselves into grizzly bears and to kill enemies. In the Cuyama River area is a cave with forty-nine bear tracks pecked on the floor, which Grant (1965: 64, Figures 81, 103) speculates might be the work of a very potent bear doctor.

Malouf (1961: 8–10) mentions that during the past 2,000 years some pictographs in Montana were made by youths to get the help of a guardian spirit to make themselves better hunters, gamblers, lovers, OR DOCTORS. He mentions "medicine rocks" both with and without petroglyphs. At one such site on the north shore of the Marias River, offerings of beads, food, etc., were made by the Assiniboin. Grant (1967: 32) mentions that among Great Basin groups a hunt shaman directing a communal hunt probably made many petroglyphs prior to the hunt. He also quotes an Eskimo informant who stated that rock drawings at Cook Inlet and Prince William Sound, Alaska, might have been made by persons who wanted to become shamans. Indian informants from Idaho ascribe rock drawings in that area to medicine men (Grant 1967: 49).

Shaman Anthropomorphs

Hoffman (1891: 174) mentions the presence of horns attached to the head of an anthropomorph as a common symbol of superior power; a wavy line extending from the head also denotes superior power (223);

a heart-to-mouth line indicates inspiration (186); a circle about the head denotes more than the ordinary amount of knowledge (255). Cadzow (1934: 40) also felt the portrayal of a face or head or horns indicated a superior being such as a chief or shaman. All humpback and horned symbols are very powerful to the Navajo (Schaafsma 1963: 60). Shaman symbols pictured by Mallery (1893: 474, Figure 653d) show rays, feathers, horns, etc. about their heads. Pictographs of various shamans, medicine men, priests, and initiates show these characteristics (see Hoffman 1891: Figure 6, number 1, Figure 7, numbers 1, 5, 12, Figure 8, numbers 1, 5, 10, 12, 13, Figure 22). The headgear of the *yei* and kachinas of the Southwest found among petroglyphs, pictographs, textiles, sand paintings, and wall paintings are excellent examples.

Two unusual historic pictographic records (Hoffman 1891: 31, 32) show shamans treating patients. One shaman treating a woman is using a bone tube and rattle. This pictograph was made on a piece of birchbark, carried in the *Mide'* sack of a shaman, and intended to record a healing event of importance. The other depicts a *Jessakkid* [shaman] using a rattle and treating a man. A wavy line from the shaman's eye to the patient's abdomen indicates that he has located the demon causing the illness. In another article comparing Eskimo pictographs with those of other American aborigines, Hoffman (1883: 18) includes a carving on ivory made by a Kaite' Yamut Indian of southeast Alaska which portrays the success of a shaman in curing two patients. A similar Alaskan native carving on a piece of walrus ivory was interpreted for Hoffman as showing a shaman exorcising a demon from a sick man (Mallery 1886: Figure 110; *M. D. Medical Newsmagazine* 1972: 229).

In the Pecos River country of southern Texas, Kirkland and Newcomb (1967: 43, 45, 65) identify the many special anthropomorphs occurring there as shamans with *atlatls*, darts, stylized projectile points, and medicine pouches. Grieder (1966: 710–720) also identifies them as shamans, but believes the fringed objects are catfish instead of medicine pouches; he believes the anthropomorphs with these objects are "fisherman" shamans belonging to an early riverine culture. Sometimes they are headless, but most are prominent in size, number, and placement. A mescaline bean society or cult is hypothesized (Grieder 1966: 75) and some of the paintings in this area are suggested to be visualizations, dreams, or hallucinations occurring in trance states induced by eating mescal beans (1966: 79–80).

Several sacred pictographs of the Ojibwa show shamans holding phytomorphs, which in *Midewiwin* ceremonies refer to medicines, herbs, medicine roots, and trees (Hoffman 1891: 195, 196, 253, 282, 283,

292, 293, 296, Figures 7, 9, Plates XXII, XVI, XIV).

Among petroglyphs and pictographs along the Angara River in Siberia, Okladnikov (1969: Plates 8, 21) found several anthropomorphs he believes are shamans or sorcerers. He compares their headgear with such diverse temporal examples as the sorcerer at Trois Frères (27), a prehistoric Siberian shaman crown with elk horns (Plate 19), and present-day shaman headgear. Dioszegi (1968: 196–198), in conjunction with Okladnikov, explored Bronze Age cliff drawings on the Oka River and noted a probable shaman anthropomorph with antlers on its head. A similar possible horned shaman's headgear has been found in the Hopewell Mound, Ohio (Wilson 1896: Plate 13). Probable shaman anthropomorphs can be identified not only by special stance, accouterments, animal disguises, and dress, but by various cephalic projections. To the list of shaman motifs mentioned previously must be added CEPHALIC PROJECTIONS and other projections.

An association with possible indicators of transcendency or flight to the supernatural (such as birds, clouds, celestial bodies, psychedelics, etc.) may also be evidence of shamanistic motif. The designation of these graphic motifs and of the use of pictography in sympathetic magic as shamanistic is not meant to exclude their possible use or origin by nonshaman artists. Graphic "tricks" used in sympathetic magic of the hunt by the hunt shaman also could be considered as shaman motifs. These would include such devices as portraying a wounded animal, fertility signs on the animal, showing it facing a trap or maze, giving it

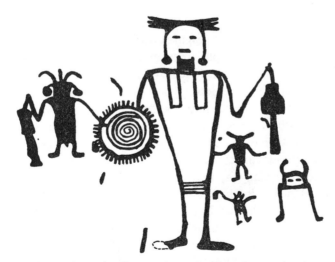

Figure 14.   Not far from the figures shown in Plate 5 are related ones such as these found at McKee Springs in Dinosaur National Monument, Utah

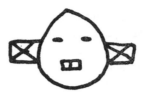

Figure 15.   At San Cristobal, New Mexico, many gods or kachinas are pecked on cliffs and boulders; some can be tentatively identified with members of the modern Puebloan pantheon. This particular figure also occurs at other sites nearby, but cannot be definitely identified as yet

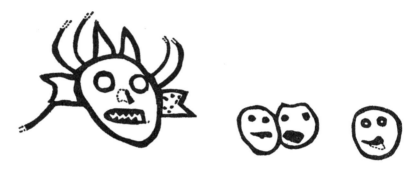

Figure 16.   Pueblo Blanco, New Mexico. This figure with two horns and dentate teeth has been identified as *Sayathlia* (also called *Hututu*) who is associated with war and medicine

two heads, and facing the animal in one direction and its tracks in the opposite (Ritter 1970: 399, Figures 195, 201, 202, 204). Other definite shaman anthropomorphs, identifiable because of special features and associations, will be mentioned subsequently.

Many anthropomorphic petroglyphs and pictographs in North America suggest medicine men, shamans, sorcerers, or their intermediaries, but it is impossible at present to differentiate them from mythical beings, ceremonial participants, culture heroes, venerated ancestors, gods, or even ordinary personages. A few that should be noted are found at Little Petroglyph Canyon, Inyo County, California (see Plate 4); the McConkie Ranch, Uintah County, Utah (see Plate 5); McKee Springs, Uintah County, Utah (see Figure 14); Sego Canyon, Grand County, Utah (see Plate 6); San Cristobal, Santa Fe County, New Mexico (see Figure 15); Pueble Blanco, Santa Fe County, New Mexico (see Figure 16); Dinwoody site, Fremont County, Wyoming (see Plate 7); and Valley of Fire, Clark County, Nevada (Ritter 1965: 1–4; see our Figure 17).

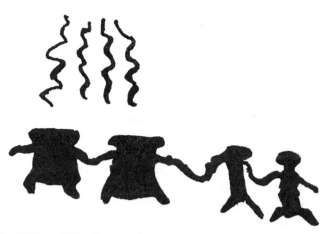

Figure 17.   Valley of Fire State Park, Nevada. These twinlike figures suggest the dichotomy or twin theme of mythology and medicine

Bark Records

Another hypothesis to be considered is that certain petroglyphs and pictographs are associated with the cure or cause of disease. Tanner, during his captivity and life with the Ojibwa (Chippewa) in the latter part of the eighteenth century, observed the use of birchbark pictographs in "medicine hunts," love making, hatred, revenge, and the cure of disease, including the sympathetic magic or "voodoo" black magic causation of illness or injury (James 1956: 179–184, 373–378; Frazer 1966: 55, 70). The Eastern tribes — "Chippewas, Mingos (Iroquois), Shawanos, and Wyandots," and others — frequently used birchbark records and dendroglyphs for similar purposes (Heckwelder 1876: 130). These were also used in the same manner but, to a lesser extent, by tribes of the upper Missouri River regions (Denig 1930: 603–605). Tanner (James 1956: 179) also records the use of a hoop, marked with a snake and the figure of a man, which was worn on the head by those who ministered to the ill.

Landes (1968: 86, 106) mentions that before a patient underwent the final public ceremony of curing, the birchbark scrolls of the *Midewiwin* doctor were produced, tobacco was offered, the scrolls were unrolled, and the doctor pointed out figures scratched on the scrolls and explained them. Various references and pictographs recorded by Hoffman (1891: 143–300) pertain not only to the primitive concept of medicine but to the curing of illness. The *Wabeno* of the *Midewiwin* [Grand Medicine Society] of the Ojibwa furnished hunting medicine and love powders, did magic tricks (e.g. handled fire), and performed medical magic. The *Jessakkid* was a seer or prophet who invoked or removed evil, whereas the *Mide'* averted evil. The *Mashkikikwinin* was an herbalist. Medical specialization apparently was valued, and in these various healing assignments, the separation of the art from the science of medicine can be recognized.

The first image appearing to an Ojibwa youth during a fast became his guardian spirit and a drawing of it was made on birchbark to be carried on a string about his neck. If he later became a *Mide'*, he carried it in his medicine bag (Hoffman 1891: 163). Sacred symbols of the society (Plate III, number 98) included the *migis*, a white shell (especially the cowrie), otter skins (211, 247, Figures 7, 8), sacred drums (Plate III, numbers 22, 23), five evil spirits (Figures 30–34), malignant bear spirits (Plate III, numbers 35, 36, 46, 47), panther spirits (Plate III, numbers 59, 60), a special stone against which the sick were placed during treatment (Plate III, number 108), and medicine lodges (Plate III, numbers 12, 56, 80). Petroglyphs of medicine lodges similar to those of the Ojibwa are found incised on the *Kejimkoojik* rocks in Nova Scotia (Mallery 1893: 424, 425, 549, Figures 717, 718). Snakeskin *Mide'* sacks which contain "life" used to prolong the life of a sick person are portrayed (185, Figure 6, numbers 1, 4, 7). Other medicine sacks are also shown (Figures 7, 8).

Tribes who had similar medicine societies and related pictography were the Menomini, Seneca, Pawnee, and Pueblo (Vogel 1970: 24; Hoffman 1891: 66, 67, 106). Many other tribes had related pictography but seemingly less structured medical societies or fraternities: e.g. Iroquois, Navajo, Potawatami, Winnebago, Sauk, Fox, Omaha, Oto, and most of the Plains Indians (Vogel 1970: 76–84; Fletcher and La Flesche 1911: 509).

The Underground Wildcat

Pictographs used as mnemonic devices in ceremonies of the Medicine Society of the Ojibwa and as cues for certain recitations, poetry, songs, and curing procedures, depicted the wild cat

to whom on account of his vigilance, the medicines for the cure of diseases were committed. The meaning probably is, that to those who have the shrewdness, the watchfulness, and intelligence of the wild cat, is entrusted the knowledge of those powerful remedies, which in the opinion of the Indians, not only control life, and avail to the restoration of health, but give an almost unlimited power over animals and birds (James 1956: 345).

These recorded facts regarding Ojibwa pictography on birchbark in Tanner's day (James 1956) suggest certain inferences and relationships regarding prehistoric or historic petroglyphs and pictographs that are reasonable and should be studied, at least as an exploratory effort.

There is an unmistakable resemblance between the birchbark drawings shown by James (1956: 345, Figures 1, 3) and a pictograph at the Agawa site on the east shore of Lake Superior, Lake Superior Provincial Park (see Figure 18) (Dewdney and Kidd 1962: 80) and a petroglyph at Blackbird Hill in the Omaha Indian Reservation near Macy, Nebraska (Grant 1967: 35; see our Figure 19). The *Piasa* pictograph near Alton, Illinois, first noted by Marquette in 1673, bears a resemblance (Armstrong 1887: 9; see our Figure 20).

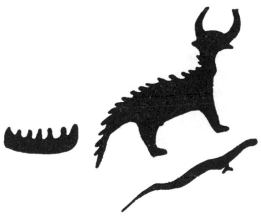

Figure 18. Agawa site, eastern shore of Lake Superior, Michigan. The large figure represents a composite or spirit animal, probably the night panther or underground wildcat of the Ojibwa

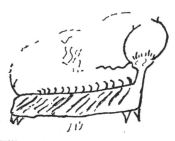

Figure 19. Blackbird Hill, Omaha Indian Reservation, Macy, Nebraska. This petroglyph has similarities to the night panther at the Agawa site and to other depictions on birchbark, wood, and quill work of Indians of the Mississippi or Great Lakes region

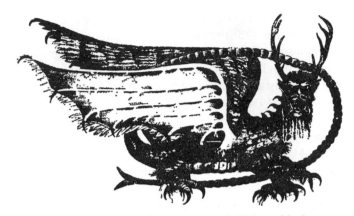

Figure 20.   *Piasa* monster (copied from Armstrong). This mythical monster, which used to be located on cliffs along the Mississippi River near Alton, Illinois, is still periodically repainted near its original location (which was quarried away over 100 years ago)

The Shell Society of the Omaha dealt with magic as well as healing by means of herbs and roots. It is most closely related to similar societies of the Winnebago, Oto, and the Grand Medicine Society of the Ojibwa. In the origin legend of the Shell Society, a mythic animal appeared as a vision in a mist and apparently gave mysterious or magical powers to the society for curing and hunting.

It seemed as big as the great lake. Its skin was covered with hair and was brown like that of the deer. The ridge of its back was serrated with tufts of hair. It had branching horns and hoofs like a deer, and a slender tail with a tuft at the end, which swept toward the sky to the farthest end of the lake (Fletcher and La Flesche 1911: 509, 515, Figure 107).

Schoolcraft (whose wife was an Ojibwa) (1852: 224), Hoffman (1891: 292), and Mallery (1893: 482) show Ojibwa pictographs of "underground wildcats" or "night panthers" which are associated with curing disease.

Similar "night panthers or underwater panthers" on artifacts from the Midwest are shown in Dockstader (1961: Plates 227, 229, 248 [possibly Plate 223, lower line, fifth figure]) on a Menomini woven yarn bag ca. 1850–1890, an Ottowa quilled medicine pouch ca. 1800–1850, a quilled buckskin robe ca. 1750–1788, and a Chippewa ceremonial box lid ca. 1850–1875. A panther with horns is mentioned by Lommel (1967:128) as a motif found in the metal art of the nomads of Siberia and southern Russia in the first millennium B.C., which is most likely connected with shamanistic ideas. Similar mythical creatures are mentioned in studies of Tagarian, Karasuk, and Pazyryk art of southern Siberia from 1300 to 400 B.C. (Okladnikov 1964: 58–66; Rudenko 1970: 108, 110, 261, Plate 142). These findings suggest the possibility that this motif could be intrusive from Siberia. It is interesting to note that a serpent (probably *Unk-ta-he* — see Emerson 1965: 41), the same or similar mythic serpent of the Inuits (Mallery 1893: 476, Figure 662), is painted below the "wildcat" at Agawa (see Figure 21). The tail of

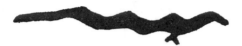

Figure 21.   Agawa site, Lake Superior Provincial Park, Canada. Beneath the night panther (see Figure 18) is found this small, footed serpent, probably *Unk-ta-he*

one of these panthers drawn for Schoolcraft by Chief Little Hill, a Winnebago, ends in a spiral (Schoolcraft 1852: 224, Plate 55, Figure 7).

Buffalo Robe Pictographs

Throughout the Great Plains the primary medium upon which pictography was practiced was animal skin, usually that of the buffalo, deer, bear, or antelope. The birchbark of the Midwest and the rock formations of the Far West were not available. Occasionally bone and other media were used. An interesting "medical record" on a flat stick or board made by the Potawatami is illustrated by Vogel (1970: 76ff.). The winter counts of the Sioux, Blackfeet, and Kiowa include numerous pictographs of medical significance. Those of Lone Dog, Baptiste Good, American Horse, The Flame, The Swan, Cloud Shield, Two Kettle, Mato Sapo, White Cow Killer, White Bull, Swift Dog, Jaw, Blue Thunder, and others of unknown authorship show many such pictographs.

Smallpox, chickenpox, measles, and similar diseases accompanied by skin lesions are represented by spots or circles on human figures. A petroglyph found on the Halleck Ranch in Picture Canyon (also called Long Canyon), Baca County, in southeast Colorado, shows a female figure covered with odd, incomplete circles (see Figure 22). Pecked in front of her mouth is an involute or scroll-like sign. Renaud (1953: 283 ff.) compares this to similar spotted anthropomorphs associated with scroll-like, involute, or spiral signs found in many winter counts of the Sioux (Dakota); these stand for those years when epidemics of small-

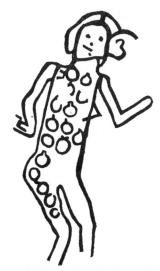

Figure 22.   Picture Canyon (Halleck Ranch), Colorado. This petroglyph with an involute cephalic projection and circular surface markings has been identified with similar figures in the Sioux winter counts as representing smallpox or measles epidemics

pox decimated the Indians (see Renaud 1953: Plate 13; Mallery 1893: Figures 291, 336, 358, 375, 407). These same signs in the winter counts are associated with other diseases, some of which are listed below (Mallery 1893: Figures 281, 355, 383, 407, 410, 417, 430). A possible corollary is an incised anthropomorph found on a kiva wall (room 529) at Awatovi, Arizona (Smith and Ewing 1952: Figure 92a; see our Figure 23). McClintock (1936: 26) records similar anthropomorphs on

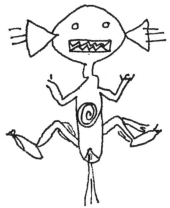

Figure 23.   This curious figure found on the kiva walls at Awatovi, Arizona, portrays an intra-abdominal involute and anal projections. When compared to Sioux winter counts of known interpretation, this figure suggests an abdominal or intestinal ailment such as diarrhea, dysentery, or cholera

robes made by the Blackfeet. Other Sioux pictographs on robes represent various epidemics — whooping cough, consumption (tuberculosis), pneumonia — and other ailments and catastrophes such as hemoptysis, freezing, burns, starvation, drowning, suicide, insanity, hermaphroditism or homosexuality, absence of skin on the penis, broken leg, broken neck, poisoning, dropsy, humpback or Potts disease, and death in childbirth (Mallery 1886: Plates XI, XII, XIX, XXIV, XXXIV, XXXV, XXXVL, XXXVII, XLVI, XLVIII; 1893: Plate XX, Figures 196–198, 203, 231, 233, 304, 335, 340, 403; Praus 1962: 2–10; see our Figures 24, 25, 26, 27).

Figure 24. Sioux winter counts. This figure has been documented as representing an illness characterized by a cough, such as whooping cough or pneumonia

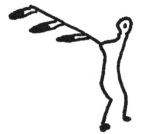

Figure 25. Sioux winter counts. This figure stands for the year a hunchbacked warrior was killed

Figure 26. Sioux winter counts. A broken leg is graphically shown by a primitive artist or shaman

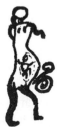

Figure 27. Sioux winter counts. This especially interesting female figure stands for "the year many women died in childbirth." Pregnancy is shown by an enlarged abdomen with a fetus inside, and illness is again indicated as in many other winter count figures by the involute — in this case as an abdominal projection

The pictographic autobiographies and war honors of Sioux chiefs such as Sitting Bull, Howling Wolf, and Making Medicine all abound with pictographic records of wounds or injuries given or received during war and exploits. Wounds are shown on anthropomorphs by splotches of red paint in the appropriate places (Mallery 1886: Plate LI). Those records of Blackfoot chiefs Big Eyes, Running Rabbit, and Mountain Chief are quite similar. A cliff site at Joliet, Carbon County, Montana, resembles these (see Plate 8).

Medicine Tipis

Another medium upon which pictographs of medical importance were painted is the skin covering of the medicine tipis of the Plains Indians, especially the Blackfoot. Other tribes of the upper Missouri River Basin had similar customs (Denig 1930: 605, Plate 74; Spinden 1957: 246–247, Figure 286). These tipis housed the sacred bundles of the tribe and were considered to have supernatural power. Both men and women made vows and invocations to them in time of danger and on behalf of the sick. Paintings of sacred objects, mythical beings, and various animals, including the plumed water serpent, were made on them. The animals were usually highly realistic, often with internal organs and heart lines. However, the more sacred objects were commonly represented by conventionalized symbols (McClintock 1936: 124–134).

Hosts and Homeopathy

Navajo sand paintings are often employed for healing, blessing, and banishing evil influences (Newcomb, et al. 1956: 6; Corlett 1935: 160). Sometimes the intent of Navajo sand painting and associated ceremonial practices is to prevent or cure illness or to be instrumental in training medicine men. The mythology and narratives of the chants mention *Kleetso*, the great snake, magic paintings, medicine, flutes, etc. The practice of sand painting illustrates a principle employed often in primitive medicine — that of transference of the illness or its cause from the patient to an intermediate or secondary host. The illness is then removed from the intermediate host or that host destroyed. In the case of the sand paintings, the illness may be transferred to the painting and then the painting (and the illness with it) cast to the four winds or otherwise destroyed. Medicine men or shamans are often considered adept at

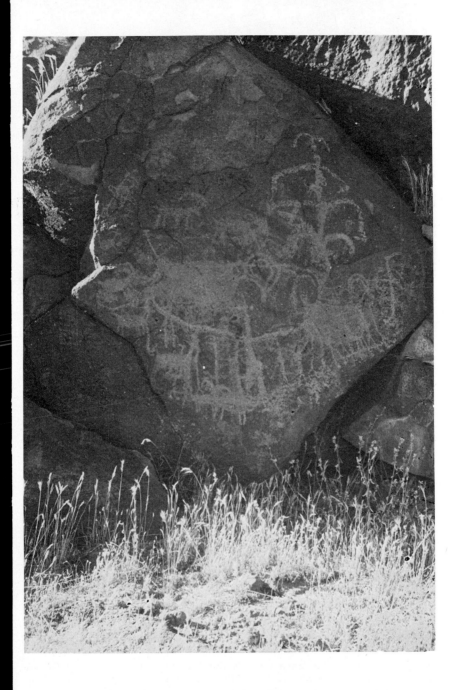

Plate 1. Coso Range, California. Repeated use of this site is evident. Shown are sheep sharing torso, tail, and horns. Additional horns have been added as a cephalic projection. Superimposition is also noted

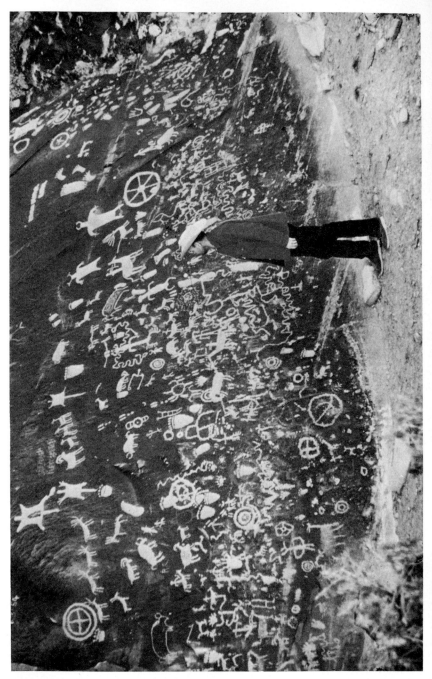

Plate 2. Indian Creek, Canyonlands National Park, Utah. Many characteristics of prehistoric art of the western United States and other areas, and of shamanistic art can be noted in this outstanding panel — superimposition, reuse, retouching, variable patination and age, hunting scenes, consanguinity lines, supernatural anthropomorphs and animals, special cephalic projections, symbolism, special enclosures, site lines, etc.

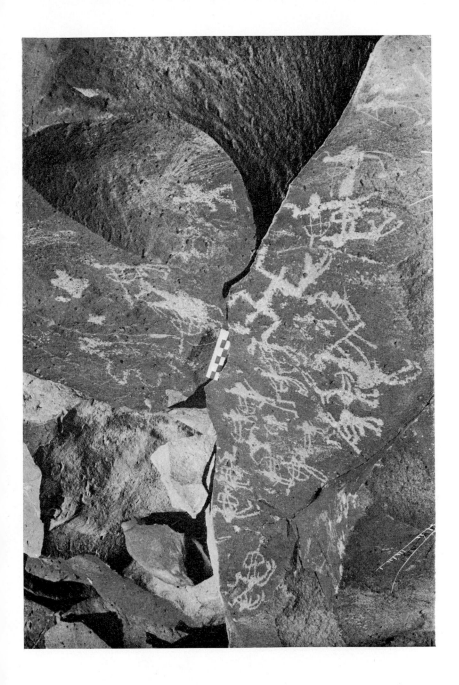

Plate 3. Cienagillos, New Mexico. *Kokopelli* is shown twenty-six times in this panel — most often as a hunter with bow and arrow

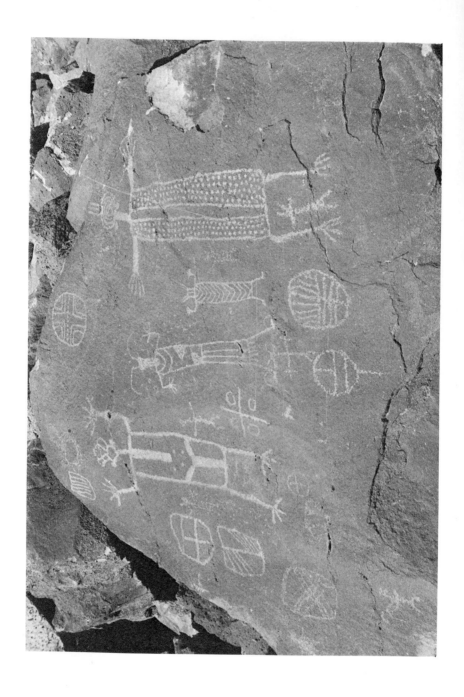

Plate 4. Little Petroglyph Canyon, Coso Range, California. Elaborate anthropomorphs with various cephalic projections are frequently found in this mountain range

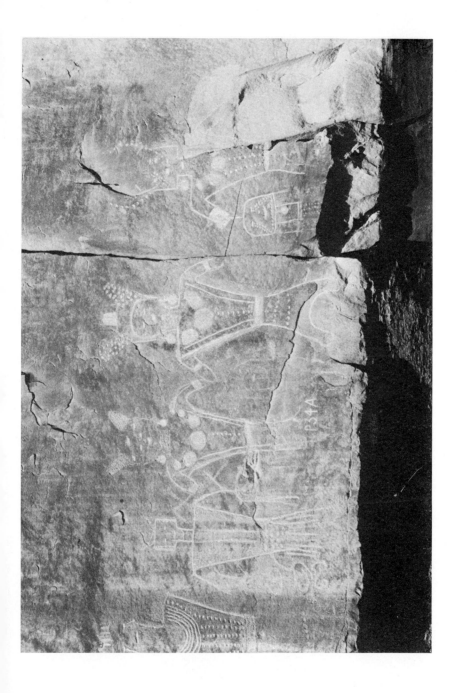

Plate 5. McConkie Ranch, near Vernal, Utah. Several panels of elaborate anthropomorphs (Fremont style) are found on this ranch

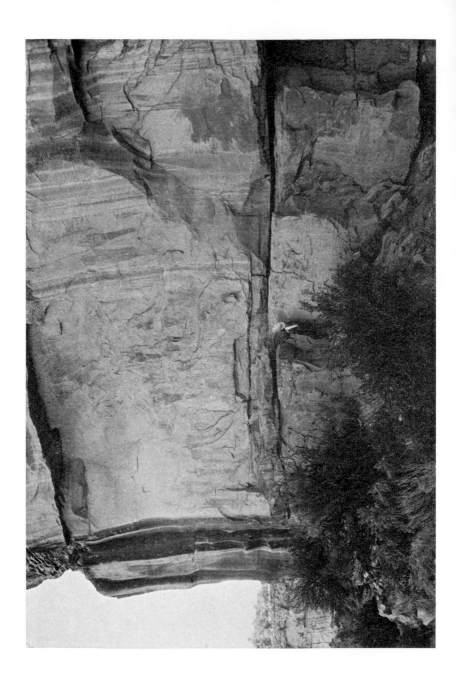

Plate 6. Large, limbless anthropomorphs such as these in Sego Canyon are frequently found in Utah

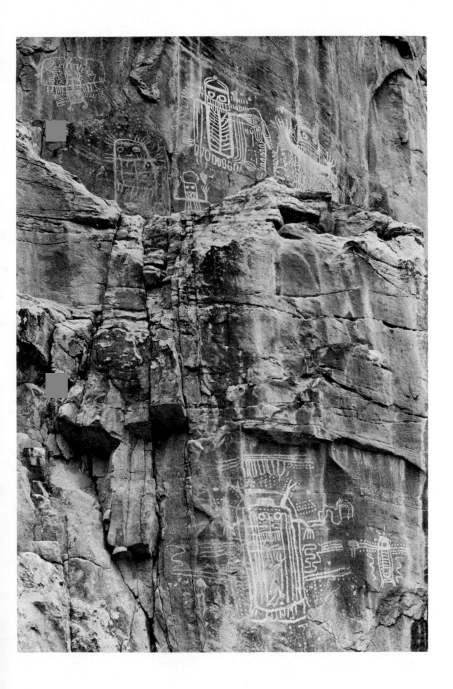

Plate 7. Dinwoody site, eastern Wyoming. These odd figures may represent supernatural beings or animals and resemble X-ray style

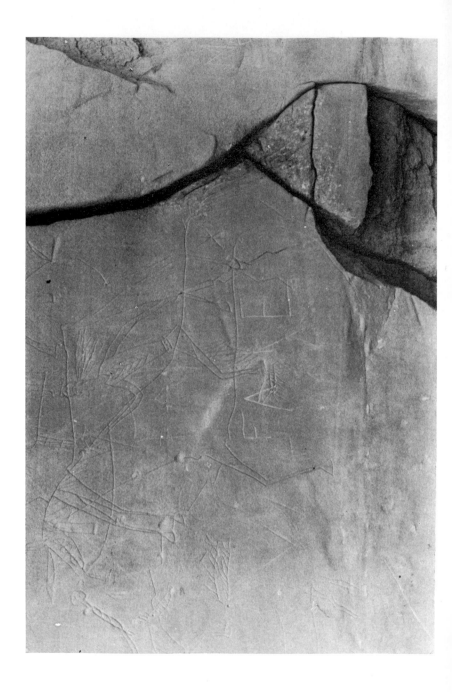

Plate 8. Joliet, Montana. The style and figures at this site resemble closely the eighteenth- and nineteenth-century pictography of the Plains Indians on robes and other media. (See also Plate 12)

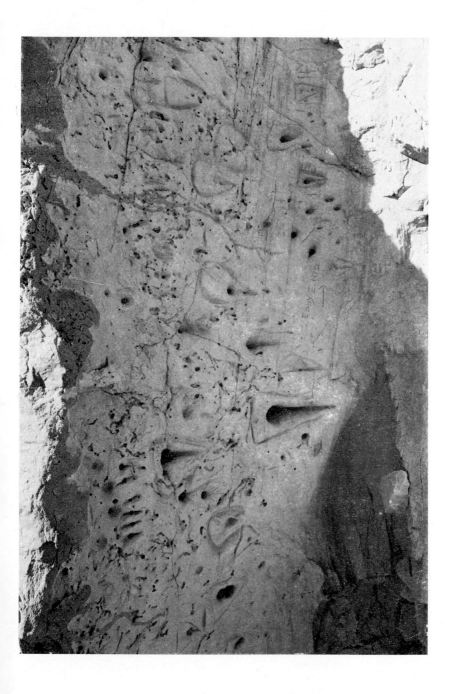

Plate 9. Mother Rock, on the southwest face of sacred Corn Mountain, near Zuni, New Mexico, is covered with genital signs made by pregnant Zuñi women

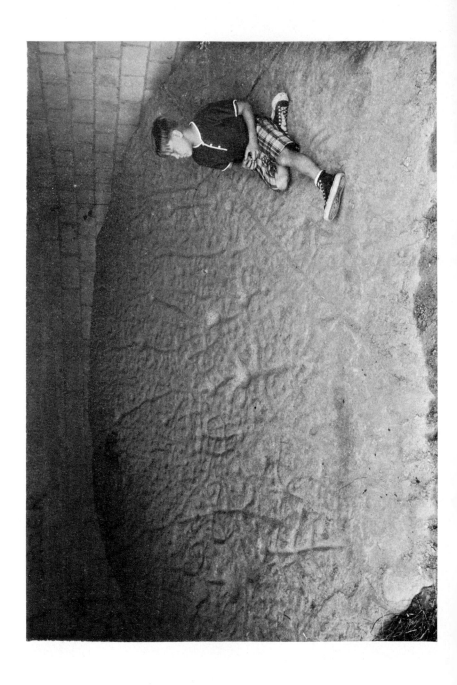

Plate 10.   Judaculla Rock, North Carolina. Cupules of various sizes are noted on this monumental boulder

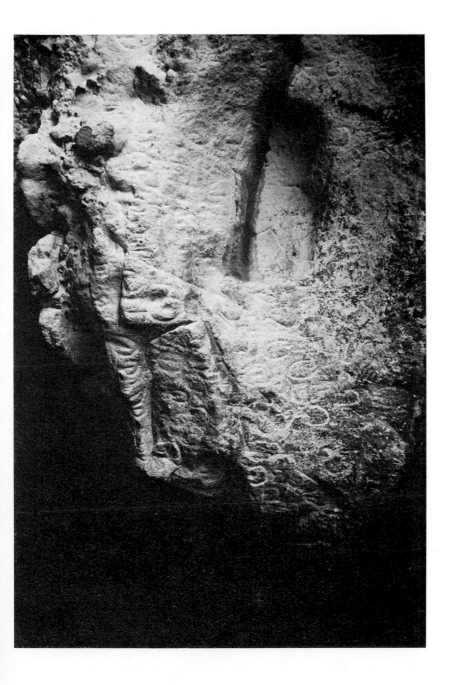

Plate 11. San Borjitas Cave, Baja Sur, Mexico. Genital signs such as these are common throughout western North America and adjacent areas

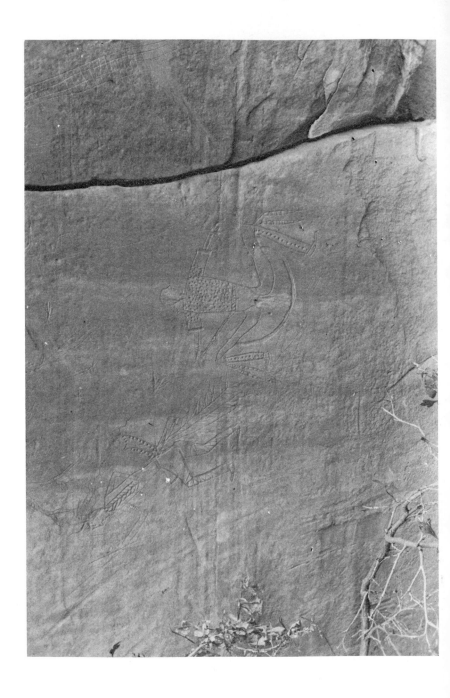

Plate 12. Joliet, Montana. Carved or etched in the nineteenth-century Plains Indian art style are these male and female figures. The latter, in the receptive female position, has the genitalia shown as an ovoid hole or irregular cupule

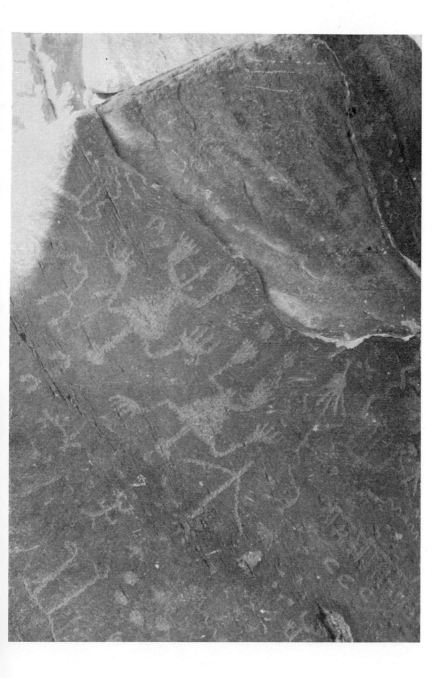

Plate 13.   Newspaper Rock, Petrified Forest National Monument, Arizona. Both male and female genital portrayals are shown

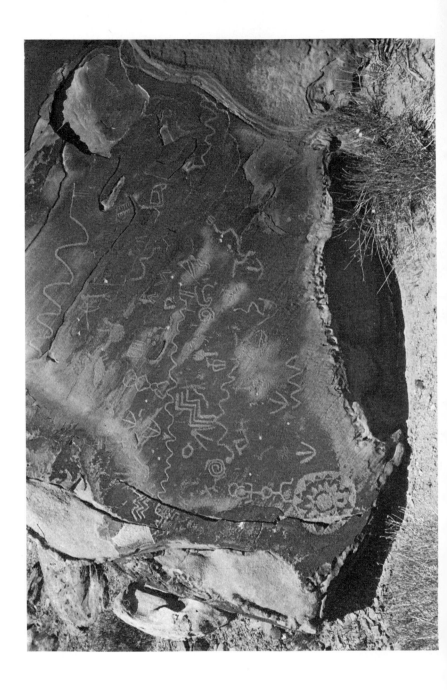

Plate 14.   Across from Ticabaa, Glen Canyon, Utah. *Kokopelli* in several poses is noted on this panel — three times with the flute, once with bow and arrow. Other associations are snakes or wavy lines and spirals

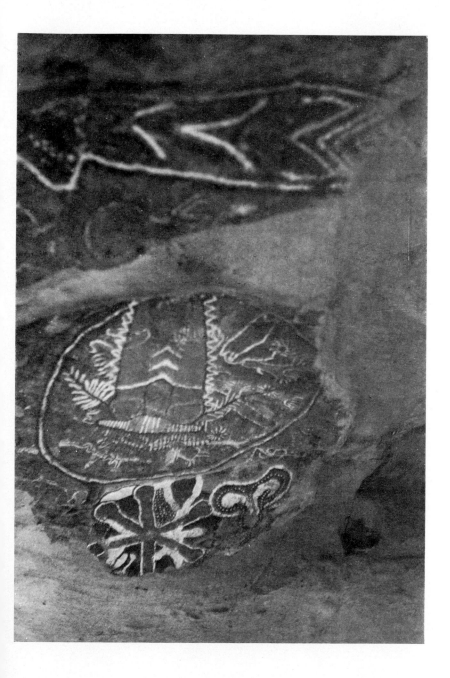

Plate 15. Pleito Creek, California. Beautiful polychrome paintings, probably of Chumash origin, are found in a small rockshelter

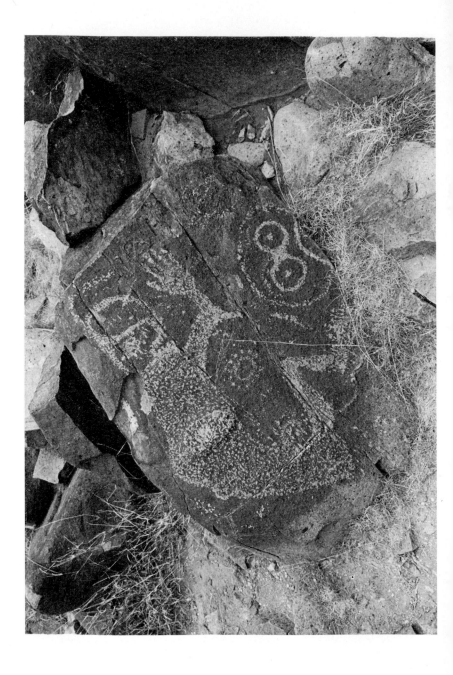

Plate 16. Three Rivers, New Mexico. *Kokopelli* is sometimes shown as insect-like, in this case with a head like a grasshopper. Of unusual interest is the incorporation of a natural rock bulge in his humpback

healing themselves and will sometimes act as the intermediate host, healing themselves and the patients through homeopathic magic (Frazer 1966: 78, 83; Lommel 1967: 53).

Healing Magic of Stone

Stones were sometimes used in this intermediate host capacity or in other ways of treating illness in addition to serving as a surface for pictographs or petroglyphs. They were rubbed to promote healing (Frazer 1966: 85) and were used as healing rests for the sick (Hoffman 1891: Plate III, Figure 108; Mallery 1893: 244; Maui Historical Society 1964: 11) like the royal birthstones used by the Hawaiian parturients (e.g. *Holo-Holo-Ku Heiau*, Kauai).

Hoffman also found that the Ojibwa used magic stones for healing (1891: 253). Vogel (1970: 76ff.) includes decorated rocks and their cases used by the Crow in healing the sick. At Kuaua, New Mexico, in Kiva III, a medicine rock is painted on the wall (Dutton 1963: 75, Figure 88). Colombian Indians [Aurohaucas] and the Inca transferred the sin causing illness to stones or large rocks, then placed them in the sun to drive away the sin or illness (Corlett 1935: 196, 227). The medicine man of the eastern Eskimo summons spirits by selecting a special grinding stone and rubbing it against the flat surface of a cliff or boulder (Corlett 1935: 87). The Cherokee had a sacred stone drum used in their dances and ceremonies. They buried it when conquest by the Delaware was imminent and attributed their subsequent misfortunes, including a smallpox epidemic, to its loss (Mooney 1900: 397, 503).

Fertility Rocks

Conception Rock and several other close locations near Ukiah, California, were used by the Pomo Indian women to promote and protect pregnancy. Those desiring pregnancy sat on this boulder and swallowed minute portions scraped from it. The surface is covered with depressions and grooves suggestive of the generative organs (Curtis 1924: 66, also see Plate 9).

Gifford and Kroeber (1937: 186) describe two baby-shaped rocks visited secretly by a Pomo couple wanting offspring. Both would run uphill to them, the woman would scratch a line on one of the rocks, and they would copulate there. At a similar rock in Pomo territory a husband and wife, accompanied by the chief, would mark it with steatite used like chalk — "V" for a desired male child, "X" for a female —

and then they would lie on the design. Later the chief came to them, they arose, and he pecked the design they had marked on the rock. In 1972 a young Pomo obstetrical patient treated by the senior author claimed she had heard her elders discuss similar fertility rocks in the region of Clear Lake, California.

Mother Rock, on the west side of Corn Mountain, Zuni, New Mexico, is covered with cupules and vulviforms (Stevenson 1904: Plate XII; see Plate 9). Pregnant Zuñi women, especially those who have been unfortunate with previous babies, visit shrines at the base of the rock pillars at this site. Their husbands and a "priest" accompany them. They deposit prayer sticks and the women scrape a bit of dust from the rock and swallow it, from one side if they desire a boy, from the other if they desire a girl (Bunzel 1932: 536). Because of the great similarity between these customs of the Pomo of California and the Zuñi of New Mexico, the possibility arises that the customs may have been more widespread in western North America.

Many sites scattered throughout western North America are also thought to be fertility rocks, sometimes associated with human fertility, but also with animal or crop fertility. In the latter capacity they are often used in sun worship or for rain production. Cup rocks, cup and groove rocks, genital symbolism (especially female), and occasionally coital scenes are found among the symbolism on fertility rocks. The association of the cup or pit and groove style with human fertility is best documented in California through the ethnographic data regarding the Pomo and through the work of Payen (1959: 80; 1968: 37), who has found a female anthropomorphic figure in the Sierra Nevada at Hawley Lake with the sexual parts represented in cupule form.

In New Mexico cup rocks were used (and manufactured by the custom of striking a boulder at daybreak) to attract the attention of the sun god (Renaud 1938: 20). The symbol on the altar at Sun Temple, Mesa Verde, Colorado, is a large shallow cupule with rays about it. Rain Rock at Fort Jones, Siskiyou County, northern California, is covered with cupules made when local aborigines pounded it to bring rain for crops. They buried it after a flood. Another flood occurred after it was dug up by highway engineers in 1955 and local Klamath Indians attributed the flood to its excavation (*Understanding* 1962: 11).

Cup rocks (with or without other petroglyphs or grooves) are most numerous in northern California, although they are very widespread throughout the world, including other areas of North America (Rau 1881: 9, 41; Payen 1968: 33). In Nevada a typical and probably very old one (Heizer and Baumhoff 1962: 234) is found at the Grimes site

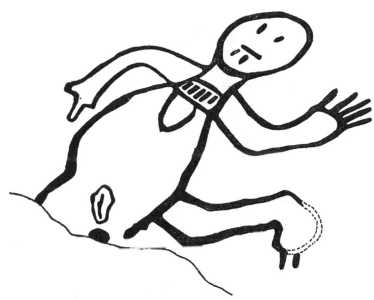

Figure 28.   Hornby Island, British Columbia, Canada. A female genital representation, usually associated with fertility or increase magic, may be shown in anatomical position, alone, or tagged on various animals

near Fallon, Churchill County, Nevada. A particularly good example is Judaculla Rock near Laport, Jackson County, North Carolina (see Plate 10). Davis (1961: 236) also mentions vulviform types which are associated with Diegueño girls' initiation ceremonies. She also states that during fertility rites aboriginal males are reported to have simulated coitus in some of the cup or pit types (Davis, personal communication).

Vulviforms (inverted or noninverted "horseshoes," "phi signs," parenthesized grooves, contoured grooves, etc.) are also widespread: e.g. Hornby Island, British Columbia, Canada (Gjessing 1958: 27; see our Figure 28); San Borjitas Cave, Coyote Bay, Cueva de las Mujeres, Baja California (see Plate 11); Track Rock Gap, Union County, Georgia (see Figure 29); Hickinson Summit, Lander County, Nevada (see Figure 30); Chalfant, Inyo County, California (see Figure 31); and Trapper Creek, Big Horn County, Wyoming (see Figure 32). Some are merely grooves, some show labia and the genital cleft, some are sculptured or in bas relief; some show pubic hair, perhaps the clitoris, and other features of perineal anatomy. The magic shell fertility symbol among the bark records of the *Bungi Midewiwin* Society (Cadzow 1926: 123–130; see our Figure 33) resembles some of these petroglyphs. (For an interesting European comparison, see Graziosi 1960: Plate 291.)

Evidence that these forms (from a mere cup or pit to more elaborate

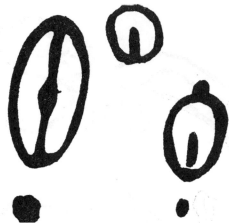

Figure 29.   Track Rock, Georgia. Many vulviforms, as well as human or animal tracks, occur here

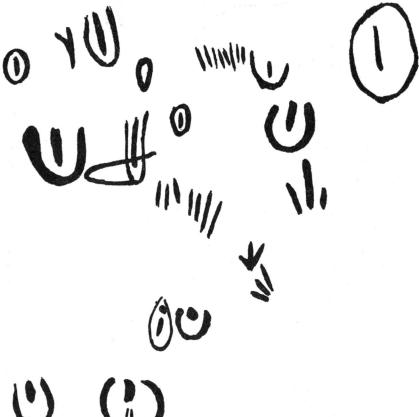

Figure 30.   Hickinson Summit, Nevada. Many vulviforms are found along this mountain pass

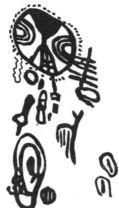

Figure 31.   Chalfant petroglyphs, California. Not far from Bishop many vulviforms can be found at several sites, including this one

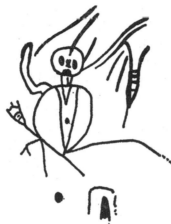

Figure 32.   Trapper Creek, Wyoming. Vulviforms and deep cupules, some of which appear to be almost tubes, are cut into the soft, red sandstone cliffs here

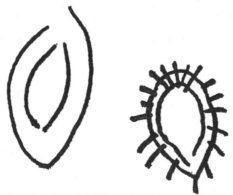

Figure 33.   Bark records, *Bungi Midewiwin* Society. The magic shell (cowrie) fertility symbol is diagramed

depictions) actually do represent the female pudenda can be inferred from a number of female anthropomorphs with their genitalia so shown. Some may be North American examples of the "hocker" or "receptive female" motif described by Covarrubias (1954: 34), or analogs of the vulviforms of Venuses of paleolithic mobiliary art of Europe (Graziosi 1960: Plates 1–12, 82, 150–153) or on cave walls (Graziosi 1960: Plates 163, 257, 258; Robert and Nougier 1961–1962: Slides 16/10, 16/11; Breuil 1952: Figures 319, 320; Leroi-Gourhan 1968: 113, 123, 244, 406, 410, 513, 517, 520, Figures 7, 52, 53, 249–251, 254, 501, 502). Other examples in western North America in which these various genital symbols are anatomically located on the anthropomorph are found on Hornby Island, British Columbia, Canada (Gjessing 1958: 271; see Figure 28); Joliet, Carbon County, Montana (see Plate 12); Big Horn River, Big Horn County, Wyoming (see Figure 34); White Mountain, Sweetwater County, Wyoming (see Figure 35); Petrified Forest National Monument, Apache County, Arizona (see Plate 13); El Morro, Valencia County, New Mexico (see Figure 36); Kenton, Cimarron County, Oklahoma (see Figure 37); and Sierra County, California (Payen 1968: Figure 4). Mammae are prominent on several female figures, such as those of Lake Canyon, San Juan County, Utah, and Carrizo Canyon, San Juan County, New Mexico, and the Halleck Ranch petroglyph of "smallpox woman" (see Figure 22).

Male anthropomorphs with prominent genitalia are found frequently and may be associated with fertility or virility, but the association is harder to prove (Renaud 1953: 289; Malouf 1961: 3). Examples from the Southwest are discussed below.

A few coital scenes probably associated with fertility rites are noted at Owl Springs, Monument Valley, San Juan County, Ariz. (see Figure 38), and Hueco Tanks, El Paso County, Texas (see Figure 39). At the former site, a birth or delivery scene is also found (see Figure 40). Animal (deer or elk) coitus is graphically portrayed at Oak Canyon, Utah (see Figure 41).

In the Northwest, Gunn (1966: front cover) illustrates a totem pole upon which Medicine Man or Shaman and Sea Dog are carved. The former helps man overcome disease and evil spirits. Sea Dog symbolized the evolution or origin of life from the sea to land forms; she is also a symbol of fertility (Gunn 1966: cover caption). A petroglyph probably representing this mythical goddess of life and fertility is found pecked on a seaside boulder at Cape Alava (within Olympic National Park, Washington). She faces the vast expanse of the Pacific Ocean, her mythical domain and origin (see Figure 42).

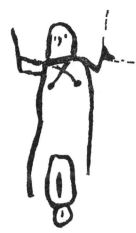

Figure 34. Big Horn River, Wyoming. The female genitalia are schematically portrayed here in a vulviform likeness

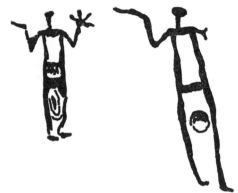

Figure 35. White Mountain, Wyoming. Sandstone cliff carvings at this site show the female genitalia as both a vulviform and a cupule

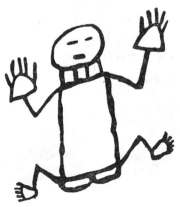

Figure 36. El Morro National Monument, New Mexico. The receptive female or "hocker" type appears at this site and several others (Figures 37, 38 and Plate 12)

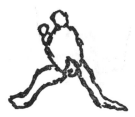

Figure 37.   Kenton, Oklahoma. Another receptive female figure is shown with a small cupule or depression

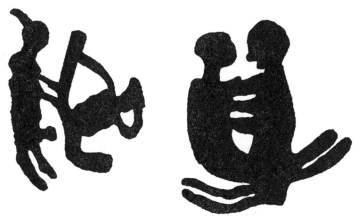

Figure 38.   Owl Springs, Monument Valley, Arizona. Coital scenes are shown as petroglyphs

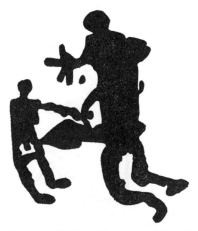

Figure 39.   Hueco Tanks, near El Paso, Texas. A white pictograph coital scene is found in a rockshelter

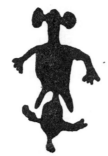

Figure 40. Owl Springs, Monument Valley, Arizona. Near the coital scenes shown in Figure 38, this delivery scene is recorded. If the parturient's hairdress conforms to modern Hopi custom, she was unmarried

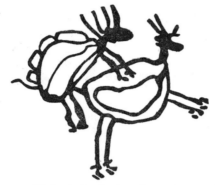

Figure 41. Oak Canyon, Utah. Animal coitus is rarely recorded, as here

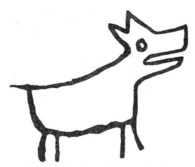

Figure 42. Cape Alava, Olympic National Park, Washington. This doglike quadruped, pecked on a rock surface facing the sea, may be the mythical god Sea Dog of the local Northwest Coast tribes

Fertility Gods

Male fertility gods of the Pueblo Indians can be identified in rock art and on kiva walls of the Southwest (Fewkes 1903: 67, Plate VII; Colton 1949: 20, 35; Smith and Ewing 1952: 63, 299; Sims 1950: 5, Plates IV, V, XIV). Near Oraibi as modern white pictographs (circa 1962) and at San Cristobal as prehistoric petroglyphs, the chief kachina or germ god and giver of life, *Ahola* [*Ahul, Aholi, Alosaka, Alosoka, Muiyinwu*; or is it *Kokopelli?*] can be found (see Figures 43, 44). Smith and Ewing (1952: 97, 304) report this particular god in the Puebloan pantheon and in kiva murals at Awatovi. This germ god and chief kachina is important enough so that he appears in six of the regular

Figure 43. Near Oraibi, Arizona, these modern (circa 1962) white pictographs probably represent *Ahola*, the Hopi germ god, who is usually shown with an up-turned nose. Perhaps one is his female counterpart and their portrayal memorializes a love tryst between Tico and Liz. *Kokopelli* and *Kokopelli Mana* are the only other Pueblo gods or kachinas shown with upturned noses, and their portrayal would also have similar implications

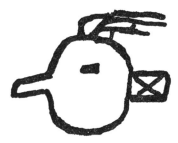

Figure 44. San Cristobal, New Mexico. This may be a portrait of *Ahola*, but it is questionable

Hopi ceremonials, including the Winter Solace, Water Serpent, and Flute ceremonies, as well as the Snake Dance. These ceremonies are concerned with crop fertility, but a concern for human fertility is also inferred because his turned-up nose is said to represent an erect phallus according to modern Hopi informants. Colton (1949: 20, 35) notes that both *Ahola* and *Kokopelli* kachinas may be shown with an upturned nose.

Kokopelli

Another Pueblo kachina or god associated with fertility of man, animals, and crops, who is also considered a powerful medicine man, shaman, healer, seducer of young girls, and hunter, is *Kokopelli* (Fewkes 1903: 86, Plate XXV; Renaud 1948: 25–40; Schaafsma 1963: 35). He (or his counterpart) is a participant in modern Hopi, Zuñi, and other Pueblo ceremonies: e.g. the Blue Flute and Drab Flute Fraternity rituals. During these ceremonies his flute is played over springs and during the preparation of certain magical medicines (Renaud 1948: 27). He is related to a female counterpart, *Kokopelli Mana,* who carries food in corn husks (Renaud 1948: 36; Smith and Ewing 1952: 299). His image among petroglyphs is similar to the Hopi kachina portrayals. *Kokopelli* or his analog can be traced back to the eleventh century on pottery (Grant 1967: 60; Gladwin, et al. 1965: 227, Plates CLVIII, CLXVII; Lambert 1967: 398; Renaud 1948: 33). His provenience can be identified as far north as Utah (see Plate 14), and as far south as Costa Rica (see our Figure 45; Mason 1945: Plate 43F), possibly even to the Andes of South America (Smith and Ewing 1952: 302; Sangines 1969: 310, 357). Among petroglyphs and pictographs he is most often depicted in Arizona, New Mexico, and Utah. He is portrayed more at the Cienagillos site, Santa Fe County, New Mexico, than at any other

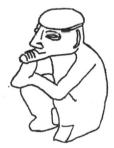

Figure 45.   Stone figurine from Costa Rica. This effigy resembles *Kokopelli* because of his pose, humped-back profile, flute, and crude genital reproduction

location, in many poses and with various associations (Renaud 1938: 55). His humpback, flute, plumed headdress, and ithyphallacism assure his identification. There is speculation that his hump or gibbous in some instances may not be kyphosis, or Potts disease, but a bag to carry gifts for maidens whom he seduces. He is shown dancing, playing the flute, hunting sheep, deer, or mountain lions, sometimes on his back in a recumbent pose. Sometimes he is found in association with water

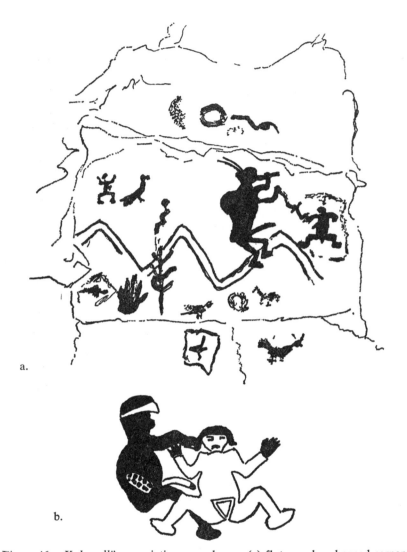

a.

b.

Figure 46. *Kokopelli's* associations are shown: (a) flute, snakes, horned serpent, birds, possible frogs, and wavy lines at Cienagillos, New Mexico; (b) a woman, either *Kokopelli Mana* or a maiden to be seduced, painted at Awatovi (room 529), Arizona

or rainfall symbols such as the cloud, rain, lightning, or netted gourds. Snakes (including the rattlesnake and plumed serpent [*Awanyu, Palulukon, Kleetso, Kolowisi*]), birds, lizards, frogs, insects, and other animals or objects which may represent fecundity, fertility, rain, or liaison with the underworld or heavens are often pecked nearby (see Figure 46).

He has been found on pottery from Aztec Ruin, Chaco Canyon, the

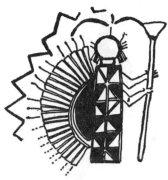

Figure 47.   Museum of Navajo Ceremonial Art, New Mexico. The Navajo *yei*, *Beganaskiddy*, now displayed in front of the museum, came from Delgadito Canyon

Great Kiva Ruins near Zuni, Hohokam sites in southeast Arizona, and sites in Chihuahua, Mexico (Renaud 1948: 33). His most common accouterment is the flute. Although there may be no relationship, among Indians of the southeastern part of the United States, Jones (1873: 29) noted that the medicine man was known to suck the painful area of a patient with a "kind of shepherd's flute." Perhaps the same or at least a closely related god or *yei* of the Navajo is the hunchbacked anthropomorph, sometimes shown with a headdress, who carries seeds in his feathered hump (Schaafsma 1965: 6, 9, 12; 1966: 14, 15; Newcomb, et al. 1956: 40, Figure 78). This *yei* is associated with animal tracks and rain cloud and corn symbols, and may carry a wand or weapon (see Figure 47).

Other Medicine Men of the Pueblo Pantheon

Among the Puebloans of the Southwest there are several other gods or societies whose major domain may or may not be medicine but who do have a medical role. Often a medicine society may recruit members from those who are cured. The clown societies of the Keres pueblos (the *Koshare*) and of the Tewa (the *Kossa*) are able to cure certain diseases, and the society membership is increased by those whom they cure (Fergusson 1957: 31, 45). The curing societies of the Keresans are similarly structured (Fox 1967: 261). *Koshare* can be identified on kiva paintings at Acoma made prior to curing ceremonies and possibly among cliff paintings and carvings southeast of this pueblo (L. White 1932: 113, 131, Plate II). A carved painting of *KoBictaiya*, a kachina who treats the ill and gives strength, is found at another cliff site near Acoma (L. White 1932: 86, 131, Plate 10). A stone figurine of *KoBic-*

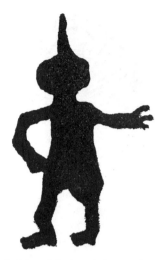

Figure 48.   San Cristobal, New Mexico. The conical headgear of this figure tends to identify him as a *Koshare*, a clown who also has a healing role

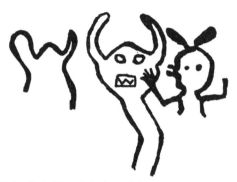

Figure 49.   San Cristobal, New Mexico. Other types of clowns with secondary medical or healing functions are the Mudheads who also cavort with the horned serpent *Palulukon Awanyu*. The figures here may portray these two

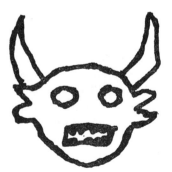

Figure 50.   San Cristobal, New Mexico. Another *Sayathlia* is found at this pueblo (see also Figure 16)

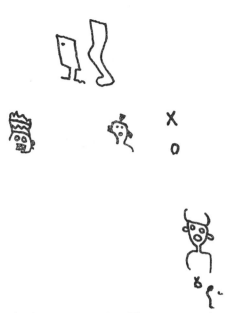

Figure 51.   Comanche Gap, New Mexico. The two top anthropomorphs have not been identified, but the lower one resembles *Tunwup* who has a healing role and represents a prehistoric shaman

taiya is used in the curing ceremony of the Flint Society of the Cochiti (and other Keresans). It is believed that the spirit of this kachina invests the figurine and aids in healing (Fox 1967: 267).

Petroglyphs of *Koshare* or his archetype are also found at San Cristobal, New Mexico (Sims 1950: Plate VII; see our Figure 48). The Mudhead (*Koyemshi*) and Galaxy (*Newewe*) kachinas of the Zuñi are also clowns. Possible Mudheads struggling with *Palululkon*, the feathered serpent, are also portrayed at San Cristobal and Comanche Gap, New Mexico (Sims 1950: 7, Plate VIII; see our Figure 49).

Fergusson (1957: 74, 128) mentions a Hopi god, *Tunwup*, the flogger kachina, who during the *Powamu* [bean planting ceremony] may whip adults and who is thought to have healing properties. She also states that the Zuñi Wood Fraternity sword swallowers have medicine especially good for sore throats, and that they use a sand painting during their ceremonies. A cured patient may request admission to this fraternity. *Sayathlia* and *Hututu* who, like *Tunwup*, have healing roles can be tenuously identified at San Cristobal (Sims 1950: 6, Plate V); possibly at Comanche Gap, Pueblo Blanco, New Mexico; Hueco Tanks; Texas (Kirkland 1940: 19, 23); and other sites in the Southwest (see Figures 50, 51).

No doubt other personages of medical import in the pantheon of Puebloan cultures will eventually be identified among rock art anthropomorphs. At present the subject is somewhat confusing, for each pueblo and language group have pictorial and nomenclatural variations for essentially the same kachina. Color clues are absent in petroglyphs. Portrayals of kachinas are sometimes sketchy, not only in rock pictographs but on wall art, pottery, textiles, and sand paintings used for such depictions. This makes specific identification difficult.

Navajo Medicine on Sand and Rock

Among the art media of the Navajo, sand paintings are the most fruitful and appropriate in the study of medical pictography. They portray many shamanistic devices such as the heart line, consanguinity lines, celestial and subterranean associations, various projections, intermediaries, continuity lines, and in themselves are special enclosures. The petroglyphs and pictographs of their rock art sometimes show a relationship to the sand paintings in style, color, and content. Many medicine men or shamans, animals gifted in curing, phytomorphs representing medicinal plants, symbols of healing (e.g. the fertility symbol of holy corn, snakes, and the flute), and magic forces (swastika, spiral, rainbow, celestial bodies, prayer sticks, wands, weapons, etc.) are shown in their sand paintings and are mentioned in the chants and mythology recited during their manufacture and use. In many respects these sand paintings are akin to the birchbark records of the Ojibwa medicine societies — both were used in healing patients, preserving the secrets and methods of healing, and training initiates; both were considered sacred mnemonic devices, even using the special pictographic devices of the heart line and spirit line (e.g. see sand paintings associated with the Male Shooting and Creation Chants).

In a description of the Night Way Chant (*Tleji* or *Yehbechai* Myth) by Wheelwright (1938: 7–11), pictographs at White House in Canyon de Chelly are mentioned as a control of the fortune of the tribe — if certain white pictographs in a cave nearby showed plainly, all would be well with the people, if dim, things would go wrong. Healing is related to the untying of knotted cords, sweating, offerings, dancing, sand paintings, masks, special robes, and medicinal plants. Diseases are represented by insects such as locusts and grasshoppers. Graphic portrayal of some of these contents occur in the sand paintings associated with the chant and myth and are recorded on slides by the Museum of

Navajo Ceremonial Art at Santa Fe, New Mexico (see slide series 1, numbers 1–5).

The Wind Chant and associated sand paintings are used to cure mental illness and snakebite, possibly blindness and paralysis. At least a score of paintings which cure by magic are mentioned in this myth. Other items and practices used in this healing ceremony are holy plants, magic symbols (snakes, sun, moon, stars, lightning, a white cross, and wind figures), corn meal, an emetic, offerings of yucca, whirling sticks, prayer plumes, cloth paintings, infusions of herbs, pellets of medicine, pollen, the use of bathing, body pressure, body and face painting, the untying of knots, massage, singing, and the setting of fires. Medicine men, shamans, or healing gods include *Kleetso* (the great snake) Wind, the Thunder People, Blue Wind, the Star People, Coyote, a bald-headed Snake Man, and Bear Medicine Man. The hero, who is also often a trial patient in this myth, overcomes, is cured by, and learns from these various practitioners and his own healing. He finally becomes a full-fledged medicine man, named *Nil-Nez-tahni*, capable of not only healing patients but of teaching others (Wheelwright 1946: 1–5; see Museum of Navajo Ceremonial Art, slide series 4, numbers 1–5).

The Feather Chant and its sand paintings are used to cure coughing. The gods encountered by the hero-initiate are the Bat, the Wind People, and *Kleetso*. Later he becomes a medicine man and goes to live near Zuni (Wheelwright 1946: 11–13; see Museum of Navajo Ceremonial Art, slide series 4, numbers 6–10).

The boy hero, *Klaha*, of the Red Ant Myth, encounters many obstacles and gods which test him and give him gifts helpful against danger and sickness. He meets Red Ant, *Kleetso*, Water Monster, Lightning, Horned Toad, Buzzard, Crow, Hawk, Bee, Wasp, and Locust. He later uses a piece of Locust and rolling weeds as medicines. Bear adopts him after *Klaha* overpowers him with divine arrows; he lives with Eagles, one of whom he marries and by whom he has a son. He is aided by Spider Woman. During one episode he is cured by being passed through hoops and another time he is brought back to life (after being crushed) by Lion, Wolf, Wildcat, and Badger (Wheelwright 1958: 1–11; see Museum of Navajo Ceremonial Art, slide series 7, numbers 1–5).

Midwifery, snakebite, toothache, antiwitchcraft, and the treatment of those struck by lightning are documented in the Male Shooting Chant. Twins born of Changing Woman and fathered by Sun and Waterfall, *Dinneh Deginneh* (a hero), Gopher, Bear, *Kleetso*, *Iknee* [Lightning],

Gila Monster, the Corn People, and the Buffalo People are figures in the myth and the sand paintings. Heart or life lines appear in some of the animals. Various medicines are mentioned, including the planting of some in a lake by *Dinneh Deginneh* and the Buffalo People (Wheelwright 1958: 15–23; see Museum of Navajo Ceremonial Art, slide series 7, numbers 6–10).

The hero of the Eagle-Catching Myth produces magic by playing a flute over a medicine bundle; later he plays four different flutes over the grinding of corn. Holy corn symbols are used to signify fertility and new life. Aside from the Eagle, two other birds contribute medicine — Owl gave medicine to the hero-medicine man, and Swallow told him what herbs to use in curing Monster Slayer. In the ceremony associated with this myth and sand painting, a medicine hogan is mentioned. A hint as to one of the main uses of the myth is suggested by the direction that beeswax was good medicine to take the pain out of wounds from eagles' claws (Wheelwright 1962: 2–9; see Museum of Navajo Ceremonial Art, slide series 3, numbers 1–5).

The Bead Myth and its associated sand paintings are used by the Navajo to treat patients for lameness. In the myth chanted during the ceremony, another boy hero becomes an important medicine man named Eagle Boy (*Keeneekee — Doneekee*). He later makes his brother a medicine man, then goes up to the sky and throws down medicine herbs. During Eagle Boy's transformation into a medicine man, offerings, dances, red and black medicines, plumed prayer sticks, and sand paintings are utilized. In addition, he is given a special ceremony and sand paintings of curative value by Spider Man (Wheelwright 1962: 11–15; see Museum of Navajo Ceremonial Art, slide series 3, numbers 6–10).

Oheedli [Water Coming Together] at the junction of the Pine and San Juan Rivers (also the border between San Juan and Rio Arriba counties, New Mexico), is a sacred spot to the Navajo. A rock wall pictographic panel representing the Twin War Gods, possibly related to the Twins of the Male Shooting Chant sand paintings, occurs here. Also represented in the pictographs are numerous *yei* with kilts, possible dance paddles and ceremonial swords, birds, deer, horses, men on horseback, and bison with arrows shot into them. Some of the bison are shown with the life line. Until recently the Navajo met here during dry years to perform ceremonies, including chanting (Dittert, et al. 1961: 230–242, Figures 71, 73; Schaafsma 1963: 60).

In discussing interpretations of Navajo rock art, Schaafsma (1963: 60) states, "The great majority of Navajo pictographs have religious or supernatural and mythical subject matter which shows Pueblo influence in form and style as well as a great likeness to modern Navajo religious art." She compares the bison impaled with feathered medicine wands found in a panel near *Oheedli* with those found in the Shooting Chant sand painting and notes that such ceremonies were held when parties were sent to hunt bison. She also states that bison became an important symbol to the Navajo and that they had ritual associations. Much bison material is used in other Navajo ceremonies. The fact that this particular rock art site was used as a shrine makes it probable that the bison at this site have ceremonial significance and were considered magic. Their use here and in sand paintings suggests that this significance involves not only sympathetic magic of the hunt or medicine hunts, but medical magic as well.

Schaafsma (1963: 60, Plate II) identifies at least one more *yei* (other than the Twin War Gods) found in both sand paintings and rock art. *Tobadsistsini* [Born-For-Water] of the Night Way and the Shooting Chants compares favorably with a pictograph in a panel of several *yei* located at the mouth of Todosio Canyon, San Juan County, New Mexico. This *yei* also closely resembles the Pueblo deity *Ahul*. Another *yei* in this panel is equivocally identified as *Hastyehogan* [the House God] perhaps paired (as in myths, ceremonies, and sand paintings) with *Hastyealti* [Talking God]. Humpback flute players made by the Navajo and representing *Kokopelli* or his homomorph *Beganaskiddy* are found in a side canyon on the east side of the Pine River Canyon (Schaafsma 1963: 42, Figure 38). Other humpback figures, perhaps related to *Kokopelli* but more likely representing *Ganaskidi* [Mountain Sheep People] or *Beganaskiddy* [Carrier of Seeds] (see Figure 47 above) are found both in sand paintings and pictographs in Todosio Canyon (Schaafsma 1963: 61, Figure 40) and the Gobernador district (Schaafsma 1966: Figures 6, 7; Newcomb, et al. 1956: 40, Figure 78). Thunderbird is represented similarly in sand paintings, at a side on the right bank of the San Juan River northeast of Cottonwood Canyon (Schaafsma 1963: 62, Figure 28), and in a rock shelter on the west side of the Pine River a mile above the junction with the San Juan (Schaafsma 1963: 19, Figures 49, 51). A horned-face petroglyph of Navajo manufacture, located on the right bank of the San Juan where Thunderbird is shown, is very much like the Horned Sun or Moon of certain sand paintings (e.g. Wind, Feather Beauty, and Male Shooting Chants) (Schaafsma 1963: 62, 66, Figure 31; Newcomb, et al. 1956: 43, Figures 80, 81).

Today only the medicine man can render a Navajo sand painting (Newcomb, et al. 1956: 44). Schaafsma (1963: 66) suggests similarly that Navajo pictographs and petroglyphs were made by medicine men because their manufacture required an artist who was skilled and versed in religious rites, both characteristics being valuable in bringing the power of a deity or natural phenomenon into close range and control through artistic representation.

Various medicine men are identifiable through both mythology and pictography, including *Kokopelli* (Hohokam, Puebloan, and Central American Indians); *Ahola, Ahul* or *Alosaka, Tunwup, Sayathlia,* and *Hututu* (Hopi, Zuñi); *KoBictaiya* (Acoma); various clowns — Mudheads, *Koyemski* (Zuñi), *Koshare* or *Kurena* (Keres), *Kossa* (Tewa), *Chiffonete* (Taos); *Tobadsistsini, Hastyehogan, Hastyealti,* or *Beganaskiddy* (Navajo); *Eshgiboga* or *Minabozho* (Ojibwa) (Hoffman 1891: 187, 224, 229, Figures 6–9; Leekley 1965: 120–121); Medicine Man and Sea Dog (Kwakiutl) (Gunn 1966: front cover); and *Nenabush* (Delaware and other Algonquians) (James 1956: 357; Rafinesque, et al. 1954: 47). However, *Kokopelli* is the most frequently portrayed and temporally durable. This is probably because of several factors — his many roles in addition to that of healer; the lesser acculturation of the Puebloans by the Euro-Americans and hence the generally better preservation of their culture; the relatively greater frequency of the use of pictographic expression by the Puebloans, especially rock art; and the portrayal of *Kokopelli* on more durable media (pottery and rock).

PROVENIENCE, SCOPE, AND SPAN

The correlation of these *Kokopelli*-like petroglyphs with modern and ancient (eleventh-century) ethnographic equivalents provides evidence that panel rock art can have continuity, order, and perhaps similar meaning over a large temporal span and geographic area.

The same could probably be said for (1) widespread genital, fertility, and increase symbols; (2) many handprints or totem symbols related to personal identification or record of visit; (3) the spatial relationship of sites illustrating hunting content (including sympathetic magic of the hunt) to special hunting places (47 percent of 900 sites studied show this content and of these 47 percent about 87 percent are found in or near special hunting areas); (4) the widespread finding in western North America of lightly patinated, fine crosshatchings superimposed on older petroglyph sites, which practice may be related to negation or acquisition of the power or "medicine" of these sites; (5) the Great Horned Serpent of North and Central America (even a double-headed serpent) which is associated with medicine, rain, and fertility, especially crop fertility; (6) the Night or Underground Panther of the Midwest who is charged with pharmaceutical knowledge and skill; and (7) the relationship of special projections, the heart line, spirit line, consanguinity line, and X-ray style to magic and medicine.

Totem Medicine

Not only are shamans reported to assume animal disguises, but among a number of the American aborigines, animals themselves are considered to have the power to cure or cause disease (Vogel 1970: 16). Among many tribes of the American Indians, totems were considered biologically and spiritually related to the individual or clan and could be invoked in disease or other need (Gunn 1966: 701). Petroglyphs or pictographs of animals in certain instances might then represent such assignments. How these can be differentiated from totem identification, hunting magic, hunting records, animal mythology, and the like is impossible to know at present. Certain inferences from mythology are possible, such as the references above to the Night Panther of the Midwest, and the Sea Dog of the Northwest Coast.

Psychedelics

Kroeber (1925: 938) postulates that the cave paintings of the Chumash and island Shoshoneans are related to the *Toloache* religion because they share a common geographic area and because this religion was worked out in certain visible symbols. He also notes that many of the pictures may have been made by shamans. Barrett and Gifford (1933: 169) record that Miwok shamans sometimes ate the root or drank a concoction of *tolguacha* [*Datura meteloides,* jimson weed] to induce delirium and give them supernatural power. At Kuaua Kiva, New Mexico, a *Grey Newekwe* holding *Datura* or jimson weed is painted on the kiva wall (Dutton 1963: 59, Figure 96). Steward (1929: 227), in referring to pictographs and petroglyphs of the Tulare-Santa Barbara area, states that they portray many realistic anthropomorphs and zoomorphs thought to be marks of shamans and their power. Grant (1965: 63–66) noted that the *Toloache* or jimson weed cult held ceremonies in which neophytes decorated bowls and pestles. The ceremony was supposed to give health, long life, prosperity, and the ability to dodge arrows.

Paintings were placed where ceremonies were performed or where ceremonial equipment was kept (Grant 1965: 91, 92). Grant believes that Chumash paintings depict not things but concepts of good and evil, which forces are also represented by the medicine man (1965: 93; see our Plate 15).

Shamanistic Accouterments and Mobile Art

The accouterments of the medical or magico-religious performer (shaman, sorcerer, or medicine man) usually included objects of artistic merit, often decorated with totemic or secret symbols thought to be useful in healing (Lissner 1961: 272). One of Steward's informants related that the Yokuts in the southern Sierra Nevada believed pictographs in that region marked "caches of medicine men or doctors" that might include sacred outfits of talismans, their wealth, and even stuffed skins of dead women adorned with valuable ornaments (Steward 1929: 135; Heizer and Baumhoff 1962: 226). Certain headgear of Siberian shamans are composed of masks and cephalic projections of feathers resembling Hopi kachina masks and headdresses of other North American Indians (Dioszegi 1968: 145, 148, 215, 292). The vast number of references and illustrations of pictographs that were made on shamanistic accouterments is a study of great scope, and their manufacture perhaps began earlier than rock art.

The most typical or characteristic accouterment of the medicine man or shaman is the drum (including the tambourine), which may have originated among the ancient Mongols of Siberia or concomitant with the origin of shamanism wherever it arose. In the Baykal region, according to Okladnikov (1964: 52), the cult of the anthropomorphous male spirit and the first shamans appeared during the Glazkovian period (1800–1300 B.C.). However, he states earlier that the specimens of paleolithic art on the Shishkino Cliffs of the upper Lena resemble those of Europe not only in subject but in specific detail. He mentions especially the treatment and poses of women, but does not mention anthropomorphs that could be sorcerers or shamans (Okladnikov 1964: 21). However, according to Lommel (1967: 149), the roots of shamanism go back to the Alpine Paleolithic (30,000 to 50,000 years ago) and existed in cave art in the Magdalenian period. Drachenlock is given as an example. The sorcerer at Trois Frères has aleady been mentioned. The early evolution if not the origin of most of the arts (music, dance, drama, medicine, graphic expression) appears to be intimately associated with shamanism (Lommel 1967: 148).

Although the exact time of the first invention of the drum is lost in antiquity, in part because of its perishable nature, there is documentation that it was widely used by aboriginal Siberian shamans: Chukchi (Antropova and Kuznetsova 1964: 821), Nanays (Levin and Potapov 1964: 719), Evens and Amur (Levin and Vasilyev 1964: 681), Evenks (Vasilevich and Smolyak 1964: 648), Nganasans (who had sets of drums; Popov 1964: 578), Shors (who placed the shaman's drum in a tree over graves; Potapov 1964a: 464), Nentsy (Prokof'yeva 1964: 564), and Buryats (Vyatkina 1964: 227). An interesting engraving of an ancient Siberian shaman's drum, dated by Okladnikov to the Bronze Age and found on the Oka River, is illustrated by Dioszegi (1968: 196). Those documented as drawing pictographs of drums or on drums are the Kets (Popov and Dolgikh 1964: 617), Altays (Potapov 1964b: 325), Khakasy (Potapov 1964c: 358), Tungus (Lissner 1961: 249, Figure 102), and other groups from Russia, Siberia, and Lapland (Lommel 1967: 60, 107, 126, Figure 41; Maringer and Bandi 1953: 154, Figure 205; Gimbutas 1956: 189).

The Eskimos of the Bering Sea, on both the Asiatic and American sides, possessed similar drums which were decorated with zoomorphs (walrus, crane, cormorant, etc.) and faces (Nelson 1899: 350–352). An Eskimo pictograph showing a masked or mythical figure playing a possible drum is illustrated by Covarrubias (1954: 155). Similar tambourine drums, four of which are in the United States National Museum and have carved handles showing faces and a walrus, have been used by Eskimos from Greenland to Siberia. They use them to drive away spirits causing illness (Wilson 1898: 561–562, Figure 203).

Among the tribes on the upper Missouri River, in particular the Assiniboin, pictographs are painted on drums, shields, medicine sacks, and lodges to ensure success in domestic affairs, to attract game, and to avert lightning and disease (Denig 1930: 605, 619). Mallery (1893: 514–517) notes that pictographs found in America resemble those on Tartar and Mongol drums and illustrates ten such painted drum heads (Figures 721, 722, 723). He states that these drums were used in ceremonies with the belief that the sounds emanating from the surface upon which the designs were made and the designs themselves could produce special influences and power. The shaman owners of the drums gave these interpretations and identified some of the figures as other shamans, spirits, gods, celestial bodies, and special animals, including the serpent. In the ceremonies of the Grand Medicine Society of the Ojibwa, the drum is considered a gift from *Kitshi Manido* [the Great Spirit] through *Minabozho*; it is to be employed at the side of the sick to assist in the expulsion of evil spirits. It is also to be used during initiation rites of the society (Hoffman 1891: 190, 191). Among the Omaha, the drum was the most important musical instrument, but the smaller, flat, hoop drum or tambourine drum was the kind used by the "doctors" in treating the sick and in magical performances (Fletcher and La Flesche 1911: 371). A medicine and dance drum of the Tlingit from Sitka, Alaska, decorated with a painting of a totemic bear, and a painted Pueblo drum are illustrated by Wilson (1898: Plate 70, Figure 224). A Tsimshian painted drum head showing a stylized eagle, masks, and ánimal figures is illustrated by Appleton (1950: Plate 27). He also shows a Mayan wooden drum carved with many figures in low relief (Plate 46).

In a synopsis of Indian "hieroglyphics," Schoolcraft (1851: Plate 58, number 45) shows the symbol used for a magic drum. He also records a work by Sheffer written in 1704 in which Lapland drum pictographs portray gods, animals, serpents, sorcerers, sickness, etc. (Schoolcraft 1851: 425). These drums were used to cure or cause disease, to influence the course and range of animals, and to produce sorcery and magic.

In summary, drum usage in shamanism reached a high peak among the American Indians, Mongols, and Siberians. It probably originated among the latter as one of the earlier musical instruments, in association with shamans, who were perhaps the first to use drums. Their sound, rhythm, and decorations were used for exorcising pathological spirits and disease, as well as for other magical results. Scientific studies show an effect on brain waves, circulation, psyche, and many physiological functions producing alertness or hypnotherapy, trance states, lessened fatigue, automatic muscle movement, peristaltic changes, and even epilepsy, depending on the talents and techniques of the musician and the conditioning, receptivity, and mental and physical state of the listener (*M. D. Medical Newsmagazine* 1959b: 149–151). These effects account in part for some of the magic attributed to the drum, but they were enhanced by the superstitious beliefs of the aborigine. The pictographs on this common accouterment of the medicine man were also credited with these real and imagined effects.

Rock art sites that show drums and possible shamans with them are found at Massacre Lakes, Nevada (see Figure 52); Little Petroglyph Canyon, California (see Figure 53); and Myer Spring, Texas (see Figure 54).

Similar observations can be made regarding the rattle and flute or flageolot, which are also commonly employed by the shaman, although they do not lend themselves so well to pictographic display. A dance rattle from Walpi, decorated with a swastika, is shown by Wilson

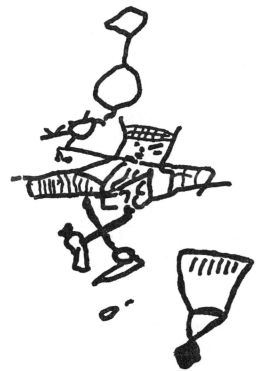

Figure 52. Massacre Lakes, Nevada. A dancer and possible drum are pecked at this site. The conical lower right-hand object, if not a drum, might be a basket

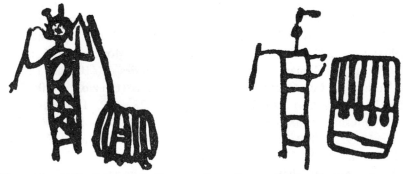

Figure 53. Little Petroglyph Canyon, Coso Range, California. These two anthropomorphs appear to be associated with drums

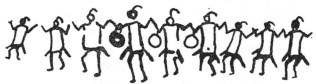

Figure 54. Myer Spring, Texas. A row of dancing figures painted in red at this site shows several who hold drums or possibly shields

(1898: Figure 225). He also illustrates Hupa, Ponca, Kiowa, and other musical instruments of these various types (1898: 567–574, 582, Figure 216, Plate 73). The flute-playing *Kokopelli* has already been mentioned.

Petroglyphs showing flutes and rattles are seen in Cienagillos, Santa Fe County, New Mexico (see Figure 55); The Needles, Canyonlands National Park, Utah (Sims 1950: Plate XIV; see our Figure 56); Myer Spring, Terrell County, Texas; Petrified Forest National Monument, Apache County, Arizona (see Figure 57); Indian Canyon, San Juan County, Utah (see Figure 58); and many others. There are many pictographs of these instruments shown on kiva walls at Awatovi (see Figure 59), Kuaua (see Figure 60), Zuni, Jemez (Tanner 1957: 23), and others (Dutton 1963: 109–112, 191; see our Figure 61).

The "mobile art" of the Old World Upper Paleolithic, especially objects such as the Baton of Montgaudier studied by Marshak (1970: 57–63), could be prime examples of shamanistic accouterments (see also Graziosi 1960: Plates 54, 60, 65, 66, 71, 88, 89; Leroi-Gourhan 1968: 395–402, 499, 500). Their association with the great cave paintings of southern France and northern Spain is well documented. The possible production of these paintings and mobile art by a shaman, medicine man, or sorcerer is suggested by the appearance on both the cave walls and mobile art of special anthropomorphs. Examples are the "Sorcerer" of Les Trois Frères (Robert and Nougier 1961: slide 2/3), the ithyphallic figure of Le Portel (1961: slides 2/2, 23/11, 23/12, 27/12), the engraved figures at Casares (1961: slide 2/4), the three anthropomorphs at Cougnac (1961: slide 2/5), the "Adam and Eve" at Rouffignac (1961: slide 2/7), the enigmatic figure at Las Monedas (1961: slide 12/1), the "bird man" of Lascaux (1961: slides 13/10 and 13/11), and others at Les Combarelles and Marsoulas (Graziosi 1960: Plate 258, 259) (see also Breuil 1952: Figures 128, 130, 139, 146, 514; Leroi-Gourhan 1968: 482, 523, Figures 57, 58, 437–446, 485, 689; Kuhn 1969: 51 009/7; 1952: 16–19, 112, 193, 195, Plate 103; Graziosi 1960: Plates 24, 25, 83–87, 257, 281–283).

We note, then, that *Kokopelli* and other shaman homologues are associated not only with the arts of painting and engraving, but also with dance, music, hunting, disguise or drama, love, and medicine.

Painted pebbles found in south Texas caves are of unknown purpose, although possibly they represent conventionalized anthropomorphs. They do not resemble the possible shaman anthropomorphs of the cave walls in that region (Kirkland and Newcomb 1967: 108–110, Plates 67, 68). The incised geometric patterns on rock slabs from Ruby Cave, Nevada, are even more difficult to interpret. These might be more re-

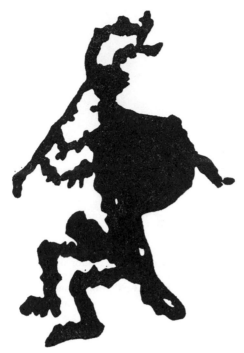

Figure 55. Cienagillos, New Mexico. A flute is being played by *Kokopelli*, who appears in typical fashion, ithyphallic and as if dancing

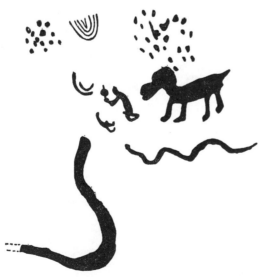

Figure 56. Windy Pictograph, The Needles, Utah. A small red pictograph figure holds a rattle as he faces four snakes

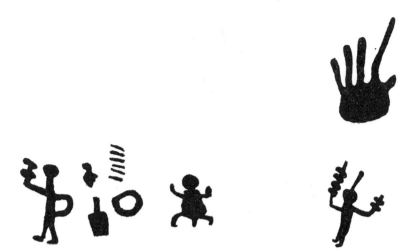

Figure 57.   Puerca Ruin, Petrified Forest National Monument, Arizona. The human figure on the right may be holding a mace or wand; the one on the left may be holding a rattle or an abbreviated version of a mace or wand.

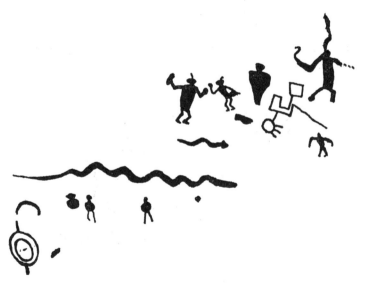

Figure 58.   Indian Creek, Utah. Two figures displayed in this panel appear to be dancing and holding rattles

Figure 59.   Awatovi, Arizona. Painted on the kiva wall at this ruin is what appears to be a flute

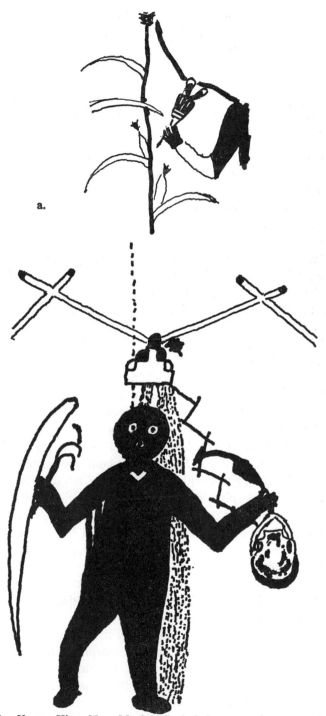

Figure 60.   Kuaua Kiva, New Mexico. Included among th many paintings of this kiva are two figures who hold rattles and other objects: (a) rattle held by some kachina associated with corn; (b) *Ka'nashkule*, a priest-clown-medicine man holds a water jug, rattle, snare, and "white worm," and is associated with cloud, rain, and lightning symbols

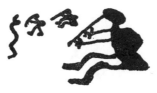

Figure 61.   El Gique, New Mexico. Pecked on a boulder along the Rio Grande
are these three *Kokopelli* figures who play the flute and are associated with a
plumed or horned serpent

vealing if studied by Marshak's discerning approach (1970) with microscopic and photographic techniques. Incised stones from Hogup
Cave, Box Elder County, Utah, show only geometric designs, but
anthropomorphic figurines of wrapped plant fibers have been identified
with the horned anthropomorphs of Fremont rock art (Aikens 1970:
83). A similar comparison and identification of clay figurines from
Pilling Cave, Emery County, Utah, with Fremont pictographs are made
by Morss (1954: 3, 6, 18, 25). Figurines from other areas of the southwestern United States show breasts, genital clefts, and "babes in
cradle"; they are compared to kachina pictographs or petroglyphs of
Basketmaker and Pueblo types (1954: 62). Other relationships and
data indicate they may be associated with fertility and increase cults
(1954: 53–61, Figures 12–22, 29, 30). One figurine shows the crying-
eye or forked-eye motif (1954: Figure 22m).

Carl Schuster was also making similar studies of mobile art, various
maze designs, and fertility symbols, but because of his death in 1969,
they are incomplete and some are unpublished. By personal communication he did indicate that he had found a few instances in which the
panel cave art in the western United States could be related to mobile
art. The association of either with shamanism was not discussed.

Engraved catlinite (pipestone) tablets from burial mounds of the
northeastern periphery of the Great Plains show animals with the heart
line. If Lommel's theory is accepted, these could be associated with a
shaman or medicine man, perhaps in the practice of medicine hunts
(Wedel 1961: Plate XIX; James 1956: 341ff.).

By the same reasoning, design elements on pottery of the Southwest
showing the heart-line motif (Dockstader 1961: Plate 166), could be
interpreted as originating from shamanism.

Bone carvings and other mobile art from the Columbia River region
often show the same X-ray style anthropomorphs as are found in the
panel rock art nearby (*Screenings* 1966: 1; Strong 1959: 123, 125).
Strong also shows a stone carving of a flute player (1959: 118) that
may or may not be related to *Kokopelli*.

In addition to the birchbark pictographs carried in the medicine bags by the *Mide'* of the Ojibwa, pictographic decorations of possible medical significance were placed on many other mobile artifacts of the American Indian such as carvings, masks, rattles, drums, soul catchers, charms, ceremonial boxes, effigies, clothing, robes, jewelry, adornments, other medicine pouches, animal parts, stones, gemstones, etc. (Boas 1951: 66, 77; Densmore 1948: 176–180; Dockstader 1961: Plates 117–120, 223, 229, 248; Gunn 1966: 705; Lommel 1967: 126, Figures 17, 18, 22, 41, 44; Mallery 1893: 515–517; 1886: 201–202; Vogel 1970: 27, illustrations following 76).

Tattoos and Skin Painting

A burial of a priest or shaman at Awatovi, Arizona, contained pigment supplies (Hrdlička 1905: 610). Sometimes the medicine man painted or tattooed his own skin or that of the patient (Corlett 1935: 143; Fox 1967: 267; Hoffman 1891: 223; Howey 1955: 282; Mallery 1893: 391; *M. D. Medical Newsmagazine* 1959b: 126; Landes 1968: 239). Among primitive peoples today, e.g. the Arunta of Australia (Spencer and Gillen 1968: 529, Figure 105) and the Omaha (Fletcher and La Flesche 1911: 519) the initiation ceremonies to become a member of a medicine society or a medicine man often include body painting. Other North American Indians did the same (Corlett 1935: 100; Hoffman 1896: 75–77). In ancient times tattoos assumed religious, magic, and social significance and were incorporated in many rituals. They were also used to identify tribes or clans, sex, various attributes such as strength, agility, or bravery, and were thought to protect against illness, prevent pain and snakebite, and to guarantee survival after death (Heckwelder 1876: 206; *M. D. Medical Newsmagazine* 1959b: 126). Unknowingly the practice of tattooing by primitive man may have transmitted such diseases as hepatitis (Australian antigen), tuberculosis, vaccinia, syphilis, and leprosy, and may have caused cellulitis, septicemia, and allergic reactions. Today its main clinical uses are for cosmetic effects to cover up scars, hemangiomas, vitiligo, and other skin discolorations. A modern observation, which does not necessarily apply to prehistoric man, is the association of tattoos with neuroses, personality disorders, criminality, and divorce *(M. D. Medical Newsmagazine* 1959b: 128–132). The Miwok of California tattooed the skin directly over an area of severe pain (Barrett and Gifford 1933: 224). The elaborate and decorative tattoos made by the Northwest Coast tribes, particularly the Haida, included totem and mythical animals, which could have been invoked for protection from harm or disease (Mallery 1893: 396–405). Other North American tribes had similar practices (Heckwelder 1876: 206). An interesting lithograph circa 1700 shows a Mohawk Indian holding an enormous snake and with one tattooed on his right breast (Josephy 1961: 191; see our Figure 62). The art of healing by tattooing was called *azhassoew* by the Ojibwa (Landes 1968: Glossary). For example, the female *Mide'* frequently tattooed the temples, forehead, or cheeks for headache and toothache. This treatment was believed to expel the malevolent causative *manido* spirit or demon (Mallery 1893: 395), but could have been effective (as with acupuncture) through counterirritant action.

The Serpent, Symbol of Healing and New Life

The serpent is associated universally with medical mythology and history — indeed the modern symbolism of the United States Army Medical Corps (also the medical corps of the British, Germans, Swedish, Filipinos, Mexicans, and French) and of the medical profession since the days of Greek ascendency has been the scepter of Aesculapius and the caduceus (Bunn 1967: 618; *M. D. Medical Newsmagazine* 1959a: 131, 1966: 12). Snakes became connected with Aesculapius because of their wisdom and ability to cure illness. Their skin-shedding ability represented healing, longevity, and immortality — the ability to slough off old age and become young again. They symbolized convalescence in their ability to change from lethargy to rapid activity (University of Colorado School of Medicine 1970). An association of serpents with the healing arts can be traced in the Near East back to 3100 B.C. (Bunn 1967: 615). Serpents in ancient myths are often said to have knowledge of life-restoring plants (Howey 1955: 89). They have also been assigned astonishingly ambivalent roles by various peoples, and worship for their life-giving powers has been documented for such diverse peoples as the Aztecs, Celts, Hindus, Phoenicians, and some African and most American Indian tribes (*M. D. Medical Newsmagazine* 1959a: 131). A relationship to phallic symbolism, eroticism, and fertility is also found among many cultures, including the use of snakes in the modern burlesque snake dance and as aphrodisiacs. Serpent myths and shaman religion of the North American Indian and Eskimo are related to those of the Finns, Laplanders, and Samoyeds (Howey 1955: 283; Squier 1851: 251). Modern Eskimos often use the serpent in their decorative art,

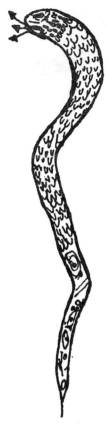

Figure 62.   This serpent held in the hands of a Mohawk warrior is also tattooed in miniature on his chest

showing the serpent *Pal-rai-yuk* and a two-headed (bipolar) serpent (Covarrubias 1954: 155). Double-headed serpents are not uncommon motifs in Central and South America (Squier 1851: 181, 198, 202; Covarrubias 1954: 45, Figures 17, 18, 19).

Hoffman (1891: Plate XXI) portrays a spiral snake on a relic formerly belonging to an Ojibwa *Mide'*. Snakes, most frequently rattlesnakes, occur on small vessels (stone and pottery) that could have been used for crushing pigment or storing paint used in making pictographs (Gladwin, et al. 1965: Plates LXII, LXV, LXVII, CI, CXXXV; *Screenings* 1964: 1; Bergen 1963: 3). Among the Ojibwa the water monster serpent played a role in their Grand Medicine Society (Emerson 1965: 43, 45; Hoffman 1891: 291; Landes 1968: 48; see our Figure 63). Five evil serpent spirits capable of causing illness are shown by Hoffman (1891: Plate III). *Meshekenabek*, the snake, is a mythical opponent to *Manabozho*, the Ojibwa culture hero and founder of the

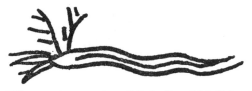

Figure 63.   The Ojibwa water monster of their Grand Medicine Society is shown in this manner on birchbark scrolls

Grand Medicine Society. The *Amphisabaena* [two-headed snake] is claimed to exist by some shamans or witch doctors in Brazil and its dried flesh used to cure dislocations and broken bones. The snake is claimed as an ancestor, god, and totem by many North American Indians, including the Cherokee, Mohican, Menomini, Leni Lenape (Delaware), Potawatomi, Ojibwa, Carolina, Seminole, Iowa, Moki, etc. (Howey 1955: 289, 291, 316) and Central or South American Indians (Squier 1851: 110, 136, 198, 251). The serpent, *Sisiutl,* is also known among the Kwakiutl, Nootka, and Tsimshian. It has been found on an ivory charm of a Tsimshian sorcerer. A double-headed snake is noted among the sand paintings at Acoma (Smith and Ewing 1952: 214) and the petroglyphs at San Cristobal (Sims 1950: 8, Plate XI). Also found among pictographs of the Coast Salish are a horned serpent and a serpentlike, double-headed animal (Gjessing 1958: 259, 260). The Kwakiutl associated the serpent with "Healing Woman," and it represented the healing power of the shaman (Locher 1932: 27).

As noted previously, *Awanyu, Palulukon, Kolowisi,* and *Kleetso* are mentioned and portrayed prominently in the ophialatric mythology and symbolism of the Pueblo and Navajo. Pictographs of snakes are found on kiva walls, slat altars, and sand painting of medicine and other religious societies at Acoma, Santo Domingo, Jemez, Isleta, Oraibi, and Zuni (Smith and Ewing 1952: 212–216; L. White 1932: 107–125). Additional authors who document this are Fewkes (1897: 2, 3), Dutton (1963: 41), and Villasenor (1963: 7, 73).

Mallery (1893: 237, 240), in discussing the symbolism of the Grand Medicine Society of the Ojibwa, mentions a horned sea monster. The Aztec solar or feathered serpent of Mexico, *Quetzalcoatl,* who served as a messenger between man and god, may be closely related to these North American serpents. Olmec paintings in Juxtlahuaca Cave, Guerrero, Mexico, described as the oldest paintings in the Western hemisphere, portray a plumed serpent, a probable predecessor to *Quetzalcoatl* (Gay 1967: 28; see our Figure 64). Symbols found in Mexico associated with this mythical serpent such as sun circles, rain, clouds,

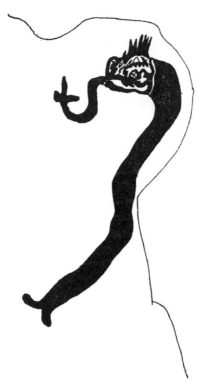

Figure 64. Juxtlahuaca Cave, Guerrero, Mexico. This red pictograph of a plumed serpent is found three-quarters of a mile beneath the surface. It is attributed to the Olmec and may be not only the earliest picture of this composite animal, but also one of the earliest paintings in the Western hemisphere

lightning, birds, and vegetation are also found among petroglyphs and pictographs of the Southwest (Howey 1955: 302–307; Squier 1851: 251). To this day, snake oil preparations are used for such complaints as rheumatism, arthritis, and other joint and muscle diseases or discomforts. A priest or shaman among one aboriginal group in the South (probably Louisiana) is described as having a serpent and sun symbol tattooed on his chest (Howey 1955: 282). One of the two degrees of the chief curing society (Flint Society) of the Cochiti and other Keresans is the snake degree (Fox 1967: 263). In this connection it appears on slat altars, kiva walls, and regional petroglyphs such as those at San Cristobal, Pueblo Blanco, and similar sites already mentioned.

A rock drawing in Segi Canyon, Arizona, shows the god *Baho-li-kong-ya*, the genius of fructification who was worshiped until the latter part of the nineteenth century by Moki priests. "It is the great crested serpent with mammae, which are the source of the blood of all animals

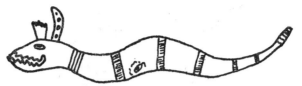

Figure 65.   *Baho-li-kong-ya*, a mythical serpent with mammae, found in Segi Canyon, Arizona, was worshiped by the Moki

and all the waters of the land" (Mallery 1893: 476, Figure 661). A reproduction of this serpent is shown in Figure 65. Corlett (1935: 179, 196) also records the medical significance of the snake among several Central and South American Indians. Of all animals, the serpent is the one most commonly associated with healing.

Among petroglyphs and pictographs of western North America, the snake is one of the most common animals portrayed, second only to the ubiquitous mountain sheep. If it is accepted that many wavy lines and spirals were intended to represent serpents and that their portrayal as totem animals may also have some medical relationship, then the snake would certainly be the most commonly represented animal associated with medicine (Renaud 1938: 51, 55).

Animal Doctors and Vectors

The Acoma, Cochiti, and other Keresans believed other animals had the power to cure; the most powerful was the bear, next most powerful the mountain lion, then the eagle. Among the paraphernalia of the Acoma and Cochiti medicine men were bear paws (Fox 1967: 267; Corlett 1935: 152). In the Zuñi cult of the beast gods, various animals are held to be givers of long life, medicinal plants, and the magic power to make them effective (Bunzel 1932: 528, 532). *Kinien*, the hawk, supplied medicine to the Ojibwa. Medicine bags of eagle and owl skins were considered especially useful in healing (Mallery 1893: 242, 246). Thunderbird brought rain which then brought plant medicines (Hoffman 1891: 203).

Gunn (1966: 705), Lissner (1961: 258, 272), and Vogel (1970: 26) also mention that many accouterments of shamans contained diverse magical symbols or numbers, as well as animal parts from which the shaman derived special abilities attributable to that particular animal.

Many accouterments of the American medicine man illustrated by Vogel (1970: following page 76) show effigies, animal parts, and pictographs of the following animals: man (scalp), thunderbird, elk, deer, eagle, horse, owl, bear, several other small animals from whose skin pouches were made, and a particularly realistic stuffed snake with a cluster of rattlesnake rattles tied to the tail. Anthropomorphs in rock art are sometimes shown with such objects (see Plate 16). This helps to identify them as possible medicine men or shamans. The many other animals or animal spirits that ethnographic evidence indicates have a role in disease, either causative or curative, would cover almost all known animals and many invented ones. Accounts of cure by the medicine man are often attended not only by the invocation of helpful animals but by the elimination of evil ones. Commonly, the practitioner is described as sucking out small snakes, worms, shells, stones, insects, etc., from the body of the patient. It was noted above that below the "night panther" at the Agawa site is a peculiar serpent. It was also noted that commonly in the Southwest where *Kokopelli* is portrayed in rock art, he is associated with snakes. The Cienagillos site where he occurs in greatest numbers best illustrates this relationship (see Figure 66). Various other serpent depictions are found throughout the Southwest.

Contagious Magic Cures and Spells

After the origin and purpose were forgotten, certain petroglyph and pictograph sites were assigned various roles by groups subsequent to the makers. They were sometimes viewed with awe, fear, suspicion, mystery, and hope, and were thought to possess various magic or supernatural powers. In some instances, these sites were avoided as malevolent, capable of causing ill health, evil, or death. Others were thought to have healing powers.

Painted Cave in the San Marcos Pass region near Santa Barbara, California, is an example of the former. Family lore of the Ogrum family, which for several generations owned the land on which the cave is located, indicates the surviving local Indians in the last century were fearful of the cave and avoided going near it. One of them, Old Pete, an elderly Chumash survivor, told Johnson Ogrum, an original owner, that a former tribal chief interpreted the pictographs in the cave according to Chumash legend. Supposedly, some of the pictographs represent funerary boats used to take the dead to the nearby islands for burial. Centipede symbols represent the cause of death (see Figures 67, 68). Judging from the age of the informant, who was seventy-two, and our data on his ancestors and Old Pete, ths story is estimated to have been over 120 years old when told in 1959.

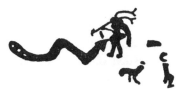

Figure 66.   Cienagillos, New Mexico. The serpent associated with *Kokopelli* at this site is a definite rattlesnake

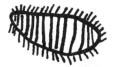

Figure 67.   Painted Cave, near Santa Barbara, California, contains beautiful polychromes which show the centipede, a sign of death according to local Chumash legend

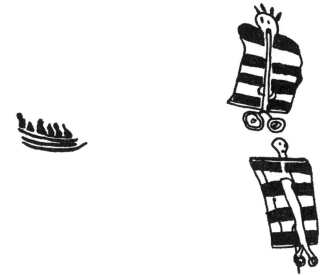

Figure 68.   Painted Cave. Figures adjacent to the centipede (Figure 67) allegedly show the dead ready for burial and the funerary boat transporting the dead to the nearby Channel Islands for burial

Contrary to this association with death, a site at Cherokee (Butte County) in northern California was used for healing. Coffin Rock, so named by pioneers because of its suggestive shape, has crude and deeply carved petroglyphs on its top (see Figure 69). Persistent Maidu legend indicates that they laid ailing members of the tribe on top of it to cure backache. This custom was still followed into the twentieth century.

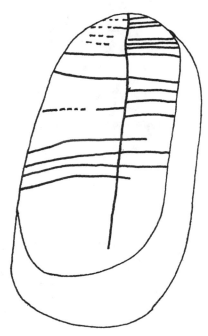

Figure 69.   Coffin Rock, Butte County, California. Until the early part of the twentieth century, Maidu Indians laid patients on this rock to cure backache

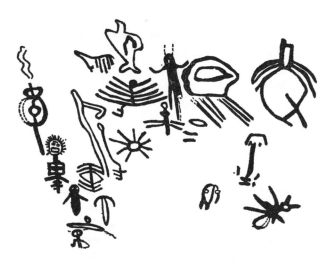

Figure 70.   Hospital Rock, Sequoia National Park, California. Ailing members of the Potwisha and, later, pioneers who were ill or injured were placed for care in rock shelters beneath pictographs painted on this boulder

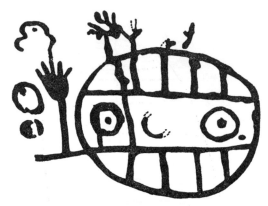

Figure 71. Ojo Caliente, New Mexico. This petroglyph is located near a former habitation site and hot springs

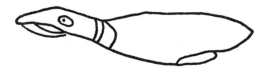

Figure 72. Seal Rocks, southern tip of Vancouver Island, British Columbia, Canada. Members of the Coast Salish placed members ill with smallpox at this site in hopes of a magic cure. Probably this large seal was originally placed here to attract seals or to assist in the hunt through sympathetic magic

Hospital Rock in Sequoia National Park was so named by Hale D. Tharp when Alfred Everton, accidentally caught in a bear trap in 1873, found shelter there, as had John Swanson when injured nearby in 1860. Other pioneers had found shelter there under similar circumstances. Prior to that, the Potwisha had used it for their sick (J. White 1952: 108; Gudde 1960: 138; Farquhar 1926: 43). Numerous pictographs are found on Hospital Rock and in adjacent rock shelter and caves (see Figure 70).

Petroglyphs are often found near hot springs or mineral springs used for treatment of various ills first by the aborigines, later by the settlers. A few examples are Richardson Springs, Butte County, California; Coso Hot Springs, Inyo County, California; Allen and Axe Springs, Churchill County, Nevada; White Arrow Hot Springs, Gooding County, Idaho; and Ojo Caliente, Rio Arriba, and Taos Counties, New Mexico (Vogel 1970: 258; see our Figure 71). At a prehistoric spa on Kulleet Bay (Vancouver Island, British Columbia, Canada), cured patients, who bathed in the spring-fed, rock basin pools, would carve their totems about the basin rims as testimonials and records of visit (Pavey, personal communication). An unusual site on the southernmost tip of Vancouver Island is called Seal Rocks because of a large seal carved there. During a smallpox epidemic in 1877, the Coast Salish placed their stricken members in front of this site in hopes of magic cures (Smith, personal communication; see our Figure 72).

Diagnostic Aids

Data regarding the health conditions of prehistoric men can be found at various sites. The many handprints, and to a lesser extent footprints, are a particularly good source for the study of injuries, mutilations, possible congenital defects such as camptodactyly, arachnodactyly, polydactyly, or syndactyly, and certain acquired diseases such as arthritis, old fractures, exostoses, Dupuytren's contracture, etc. The positive pictographic impressions or prints are more revealing, whereas the petroglyphs, being manufactured, are suspect of artistic license — an extra digit or a deficient digit may merely reflect the whims of the maker (see Figures 73, 74).

At many sites, including the House of Many Hands in Mystery Valley, Arizona, and the Cave of Two Hundred Hands near The Needles (Canyonlands National Park) of southeastern Utah, prehistoric men left an impressive handprint registry. In most instances they dipped their palms in paint, then imprinted positive handprints on the stone walls. In other instances they painted stripes on their hands and then made the imprints. Sometimes they held the hand against the wall, then blew or sprayed paint about the hand, leaving a negative print. With the former technique some are clear enough that fingerprints and other dermatoglyphics show well. Potentially these could be used to classify and identify fingerprint types, anthropological relationships, chromosome variants, and special diseases. The use of dermatoglyphics in diagnosis is a relatively new scientific study, not to be confused with or related to palmistry. In the medical literature the list of dermatoglyphic abnormalities associated with disease is growing; these include mongolism, Turner's syndrome, Klinefelter's syndrome, trisomy autosome anomalies, pseudohypoparathyroidism, Wilson's disease, psoriasis, neurofibromatosis, phenylketonuria, certain congenital heart diseases, schizophrenia, epilepsy, and some cases of undifferentiated mental deficiency (*Medical Tribune* 1965: 9, 29). Many of these individuals could not survive under conditions of primitive existence and barely do so supported by modern medical technology. However, palmar "mapping"

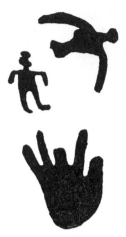

Figure 73.   Cienagillos, New Mexico. This petroglyph indicates that the two distal phalanges of the middle finger were missing

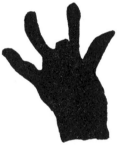

Figure 74.   Abo Gap, New Mexico. A pictograph in a rock shelter at this site portrays a hand with the two distal phalanges and perhaps part of the proximal phalanx missing from the middle finger. Compare with Figure 73

ridge counts, and triradial angulation studies applied to the many hand-prints of prehistoric man throughout the world would no doubt reveal new medical facts about him as they have about modern man.

Most of these handprints were probably made as a record of visit or as personal identification, but a curious use has been described by Keams. The Hopi considering candidates for the *Salyko* fraternity selected only those whose handprints dried immediately (Mallery 1886: 222). Emotionally unstable, tense, nervous individuals tend more to have moist, sweaty palms, and their handprints would not dry as fast. Could it be that this requirement served to eliminate such individuals and hence was useful as a rough physiological and psychological test?

CONCLUSION

We have presented an explanatory framework based on the interpretation of pictography (emphasizing petroglyphs and pictographs) in western North America. Our main hypothesis is that many, probably a majority, of the petroglyph and pictograph sites in (western) North America have medical significance. Medical significance employs both the primitive and modern concepts, the latter being more restrictive. Secondary hypotheses suggested are that many are made by, or under the influence of, medicine men or shamans and that certain themes, motifs, and graphic devices can be linked to these manufacturers. Some of these themes, motifs, representations, and "supernatural" content can be differentiated from the natural or secular.

It is not enough to present hypotheses. One must also present a testing procedure to assess their validity or lack thereof.

In terms of sampling, we believe that a culling of the literature coupled with a field study of over 900 sites provides an adequate data base.

The arguments and inferences presented are speculative (often embryonic and exploratory), but the degree of probability increases with the use of ethnographic analogy, archaeological and environmental associations, and covariation of site elements and motifs. These provide a testing mechanism. Within this report we have presented such data concerning the hypotheses. It should be noted, however, that some rock art was multifunctional to the maker, the beholder, or their respective groups. Also, the generality of our hypotheses provides for additional, equally valid hypotheses (e.g. Heizer and Baumhoff 1962; Ritter 1970). An explanatory base has nevertheless been presented which may have implications regarding aboriginal man's behavior throughout the world.

For a number of rock art sites we can neither prove nor disprove our hypotheses. Here, ethnographic analogy, the direct historical approach, site associations, or site content provide few clues as to their meaning. Only by reference to those where inferences have more probability or by examination of site associations and content in order to develop new or additional hypotheses will their explanation be manifested.

Through this study we have also noted that some of the portrayed "supernatural" animals (plumed serpent, two-headed serpent, night panther, water monsters, totem animals); a select few anthropomorphs (*Kokopelli* and his homomorphs); mask types; large, limbless figures; genital or fertility symbols (cupules, vulviforms, hocker-type female figures, clouds); and sympathetic magic of the hunt (hunting scenes, wounded animals, traps, weapons) illustrate that the content of rock art can have continuity and order — perhaps with similar meaning or function — over a long temporal span, transcending cultural boundaries and large geographic areas. Further studies along these lines may provide insights into intergroup communications, style drift, population movements, and the like.

The discussion of other subjects would be appropriate to the title of this paper. Study of Tables 1–5 shows many subjects inadequately covered or not covered at all and suggests further study, communication, and research. The selection of sites, their primary use, reuse, continuum of use, secondary functions, site ecology and associations — for example, associations with ritual, ceremonial structures, certain animals and plants — should be explored further. The content within sites such as special groupings, symbolism, ideographs, other sympathetic magic, and phytomorphs — for example the swastika, sun disc, "black magic," puberty pictographs, and color use — should be further researched.

Examination of petroglyph and pictograph sites in North America using the suggested hypotheses should be considered only a step toward culture reconstruction. What is needed is correlation with other aspects of the culture and surrounding environment through proper archaeological and environmental studies. The goal is explanation of culture process, culture history, and group behavior. Studies presented here provide only a small view, but do provide a paradigm for investigation of the magico-religious subsystem. Integration with the adaptive responses of the maker's group and the economic-subsistence and sociopolitical subsystems is also needed. The end goal is the presentation of generalities or (statistical) laws of human behavior with application to present and future peoples.

In this manner a prediction of certain aspects of behavior will follow. If our hypotheses can be more completely validated with more rigorous testing procedures, and perhaps narrowed down or coupled with other data mentioned, then we may be able to discern more of man's relation with his environment, and perhaps more of his emotional or cognitive responses to it.

REFERENCES

AIKENS, C. MELVIN
1970 *Hogup cave.* University of Utah Anthropological Papers 98:83. Salt Lake City: University of Utah Press.

ANONYMOUS
1970 "The vase of Gudea." Descriptive folder. Chicago: American Medical Association.

ANTROPOVA, V. V., V. G. KUZNETSOVA
1964 "The Chukchi," in *The peoples of Siberia.* Edited by M. G. Levin and L. P. Potapov, 799–835. Chicago: University of Chicago Press.

APPLETON, LE ROY H.
1950 *Indian art of the Americas.* New York: Charles Scribner's Sons.

ARMSTRONG, P. A.
1887 *The Piasa or devil among the Indians.* Morris: E. B. Fletcher.

BARRETT, S. A.
1952 Material aspects of Pomo culture. *Bulletin of the Public Museum of the City of Milwaukee* 20:261–508.

BARRETT, S. A., E. W. GIFFORD
1933 Miwok material culture. *Bulletin of the Milwaukee Public Museum* 2:169–224.

BERGEN, HAROLD G.
1963 Salvage archaeology. *Screenings* 12:3.

BINFORD, L. R.
1968 "Archaeological perspectives," in *New perspectives in archaeology.* Edited by S. R. Binford and L. R. Binford, 5–33. Chicago: Aldine.

BLACK, ROMAN
1964 *Old and new Australian aboriginal art.* Sidney: Angus and Robertson.

BLUM, HAROLD F.
1970 "On growth of art," in *Valcomonica symposium, acts of the international symposium on prehistoric art.* Edited by Emmanuel Anatit, 531–536. Capo di Ponti: Centro Camuno di Studi Preistorici.

BOAS, FRANZ
1951 "Representative art," in *Primitive art, 64–87.* Irving-on-the-Hudson: Capitol.

BREUIL, HENRY
1952 *Four hundred centuries of cave art.* Dordogne: Fernan Windels.

BUNN, JOHN T.
1967 Origin of the caduceus motif. *Journal of the American Medical Association* 202:615–619.

BUNZEL, RUTH
1932 "Introduction to Zuñi ceremonialism," in *Forty-seventh annual report of the Bureau of American Ethnology,* 473–544. Washington: United States Government Printing Office.

CADZOW, DONALD A.
1926 Bark records of the Bungi Medewin Society. *Indian Notes and Monographs, Museum of the American Indian, Heye Foundation* 3:123–140.

1934   Petroglyphs (rock carvings) in the Susquehanna River near Safe Harbor, Pennsylvania. *Publications of the Pennsylvania Historical Commission* 3:5–51.

CARTWRIGHT, WILLIAM D., FREDERIC H. DOUGLAS
1934   *Symbolism in Indian art and the difficulties of its interpretation.* Denver Art Museum Leaflet 61:42–44.

CHENG TEK'UN
1966   "Prehistoric China," in *Archaeology in China*, volume one (second edition), 1–250. Cambridge: W. Heffer and Sons.

COLTON, HAROLD S.
1949   *Hopi kachina dolls.* Albuquerque: University of New Mexico Press.

CONNOR, STUART W.
1962   *A preliminary survey of prehistoric picture writing on rock surfaces in central and south central Montana.* Billings Archaeological Society Anthropological Paper 2:1–31.

CORLETT, WILLIAM THOMAS
1935   *The medicine man of the American Indian and his cultural background.* Springfield: Charles C. Thomas.

COVARRUBIAS, MIGUEL
1954   *The eagle, the jaguar, and the serpent.* New York: Alfred A. Knopf.

CURTIS, EDWARD S.
1924   The Pomo. *The North American Indian* 14:66.

DAVIS, EMMA LOU
1961   The Mono Craters petroglyphs. *American Antiquity* 27:236–239.

DENIG, EDWIN T.
1930   "Indian tribes of the upper Missouri," in *Forty-sixth annual report of the Bureau of American Ethnology*, 395–628. Washington: United States Government Printing Office.

DENSMORE, FRANCES
1948   A collection of specimens from the Teton Sioux. *Indian Notes and Monographs, Museum of the American Indian, Heye Foundation* 11:158–204.

DEWDNEY, SELWYN, KENNETH E. KIDD
1962   *Indian rock paintings of the Great Lakes.* Toronto: University of Toronto Press.

DIOSZEGI, VILMA
1968   *Tracing shamans in Siberia.* New York: Humanities Press.

DITTERT, ALFRED E., JIM J. HESTER, FRANK W. EDDY
1961   *An archaeological survey of the Navajo Reservoir District, northwestern New Mexico.* Monographs of the School of American Research and the Museum of New Mexico 23:1–277.

DOCKSTADER, FREDERICK
1961   *Indian art in America.* London: New York Graphic Society.

DUTTON, BERTHA P.
1963   *Sun father's way, the kiva murals of Kuaua.* Albuquerque: University of New Mexico Press.

EMERSON, ELLEN RUSSELL
1965   *Indian myths.* Minneapolis: Ross and Haines.

ERWIN, RICHARD P.
1930   "Indian rock writings in Idaho," in *Twelfth biennial report, State Historical Society of Idaho*, 35–111.

FARQUHAR, F. P.
1926   *Place names of the High Sierras.* San Francisco: Sierra Club.

FERGUSSON, ERNA
1957   *Dancing gods.* Albuquerque: University of New Mexico Press.

FEWKES, JESSE WALTER
1897   Tusuyan totemic signatures. *American Anthropologist*, o.s. 10:1–11.
1903   "Hopi katcinas," in *Twenty-first annual report of the Bureau of American Ethnology*, 3–126. Washington: United States Government Printing Office.

FLETCHER, ALICE, FRANCIS LA FLESCHE
1911   "The Omaha tribe," in *Twenty-seventh annual report of the Bureau of American Ethnology*, 17–654. Washington: United States Government Printing Office.

FOX, ROBIN J.
1967   "Witchcraft and clanship in Cochiti therapy," in *Magic, curing, and witchcraft.* Edited by John Middleton, 255–283. Garden City, New Jersey: Natural History Press.

FRAZER, SIR JAMES GEORGE
1966   "Sympathetic magic," in *The golden bough* (third edition). New York: St. Martin's Press.

GAY, CARLO T. E.
1967   Oldest paintings of the New World. *Natural History* 76:28–30.

GIFFORD, E. W.
1936   Northeastern and western Yavapai. *University of California Publications in American Archaeology and Ethnology* 34:290 ff.
1940   Cultural elements distribution: XII Apache-Pueblo. *University of California Anthropological Records* 4:154 ff.

GIFFORD, E. W., A. L. KROEBER
1937   Cultural element distribution: IV Pomo. *University of California Publications in American Archaeology and Ethnology* 37:117–254.

GIMBUTUS, MARIJA
1956   *The prehistory of Eastern Europe.* American School of Prehistoric Research, Peabody Museum, Harvard University Bulletin 20.

GJESSING, GUTORM
1958   "Petroglyphs and pictographs in the Coast Salishan area of Canada," in *Miscellanea Paul Rivet octogenario dicata.* Mexico City: Universidad Nacional Autónoma de Mexico.

GLADWIN, H. S., E. W. HAURY, E. B. SAYLES, N. GLADWIN
1965   *Excavations at Snaketown.* Tucson: University of Arizona Press.

GRANT, CAMPBELL
1965   *The rock paintings of the Chumash.* Berkeley: University of California Press.
1967   *Rock art of the American Indian.* New York: Thomas Y. Crowell.

GRAZIOSI, PAOLO
1960   *Paleolithic art.* New York: McGraw-Hill.

GRIEDER, TERENCE
1966 Periods in Pecos style pictographs. *American Antiquity* 31:710–720.
GUDDE, E. G.
1960 *Caifornia place names.* Berkeley: University of California Press.
GUNN, SISVAN W. H.
1966 Totemic medicine and shamanism among the northwest American Indians. *Journal of the American Medical Association* 196: 700–706.
HECKWELDER, JOHN
1876 History, manners, and customs of the Indian nations. *Memoirs of the Historical Society of Pennsylvania* 12:47–432.
HEIZER, ROBERT F., MARTIN A. BAUMHOFF
1959 Great Basin petroglyphs and game trails. *Science* 129:904–905.
1962 *Prehistoric rock art of Nevada and eastern California.* Berkeley: University of California Press.
HOFFMAN, W. V.
1883 Comparison of Eskimo pictographs with those of other American aborigines. *Transactions of the Anthropological Society of Washington* 2:1–19.
1891 "The Midewiwin or Grand Medicine Society of the Ojibwa," in *Seventh annual report of the Bureau of Ethnology.* Washington: United States Government Printing Office.
1896 "The Menomi Indians," in *Fourteenth annual report of the Bureau of Ethnology.* Washington: United States Government Printing Office.
HOWEY, M. OLDFIELD
1955 *The encircled serpent.* New York: Arthur Richmond.
HRDLIČKA, ALEŠ
1905 "The paintings of human bones among the Indians," in *Annual report of the Smithsonian Institution, 1904.* Washington: United States Government Printing Office.
JAMES, EDWIN
1956 *A narrative of the captivity and adventures of John Tanner during thirty years' residence among the Indians* (second edition). Minneapolis: Ross and Haines.
JONES, CHARLES C., JR.
1873 *Antiquities of the southern Indians.* New York: D. Appleton.
JOSEPHY, ALVIN M., JR., editor
1961 *The American Heritage book of Indians.* Photograph and caption: 156. New York: Simon and Schuster.
Journal of the American Medical Association
1960 Asclepius — man or myth? *J. Amer. Med. Ass.* 172:245.
KEITHAHN, E. L.
1940 The petroglyphs of southeastern Alaska. *American Antiquity* 6: 123–132.
KILGAUER, FREDERICK G.
1959 Medicine in art. *What's New* 215:43–45.

KIRKLAND, FORREST
1940 Pictographs of Indian masks at Hueco Tanks. *Bulletin of the Texas Archaeological and Paleontological Society* 12:9–29.

KIRKLAND, FORREST, W. W. NEWCOMB, JR.
1967 *The rock art of Texas Indians.* Austin: University of Texas Press.

KROEBER, A. L.
1925 *Handbook of the Indians of California.* Bureau of American Ethnology Bulletin 78. Washington: United States Government Printing Office.

KUHN, HERBERT
1952 *Die Felsbilder Europas.* Stuttgart: W. Kohlhammer.
1969 *Kunst der Eiszeit.* (Color slides.) Slide number 7. Heidelberg: V.-Dia Verlag.

LAMBERT, MARJORIE F.
1967 A Kokopelli effigy pitcher from northwestern New Mexico. *American Antiquity* 32:398–400.

LANDES, RUTH
1968 *Ojibwa religion and the Midewiwin.* Madison: University of Wisconsin Press.

LEEKLEY, THOMAS B.
1965 *The world of Manabozho.* New York: Vanguard Press.

LEROI-GOURHAN, ANDRE
1968 *The art of prehistoric man in Western Europe.* London: Thames and Hudson.

LEVIN, M. G., L. P. POTAPOV
1964 "The Nanays," in *The peoples of Siberia.* Edited by M. G. Levin and L. P. Potapov, 691–720. Chicago: University of Chicago Press.

LEVIN, M. G., B. A. VASILYEV
1964 "The Evens," in *The peoples of Siberia.* Edited by M. G. Levin and L. P. Potapov, 670–684. Chicago: University of Chicago Press.

LISSNER, IVAR
1961 *Man, god, and magic.* New York: G. P. Putnam's Sons.

LOCHER, G. W.
1932 *The serpent in Kwakiutl religion.* Leiden: E. J. Brill.

LOMMEL, ANDREAS
1967 *Shamanism: the beginning of art.* New York: McGraw-Hill.

MALLERY, GARRICK
1886 "Pictographs of the North American Indians," in *Fourth annual report of the Bureau of Ethnology,* 13–256. Washington: United States Government Printing Office.
1893 "Picture-writing of the American Indians," in *Tenth annual report of the Bureau of Ethnology,* 3–882. Washington: United States Government Printing Office.

MALOUF, CARLING
1961 Pictographs and petroglyphs. *Archaeology in Montana* 3:1–13.

MARINGER, JOHANNES
1960 *The gods of prehistoric man* (first American edition). New York: Alfred A. Knopf.

MARINGER, JOHANNES, HANS-GEORG BANDI
1953   *Art in the Ice Age*. London: George Allen and Unwin.

MARSHAK, ALEXANDER
1970   The Baton of Montgaudier. *Natural History* 79:57–63.

MASON, J. ALDEN
1945   Costa Rican stonework (the Minor C. Keith Collection). *Anthropological Papers of the American Museum of Natural History* 39:189–318.

MAUI HISTORICAL SOCIETY
1964   *Lahaina historical guide*, 1–52. Honolulu: Star-Bulletin.

MC CLINTOCK, WALTER
1936   Painted tipis and picture-writing of the Blackfoot Indians. *Masterkey* 10:123–124.

M.D. Medical Newsmagazine
1959a   Reptilian record. *M.D. Medical Newsmagazine* 3(4):131–134.
1959b   The epic of medicine: epidermal art, drum data. *M.D. Medical Newsmagazine* 3(5):89–161.
1966   Grandeur and misery of the symbols: symbols of medicine. *M.D. Medical Newsmagazine* 10:9–181.
1972   Men of magic. *M.D. Medical Newsmagazine* 16:227–232.

Medical Tribune
1965   Medicine in the making. *Medical Tribune* (December 25-26):9–29.

MOONEY, JAMES
1900   "Myths of the Cherokee," in *Nineteenth annual report of the Bureau of American Ethnology*, 3–548. Washington: United States Government Printing Office.

MORSS, NOEL
1954   *The clay figurines in the American Southwest*. Papers of the Peabody Museum of American Archaeology and Ethnology, Harvard University 49.

NELSON, EDWARD W.
1899   "The Eskimo about Bering Strait," in *Eighteenth annual report of the Bureau of American Ethnology*, 3–518. Washington: United States Government Printing Office.

NEWCOMB, FRANC JOSEPH, STANLEY FISHER, MARY C. WHEELWRIGHT
1956   A study of Navajo symbolism. *Papers of the Peabody Museum of Archaeology and Ethnology, Harvard University* 32:6–33.

OKLADNIKOV, A. P.
1964   "Ancient populations of Siberia and its culture," in *The peoples of Siberia*. Edited by M. G. Levin and L. P. Potapov, 13–98. Chicago: University of Chicago Press.
1969   Die Felsbilder am Angara-Fluss bei Irkutsk, Siberien. *Jahrbuch für Prähistorische und Ethnographische Kunst* 22:18–20.
1970   *Yakutia, before its incorporation into the Russian state*. Arctic Institute of North America, Anthropology of the North: Translations from Russian Sources 8. Montreal: McGill Queens University Press.

PAYEN, LOUIS A.
1959   Petroglyphs of Sacramento and adjoining counties, California.

University of California Archaeological Survey Report 48:66–83.
1968 A note on the cupule sculptures in exogene caves from the Sierra Nevada, California. *Caves and Karst* 10:33–40.

POPOV, A. A.
1964 "The Nganasans," in *The peoples of Siberia.* Edited by M. G. Levin and L. P. Potapov, 571–581. Chicago: University of Chicago Press.

POPOV, A. A., B. O. DOLGIKH
1964 "The Kets," in *The peoples of Siberia.* Edited by M. G. Levin and L. P. Potapov, 607–619. Chicago: University of Chicago Press.

POTAPOV, L. P.
1964a "The Shors," in *The peoples of Siberia.* Edited by M. G. Levin and L. P. Potapov, 440–473. Chicago: University of Chicago Press.
1964b "The Altays," in *The peoples of Siberia.* Edited by M. G. Levin and L. P. Potapov, 305–341. Chicago: University of Chicago Press.
1964c "The Khakasy," in *The peoples of Siberia.* Edited by M. G. Levin and L. P. Potapov, 342–379. Chicago: University of Chicago Press.

PRAUS, ALEXIS
1962 The Sioux, 1798–1922, a Dakota winter count. *Cranbrook Institute of Science* 44:1–10.

PROKOF'YEVA, E. D.
1964 "The Nentsy," in *The peoples of Siberia.* Edited by M. G. Levin and L. P. Potapov, 547–570. Chicago: University of Chicago Press.

RAFINESQUE, CONSTANTINE, C. F. VOEGELIN, ELI LILLY, ERMMIE VOEGELIN
1954 *Walum Olum.* Indianapolis: Indiana Historical Society.

RAU, CHARLES
1881 *Observations on cup-shaped and other lapidarian sculptures in the Old World and in America.* Washington: United States Government Printing Office.

RENAUD, ÉTIENNE B.
1938 Petroglyphs of north central New Mexico. *Archaeological Survey Series* 11:20–36.
1948 Kokopelli, a study in Pueblo mythology. *Southwestern Lore* 14: 25–40.
1953 Some anthropomorphic petroglyphs and pictographs. *El Palacio* 60:283–295.

RITTER, DALE W.
1961 X-ray petroglyph in Nevada. *Screenings* 10:4.
1965 Petroglyphs, a few outstanding sites. *Screenings* 14:1–4.
1970 "Sympathetic magic of the hunt as suggested by petroglyphs and pictographs of the western United States," in *Valcamonica Symposium, Acts of the International Symposium on Prehistoric Art.* Edited by Emmanuel Anati, 397–421. Capo di Ponte: Centro Camuno di Studi Preistorici.

RITTER, DALE W., ERIC W. RITTER
i.p. *Medicine men and spirit animals in the rock art of western North America.* Publication of the Institute for Comparative Research in Human Culture, Norway.

ROBERT, ROMAIN, L. R. NOUGIER
1961–1962 *Art treasures of prehistoric man.* (Color slide series with caption cards.) New York: Cultural History Research.

RUDENKO, SERGEI I.
1970 *Frozen tombs of Siberia, the Pazyryk burials of Iron Age horsemen.* Berkeley: University of California Press.

SANGINES, CARLOS PONCE
1969 *Tunupa y Ekako.* Academia Nacional de Ciencias de Bolivia, Publicación 19, 5–288. La Paz.

SCHAAFSMA, POLLY
1963 Rock art in the Navajo Reservoir District. *Museum of New Mexico Papers in Anthropology* 7:34–66.
1965 "Southwest Indian pictographs and petroglyphs." Pamphlet. Santa Fe: Vergara Printing Co.
1966 "Early Navaho rock paintings and carvings." Museum of Navajo Ceremonial Art pamphlet. Santa Fe.

SCHOOLCRAFT, HENRY R.
1851 *Antiquities, history, conditions, and prospects of the Indians of the United States,* part one. Philadelphia: Lippincott, Grambo.
1852 "Art of recording ideas (pictography)," in *Antiquities, history, conditions, and prospects of the Indian tribes of the United States,* part two. Philadelphia: Lippincott, Grambo.

Screenings
1964 Illustration and caption. *Screenings* 13:1.
1966 Illustration and caption. *Screenings* 15:1.

SIMS, AGNES
1950 *San Cristobal petroglyphs.* Santa Fe: Southwest Editions.

SMITH, WATSON, LOUIE EWING
1952 *Kiva mural decorations at Awatovi and Kawaika-a.* Papers of the Peabody Museum of American Archaeology and Ethnology, Harvard University 37.

SPENCER, BALDWIN, F. J. GILLEN
1968 *The native tribes of central Australia* (originally published 1899). New York: Dover.

SPINDEN, HERBERT JOSEPH
1957 *Maya art and civilization.* Indian Hills: Falcon's Wing Press.

SQUIER, E. G.
1851 *The serpent symbol in America.* American Archaeological Researches 1.

STEVENSON, MATILDA COXE
1904 "The Zuñi Indians, their mythology, esoteric fraternities, and ceremonies," in *Twenty-third annual report of the Bureau of American Ethnology, Smithsonian Institution.* Washington: United States Government Printing Office.

STEWARD, JULIAN H.
1929 *Petroglyphs of California and adjoining states.* Berkeley: University of California Press.

STRONG, EMORY
1959 *Stone Age on the Columbia River.* Portland: Metropolitan Press.

1969   *Stone Age in the Great Basin.* Portland: Binfords and Mort.
Sunset Magazine
1968   Photograph and caption. *Sunset Magazine* (August): 30.
SWAUGER, JAMES L.
1962   An X-ray figure on the Timmons Farm petroglyph site. *West Virginia Archaeologist* 14:34–35.
1964   The Timmonh Farm petroglyph site 46-Oh-64. *West Virginia Archaeologist* 17:1–8.
1968   The dam no. 8 petroglyph site 33 Co. 2. *Ohio Archaeologist* 18: 4–11.
TANNER, CLARA LEE
1957   *Southwest Indian painting.* Tucson: University of Arizona Press.
Understanding
1962   The rock that made rain. *Understanding* (November): 10–11.
UNIVERSITY OF COLORADO
1970   School of Medicine brochure. Boulder: University of Colorado Press.
VASILEVICH, G. M., A. V. SMOLYAK
1964   "The Evenks," in *The peoples of Siberia.* Edited by M. G. Levin and L. P. Potapov, 620–654. Chicago: University of Chicago Press.
VILLASENOR, DAVID
1963   *Tapestries in sand.* Healdsburg: Naturegraph.
VOGEL, VIRGIL J.
1970   *American Indian medicine.* Norman: University of Oklahoma Press.
VYATKINA, K. V.
1964   "The Buryats," in *The peoples of Siberia.* Edited by M. G. Levin and L. P. Potapov, 203–242. Chicago: University of Chicago Press.
WEDEL, WALDO R.
1961   *Prehistoric man on the plains.* Norman: University of Oklahoma Press.
WELLES, RALPH E., FLORENCE B. WELLES
1961   *The big horn of Death Valley.* Fauna of the National Parks of the United States, Fauna Series 6. Washington: United States Government Printing Office.
WELLMAN, KLAUS F.
1970   Kokopelli of Indian paleology, hunchbacked rain priest, hunting magician, and Don Juan of the old Southwest. *Journal of the American Medical Association* 212:1678–1682.
WHEELWRIGHT, MARY C.
1938   *Tleji or Yehbechai myth.* Museum of Navajo Ceremonial Art Bulletin 1.
1946   *Wind chant and feather chant.* Museum of Navajo Ceremonial Art Bulletin 4.
1958   *Red Ant myth and shooting chant.* Museum of Navajo Ceremonial Art Bulletin 7.
1962   *Eagle catching myth and bead myth* (revised edition). Museum of Navajo Ceremonial Art Bulletin 3.

WHITE, J. R.
1952   *Sequoia and Kings Canyon National Parks.* Palo Alto: Stanford University Press.

WHITE, LESLIE A.
1932   "The Acoma Indians," in *Forty-seventh annual report of the Bureau of American Ethnology,* 17–192. Washington: United States Government Printing Office.

WILDSCHUT, WILLIAM
1960   *Crow medicine bundles.* Contributions from the Museum of the American Indian, Heye Foundation 17.

WILSON THOMAS
1896   "The swastika," in *Report of the United States National Museum, 1894,* 757–1017. Washington: United States Government Printing Office.

1898   "Prehistoric art," in *Report of the National Museum, 1896,* part two, 331–664. Washington: United States Government Printing Office.

WINCHELL, N. H.
1911   "Pictographs and carvings," in *The aborigines of Minnesota.* Minnesota Historical Society: 564 ff. Saint Paul: Pioneer.

Cross-Cultural Perspectives on Midwifery

SHEILA COSMINSKY

All human societies have patterned sets of beliefs and practices concerning pregnancy, delivery, and the puerperium. Some societies have a specialist who is primarily concerned with these matters. This specialist is referred to as a "midwife."

This paper examines the variations that exist in the status and role of the midwife, primarily in non-Western societies, and considers some of the changes occurring with the spread of Western or modern medicine. Specific aspects that are analyzed are recruitment, acquisition of skills and knowledge, training, status, the midwife's role in prenatal care, delivery, and postnatal care.

The United States has witnessed the decline of midwifery with the rise of the obstetrician and other medical specialists (Stern 1972). Today, however, a renewed interest and the beginning of a resurrection of the midwife, or nurse-midwife, seem to be gradually occurring. Another is the realization that the United States' infant mortality rate is higher than at least fourteen other countries. Haire (1972) has made a comparative study of obstetric techniques and procedures in these countries and suggests that highly trained midwives are an important source of obstetrical care for normal women in countries which have a lower rate of infant mortality, e.g. in Norway, 96 percent of deliveries are by midwives. The emotional support given to mothers during the prenatal and labor stages seems to be accompanied by a lessened need for obstetrical intervention and medication during labor. Questions are being raised about various obstetrical practices used in the United States, such as the value of the supine position for delivery, the separation of the mother from her family, pathologic effects of chemical stimulation of labor, use of forceps, and performing routine episiotomies. Some of the questions that are raised in this paper concern the implications of the spread of certain of these practices to other parts of the world.

DEFINITIONS

The use of the term "midwife" ranges from referring to anyone who assists at birth, whether a specialist or not, to that employed by the World Health Organization (W.H.O.), which stresses professional training and formal education. Qualified and trained, according to a committee report (W.H.O. 1966) means at least secondary school education and training in scientific medicine. W.H.O. considers indigenous midwives together with any birth attendant as a "traditional birth attendant," who "mostly have no training at all in midwifery, but are usually well versed in folklore relating to maternal and infant care and are likely to be among the most highly respected members of their communities" (1966: 16). W.H.O. is developing programs for bringing the traditional birth attendant into the cadre of health personnel. However, the amount of training and education that they recommend is not feasible in many parts of the world and thus the traditional attendant, including indigenous specialists, will never attain the status of midwife according to W.H.O. standards.

Many ethnographic reports also do not differentiate a specialized status of midwife from any birth attendant. It is often difficult to ascertain whether such a status even exists. One of the problems in doing a cross-cultural study is the comparibility of these categories. For example, among the Navajo, Lockett (1939) says that the midwife was a special status referred to by a special name. Leighton and Kluckhohn (1947) say that any female, although usually a relative, may attend birth; sometimes a "semi-professional" person is summoned. What does "semi-professional" mean? Is this the same status to which Lockett refers? What are the qualifications and training of such a person that make him or her "semi-professional?"

The indigenous midwife (e.g. *partera, comadrona, bidan, dai*) is referred to in the literature by a variety of terms, such as "empirical midwife" (Kelly 1965) or "lay midwife" (Osgood, et al. 1966), to distinguish them from licensed midwives who have formal medical education or degrees. Various societies also use different terms to distinguish them. In Vietnam, *ba mu vuon*, the traditional midwife, is distinct from the *nu ho sinh*, the government licensed midwife (Coughlin 1965). In

Ica, Peru, native midwives are called *parteras*, whereas hospital-trained and licensed midwives are known by rural women as *profesoras*, the general term for people who deal in book knowledge (Wellin 1956).

For purposes of this paper, the term midwife refers to a position which has been socially differentiated as a specialized status by the society. Such a person is usually regarded as a specialist and a professional in her own eyes and by her community.

The main emphasis in this paper is on general statements, problems, and trends concerning midwives in different societies, especially non-Western ones. Only a few selected ethnographic examples will be presented.

CHARACTERISTICS, RECRUITMENT, AND TRAINING

Ford (1945) found elderly women assisting at birth in fifty-eight cultures and not assisting in only two. Most midwives are females. A few cases of male midwives, however, have been reported (Mexico, Philippines, Appalachia).[1]

Midwives also tend to be elderly and/or to have had children of their own. The majority are past the childbearing age, which means they are freer to assume midwifery responsibilities. In contrast, the government midwifery programs tend to train younger people. This person may also be unmarried and have no children, which might negatively affect her status in the community, especially as an expert on childbirth (Blum and Blum 1965: 154). In areas where both types of midwives exist, the formally trained one may be put in a supervisory position (Greece, India). Where age confers respect, this can and does create problems.

Some programs have recommended an age limit for midwives, such as 65 (Lamson 1934), or 70 (Mongeau, et al. 1960). It is at this age, however, when the midwife is often at the peak of her career. She is also probably training a younger assistant. The average age of "granny" midwives in a rural southern U.S. community was 66 (Mongeau, et al. 1960) and in Appalachia it was 70 (Osgood, et al. 1966). This age restriction would effect another change in the pattern of the midwife's status. The implications of such changes in age characteristics should be investigated.

A person may become a midwife through supernatural calling, inheritance, or voluntarily by her own means. In societies where supernatural agents are important in the selection and training of midwives, they

[1] Since most midwives are females, although a few males do practice midwifery, the feminine pronoun will be used in this paper when referring to midwives.

usually appear in dreams or visions (Guatemala, Ojibwa, Philippines, rural southern United States). In some cases, these visions are interpreted by a diviner as indicating the person should be a midwife. The midwife claims that her skills and knowledge are taught in a dream or vision. In Guatemala, a midwife has usually been sickly, and the shaman divines the cause as a warning from God to take up her calling or destiny as a midwife. If she refuses, she or her family will be punished more severely by God. Other signs of her calling include having been born with a caul and finding certain objects, such as oddly shaped stones and a knife or scissors. Hart (1965: 26) points out that the supernatural source and validation of the midwives' skills give them an increased sense of adequacy and protect them by minimizing their liability.

Supernatural training may be combined with a pattern of inheritance. In some parts of the Philippines, the visions bringing knowledge of midwifery come from third-generation relatives, such as one's parents' grandparents (Hart 1965). Inheritance is the primary means of recruitment and training in some societies (Sudan, Vietnam, Peru).

A special variation of the inheritance pattern occurs in India, where the position of midwife (*dai*) is relegated to the lowest castes or the untouchables, and caste membership is inherited.

The most common pattern of training and acquiring skills is apprenticeship or assistant status to another midwife, often a relative (Ojibwa, Peru, Mexico, Appalachia, rural southern U.S.). Even where the midwife claims to receive her knowledge from dreams or vision, she has also often been an apprentice to another midwife (Philippines, Ojibwa). In some societies, as in parts of the Philippines, various combinations of recruitment and training patterns occur (Rubel, et al. 1971).

W.H.O. reports that two-thirds of the babies in the world are delivered without a trained attendant (W.H.O. 1966). They do not consider apprenticeship as training. Only formal Western medical training is acceptable. Much of the literature stresses the lack of any "professional" training of scientific knowledge. The bias in the use of the term "training" is reflected in the following comment by an Indian villager, who was visited by a government health visitor encouraging antenatal clinic visits. The health visitor said that the midwife was all right, "but she had no training." The villager was amazed "and asked how any person could be untrained if she had delivered babies all her life" (Gideon 1962).

Kelly (1956) has suggested that the main areas in which the traditional midwife needs training are: (1) basic principles of hygiene and asepsis, (2) prenatal and postnatal advice and care, and (3) recognition of cases beyond her capacities, which, if possible, should be referred to a doctor. However, the midwife, through extensive experience, is often skillful in calculating the month of pregnancy, gauging the position of the fetus (Kelly 1956), and in dealing with the anxieties of her clients. Landes (1938) says that the Ojibwa midwife is a "highly skilled occupation, depending on an extensive herbal knowledge, detailed knowledge of female anatomy and physiology, varied massage techniques, and a cool and resourceful intelligence." As Wellin has emphasized (1956), native midwives do not lack education but possess a certain kind of education and command certain kinds of knowledge and understanding, which are integrated into the whole fabric of social life.

Nevertheless, W.H.O. states that "it is recognized that, without a system for regular supervision, the traditional birth attendant CANNOT [emphasis added] maintain a level of ACCEPTABLE performance. For this reason, it is essential that provision for supervision and guidance be an integral part of any programme destined to train and utilize the traditional birth attendant" (1966: 16). Although it may be beneficial to have some guidance and supervision, such a statement is patronizing and condescending and should be questioned. When such attitudes are exhibited in attempted programs, they may lower the status and authority of the traditional birth attendant or midwife and make her doubt her own sense of adequacy, although the aim of the program may be to raise it. Mongeau, et al. (1960) point out in their study of the "granny" midwife that changes brought about by the government training program have made her overcautious. This brings approval from the Health Department, but increases anxiety on the part of the patient.

STATUS

The midwife usually occupies a respected position, although variation does exist in her status in different societies. With the influence of modern medical programs, her position often becomes an ambiguous one. Hospital personnel, medical practitioners, and the educated classes tend to assign her a low status, regarding her as superstitious, ignorant, and dangerous (Wellin 1956). Within her community, however, she is usually respected and enjoys considerable status. In some cases, her use of modern techniques and medicines increases her prestige.

Kelly (1956) reports that the midwife enjoys a moderately high status in some *mestizo* areas of Mexico, but in indigenous areas, she sometimes has little personal prestige and is selected for her alleged esoteric powers, rather than for her skills. The reverse is generally true in Guatemala. Ladinos express distrust and fear of midwives, pointing out that many women die during childbirth in the village and desire to go to the city hospital (Solien de González 1963). On the other hand, in Indian communities, the midwife has comparatively high prestige and is respected for her skills, although supernatural sanctions may add to her status.

The position of the midwife has varied in the Western world, as shown by her decline in the United States and the present highly developed midwifery programs in England and several European countries. In the fifteenth, sixteenth, and seventeenth centuries, however, the midwife was criticized by the church and state, and frequently considered as a witch and condemned. The use of any spells or traditional rituals was interpreted as witchcraft. Midwives were accused of infanticide and giving unbaptized babies to the devil. Municipal ordinances were enacted to regulate the practice of midwifery and enforce training (Forbes 1966).

Times have not changed very much in this respect. In Peru, native midwives are classed with "native curers," "witches," or "sorcerers" as a species of empiricism or quackery and are outside the legal pale. On the local level, however, no one interferes with their practice (Wellin 1956). In a recent study of medical practices in Mexico, Schendel (1968: 145) writes: "The majority of quack-curers [his translation of *curanderos*] — many of them part-time street vendors or dirty old crones — function basically as midwives." Although he says only a small number of these "quacks" are self-styled witches or *brujos*, according to Public Health doctors and the Mexican Secretary of Public Health, Dr. Amézquita, "They are all witchdoctors." However, for the sake of better public relations, these unlicensed practitioners are officially referred to not as quacks or witchdoctors, but as untrained midwives. Midwifery is after all, one of their most active roles. It is also probably the role in which they possess the greatest potentiality for harm" (Schendel 1968: 169). The lumping together of curers, witches, and midwives for these Mexican societies not only goes against most anthropological evidence, which indicates these are highly specialized statuses, but is also very ethnocentric and should be avoided.

Mexico, nevertheless, recognizing the importance and influence of the midwife, has started several training centers. Both old midwives and young girls who want to enter the profession are given a free one-year training course, living on the premises and receiving free room and board. They are then certified to serve as auxiliary nurses. Kelly (1965) has made a proposal of an anthropological approach to midwifery programs in Mexico. When programs are run by the Public Health doctors and nurses who have the attitude that native midwives are all quacks and witches, one wonders to what degree the suggestions that Kelly made are being taken into account. To my knowledge, there have been no anthropological studies of these programs, and this is a vital area for future investigation.

The indigenous midwife in India (the *dai*) occupies a status at the low end of the scale. Due to the belief that birth is an unclean and polluting process, only a person of low caste or an untouchable is allowed to deliver the baby, cut the cord, dispose of the placenta, and change the bandages. Midwifery is the traditional occupation of the castes of Chamars or leatherworkers (Briggs 1920), sweepers (Minturn and Hitchcock 1963), and barbers (Ghosh 1968). The nurse midwife, who has had about eighteen months of hospital training in midwifery and nursing, usually belongs to one of the higher village castes, for example the Jat or a farmer caste. However, she will not dispose of the placenta or cut the cord. She either brings an untouchable woman to do that, or the family has to get one, so that it is necessary to pay another person. Consequently, the pregnant woman is reluctant to use the nurse-midwife (Ghosh 1968; Gordon, et al. 1964). There are an increasing number of indigenous midwives who have received some scientific training in midwifery programs and also perform the traditional duties because of their low caste.

One of the problems in the spread of Western medicine is exporting the same status consciousness which American obstetricians and physicians exhibit. Some examples were mentioned above. This problem is also illustrated by changes currently taking place in Japan, where various types of formal midwifery training have existed since A.D. 772, incorporating new medical knowledge when necessary. A law was passed in 1947 which will in time eliminate all practitioners who are not high-school and nursing-school graduates, and who have not taken a supplementary course in their specialty. The emphasis on midwifery reforms developed partly from criticism by the Occupation Forces of Japanese medical service qualifications. Standlee warns that these changes "may in time remove the nurse from the bedside care of the patient . . . it is to be hoped that it will not create the unrest, dissatisfaction, and personnel poverty that followed the imposition of an academic caste system among nurses in the United States" (1959: 139). The enforced grafting of a Western doctrine on a midwifery pattern that has served a society satisfactorily for over a thousand years should be questioned.

PRENATAL CARE

The role of the midwife during the prenatal period may vary from a minimal one, as in the Punjab (Gordon, et al. 1964) where the midwife usually does little until labor begins, to a more active one, as in Mexico and Guatemala. There the midwife is selected between the fourth and seventh month and visits the woman weekly or monthly. Time and frequency of visits vary between villages and may depend on the health of the mother and whether she is a primapara or a multipara.

The most common prenatal practice is that of ABDOMINAL MASSAGE. Massage is thought to make birth easier and allows the midwife to determine the position of the fetus and change it if necessary. One Guatemalan midwife told the author that she massages the woman, "little by little, not forcefully. If you rub with force, she will die." In some areas, however, massaging is heavier, and Foster attributes many miscarriages in Tzintzuntzan, Mexico, to heavy massaging. Hart (1965) stresses that vigorous massage or extreme manual rotation performed less than six weeks before labor can cause premature separation of the placenta from the uterus.

In some African societies, during the last month, the midwives manually dilate the passages to prevent obstructed labor. Gelfand (1964) suggests that one possible advantage of manual dilation is the apparent rarity of peritoneal tears. He suggests that despite the increased risk of infection, childbed fever is rare amongst African mothers. Unfortunately Gelfand generalizes about African mothers without making it clear to which specific societies he is referring, and such generalizations are open to serious question. He may be referring primarily to the Shona, among whom he worked.

The midwife often administers medicines, usually herbal teas, and gives advice on proper diet and exercises. In many societies certain foods are proscribed because they will make the body "cold" or harm the fetus (Philippines, Vietnam, Mexico, Guatemala).

Pregnancy is regarded as normal and not a cause for anxiety in some societies; in others, it is regarded as a "sickness" or as a period of danger, both physically and supernaturally. In some cases, modern medical practitioners have increased this anxiety. A government midwife in a Greek town said only if women are afraid will they go to a doctor (Blum and Blum 1965). The Hutterites in the United States are non-anxious about pregnancy and have their own midwives. Thus there is no motivation for prenatal examinations by physicians. Certain doctors have tried to secure patient interest in regular obstetric care by impressing upon them the hazards of pregnancy. Eaton points out (1958) that this may function to prevent a few cases of infant mortality and maternal deaths, but is "paid" for in part by an increase in anxiety among Hutterite women. One can raise the question as to whether this anxiety contributes to a more difficult labor and causes other problems.

Antenatal clinics are increasingly being included in medical programs for health education and to prevent birth complications. People at first do not consider such clinics necessary (Turtell 1965; Kendall 1953; Ghosh 1968) but through the influence of successful patients, acceptance is gradually increased. In Accra, Ghana, Goodman (1951) reports that people regard the clinics as social gatherings with the opportunity of obtaining free or cheap medicines. Where attendance is sporadic, the medical effects on the patients are doubtful (van Amelsvoort 1964). Nevertheless, they provide the opportunity of treating anemias, chronic malaria, helminthiasis, and of detecting possible birth complications (Goodman 1951; Turtell 1965).

In some societies, midwives perform abortions (Mexico, India, Greece). These may be for unwanted pregnancies or as a method of birth control. Midwives are also called if a spontaneous abortion or miscarriage is feared and may administer herbal infusions or other treatments to prevent miscarriages. Midwives also administer various medicines and perform rituals believed to help barren women (Beals 1946).

DELIVERY

In many societies, the mother is secluded in either a special hut or a partitioned part of the house (Ford 1945). This isolation may be due to the belief that the mother is in a polluted state or that the mother and newborn are highly susceptible to physical and supernatural dangers. In some places, as in parts of India, birth is highly secretive: the house is shut, and the woman is not supposed to cry out (Gordon, et al. 1964). This is to protect her from spirits and people who might want to do her harm. In a few societies (Navajo, Iban) birth is a more communal and public affair, there is no seclusion, and relatives and neighbors may attend.

Labor and delivery usually occur in the same location. Generally, in the United States, however, the mother is moved to a delivery room separate from the one in which she was in labor. Doris Haire (1972), while visiting hospitals in different parts of the world, saw a tendency to increase moving. For example, in the Orient, new hospitals tend to have delivery rooms built separate from labor rooms so that the woman must be moved as she approaches birth. Experiments on mice have shown that subjection to environmental disturbances during labor caused significantly longer deliveries and the disturbed mice gave birth to 54 percent more dead pups than did the control group. The effect on humans of environmental disturbance has not been studied (Haire 1972).

One or more persons usually assist the midwife. These attendants are most frequently elderly females, although some societies require the husband to assist and support the parturient (Mexico). The presence of relatives as birth assistants gives emotional support to the woman.

Patterns of management of labor range from "laissez faire" to an extreme speeding up of labor (as in the United States). As with prenatal care, the most commonly reported pattern is abdominal massage and pressure, often rubbing on some type of oil or herbal mixture. The dangers of placental separation or ruptured uterus were mentioned above (Hart 1965). However, Norman Casserly, a male midwife in the United States,[2] points out that massage during delivery keeps the blood flowing and the pelvic musculature relaxed, and neither external nor internal tearing occurs. The hormone relaxin renders joints and muscles flexible, rubbery, and there is no need for episiotomy (*Prevention* 1972).

Haire (1972) has summarized the disadvantages of routine episiotomies as practiced in the United States and says that obstetricians and gynecologists in many countries tend to agree that a superficial first degree tear is less traumatic to the perineal tissue than an incision which requires several sutures for reconstruction. Such operations are rare in non-Western societies, but crude episiotomies are carried out by village midwives in the northern Sudan because of labor difficulties due to female circumcision (Jeliffe and Bennett 1962: 69).

A particular type of manipulation known as heeling is reported for the Punjab (Gideon 1962: Gordon, et al. 1965). The midwife exerts pressure and countertraction with each labor pain with her feet on either side of the birth canal. The midwife also lubricates the vaginal canal with clarified butter or oil.

Midwives can be important agents of change, through which various Western practices are spread. One such change that has been occurring in some places is the substitution of the supine position for delivery for the traditional one of kneeling, sitting, or squatting (Kelly 1965; Madsen 1965: 89–138). One Guatemalan ladino midwife said that she

---

[2] Norman Casserly is a male midwife in the United States who practices the methods of natural childbirth. He has been barred from practice on the grounds of practicing medicine without a license. He is appealing his case claiming that pregnancy is a normal condition, not a pathological one, and consequently he was not practicing medicine.

"has not been able to change the position of delivery and considers it very unbecoming for her, as a practical nurse, to follow the Indian pattern" of kneeling (Reina 1966). Although most American doctors advocate the flat supine position, research suggests that it makes spontaneous delivery more difficult, and thus increases the use of forceps, episiotomies, chemical induction of labor, and other forms of interference (Haire 1972; Mead and Newton 1967). Such substitutions may therefore be more harmful if they abolish a practice which actually may be a safer one.

Herbal and patent medicines are frequently used by midwives to ease labor pains and/or to speed up labor (Arikara, Cherokee, Buganda, Guatemala, Mexico). Some medical personnel feel that the use of herbs, some of which have been shown to have oxytocic effects, whether for normal or delayed labor is dangerous (Jeliffe and Bennett 1962; Billington, et al. 1963; Schendel 1968). An underlying assumption is that the midwife uses these herbs indiscriminately and ignorantly. However, in many cases, part of the midwive's special knowledge is the amounts of such herbs to be used for various purposes and the effects of these amounts. The condemnation of indigenous herbal medicines, while using other forms of oxytocic agents, analgesics, and anaesthetics, which have unknown effects and some of which research is showing are harmful to the mother and fetus (Haire 1972) is hypocritical, ethnocentric, and dangerous.

Attempts to induce gagging, vomiting, sneezing, blowing in a bottle in order to make the muscles contract are frequently used in cases of difficult or prolonged labor. The midwife may also employ techniques based on a sympathetic magical connection, such as unlocking bolts and locks, opening drawers and doors, untying the mother's hair, and using charms made from molts of animals. The midwife may also perform various rituals, say prayers, and listen to confession from the parturient. In some societies, difficult labor is regarded as a sign of marital infidelity and the mother is urged to confess (Gelfand 1964).

Abnormal presentations and multiple births usually present complications, which may result in infection or death. Some midwives manipulate the fetus externally (Mexico) or use techniques of oiling and attempting to extend the vagina and manipulate the fetus internally (India). Surgery seems to be rare. Where medical assistance is available, midwives are urged to either send for a doctor or send the patient to the hospital if they suspect complications. In some societies, the midwife performs infanticide, particularly in cases of multiple births or deformed babies.

In most societies, the midwives give encouragement, emotional support, relieve pain, and allay anxiety; in a few groups (Buganda), the opposite seems to be the case — midwives increase the pain and discomfort, especially in the attempt to speed up labor (Ford 1964). The effects of these activities are a matter on which little research has been done and should be pursued.

W.H.O. has reported that one of the outstanding developments in maternity care is the increase in the number of deliveries taking place in hospitals or maternity centers. Where this has occurred, domiciliary deliveries have decreased and the midwife is used mostly for prenatal and postnatal care. Ghosh (1968) suggests that where this is the case, midwives be asked to take more active part in health education, family planning, and immunization programs. Van Amelsvoort (1964) raises the question of the extent to which hospital deliveries actually reduce mother and child mortality. In the Asmat region of New Guinea, he says they had no figures or estimates to show whether normal delivery in the village was an important cause of mortality or that hospital delivery actually reduced mortality. Figures from a nearby area indicate that home delivery is not the main cause of fatalities of mother and child.

In most parts of the world, there is a shortage of medical personnel and hospitals are overcrowded. An increase in normal hospital deliveries puts an additional drain on hospital personnel and budget (van Amelsvoort 1964). Several authorities advocate home deliveries in a familiar environment with trained midwives, improved antenatal work, and better cultural contact rather than routine hospital admissions. Hospital deliveries should be recommended only if there are indications of complications (Stein and Susser 1959; Roberts 1960; Killen 1960; van Amelsvoort 1964).

In areas where homes are scattered and transportation difficult, midwives may have difficulty practicing domiciliary midwifery. Another alternative is practiced by some "qualified" and "trained" Buganda midwives. They run private maternity centers in their own homes. Women come to stay in the midwife's house to await delivery, where they enjoy a homey atmosphere and help around the house. The mother usually stays with the midwife for about three days after delivery (Billington, et al. 1963).

THE PLACENTA AND UMBILICAL CORD

The placenta is usually expelled without manual assistance. In cases of delayed expulsion, many of the same techniques for delayed labor are used — e.g. massage or abdominal pressure, medication, rituals, attempts to make the woman gag, sneeze, or vomit.

In societies where the placenta is believed to affect the future life of the child, the disposal of the placenta and cord may be a cause of anxiety in hospital deliveries (Wellin 1956). A few hospitals in northern Mexico deliver the placenta to the family upon request. Kelly (1956) suggests that this practice could be adopted elsewhere.

In most non-Western societies, the placenta is expelled before the umbilical cord is cut. Occasionally, the midwife squeezes the blood in the cord toward the infant's navel before cutting (Cherokee, Guatemala). The cord is usually tied with thread, string, or plant fiber, at a specific length which varies widely in different societies. Where the cord is customarily not tied (Buganda), the danger of hemorrhage exists.

Traditional methods of cutting and dressing the cord have been criticized as possible factors causing tetanus neonatorum, either because the cutting instrument is not clean or the dressing material is contaminated. Cutting tools include bamboo, shell, broken glass, knife, scissors, shears, sickles, trowels, and razors. Coughlin (1965) reports that in Vietnam, considerable numbers of tetanus cases result, according to medical sources, from the use of bamboo or glass. Custom forbids the use of any metal instrument for cutting the cord, lest the child be mute. No statistics are given, however. What is the rate of tetanus? How does this compare to the rate when other methods are used? In parts of Mexico and Guatemala, the midwife cauterizes the cord with either a candle flame, a burning end of a stick, or a red-hot blade, and applies hot candle wax (McKay 1933; Gerdel 1949; Romney and Romney 1963; Solien de González and Béhar 1966).

A study made by Gordon, Gideon, and Wyon (1964, 1965) in the Punjab attempts to determine which specific techniques of cutting and dressing the cord, employed by the various categories of midwives (untrained midwives, trained midwives, and nurse-midwives), are statistically associated with neonatal deaths, especially from tetanus. In nine out of twelve cases of tetanus, the dressing was ash made from cow dung and earth. While ash itself has some aseptic properties, the cow dung may have unburned particles or chance contamination. The sickle was the cutting instrument associated with the highest death rate. This study is a model which should be followed to investigate the actual effects of various methods used by midwives, rather than the blanket condemnation of these practices without evidence of detrimental effects.

TREATMENT OF THE NEWBORN

The newborn is sometimes slapped on the buttocks, held upside down, or sprinkled with water to make it cry. Various rituals are also performed. The child may be cleaned with oil or washed in lukewarm water. Usually the midwife visits and cleans the baby several times during the first week or two. The midwife may clear the baby's throat and nose of mucus and blood with her fingers, which could be a source of infection. The baby's eyes may be wiped with a rag or cotton, treated with a drop of lemon juice, oil, onion, flowers of Castille and San Juan, boric acid, or patented eye drops. Medicines are often given to prevent illness (Buganda) and purgatives administered to clean the meconium (Philippines, Mexico, Peru, India).

Various amulets may be used and the midwife may perform various rituals to protect the baby from diseases such as the evil eye (India, Peru, Mexico). Curing such illnesses of the infant is often another function of the midwife (Guatemala, Mexico, Peru). Rituals may also be performed which symbolize the sex identity of the baby (Mexico). The midwife may read certain signs of the child's and mother's fate, such as caul births, position of birth, lines on the umbilical cord, and the time of birth (Mexico, Guatemala, Thailand, Philippines). Shaping of the baby's head, nose, and limbs is also a function of the midwife in some societies (Zuñi, Chagga).

POSTNATAL TREATMENT OF THE MOTHER

Little information is available on the immediate treatment after birth, especially concerning treatment of wounds of the birth canal and the vaginal area. Alcohol, salt, and various herbs are sometimes used to prevent infection (Thailand, Vietnam).

One of the most widespread postnatal practices is the binding of the mother's abdomen (abdominal binders are also often used prenatally). Patent medicated plasters may also be applied (Guatemala). Medicines of various kinds are often taken to recover strength and decrease soreness and pains. In many areas, the midwife massages the abdomen and the uterus area to ease after-pains, and massages the breasts to stimulate the flow of milk. This pattern is often combined with the application of heat. In indigenous parts of Guatemala and Mexico, the sweatbath is used. Throughout Southeast Asia (Thailand, Vietnam, Philippines, Iban, India) heat is applied by "mother roasting" or "lying by the fire."

At the end of the convalescent period, various rituals may be held in which the midwife plays an important part. In addition to restoring the mother's relationships with relatives and friends, and marking the return of the mother to normal activities, these rituals usually mark the end of the midwife's duties (Guatemala, Philippines).

CONCLUSION

Maternal and child health programs and midwifery training programs should have as fundamental points of reference the local body of beliefs and practices associated with pregnancy, birth, and postnatal care and the role played by the indigenous or local specialists. Kelly (1965) says that the cultural background can be analyzed in terms of three interrelated areas: (1) avoidance of unnecessary conflict with existing culture patterns, (2) exploitation of elements of the local culture which are favorable or neutral, and (3) delineation of harmful practices, which should be combated. Jeliffe and Bennett (1962), along similar lines, suggest an unprejudiced analysis of these beliefs to physical and psychological health, on the basis of current scientific principles.

As I have tried to point out in this paper, these are programmatic statements which have yet to be followed, hopefully by an unprejudiced analysis. Most of the literature dealing with either proposed or developed programs condemn many of the traditional beliefs and practices concerning childbirth and blame infant and maternal mortality on the midwives. Few systematic studies have been made demonstrating the actual effects of specific practices, especially in terms of morbidity and mortality rates. Hardly any anthropological studies exist of midwifery training programs, or maternal and child health programs, their effects and their relationship to traditional midwifery. An important need exists for anthropological research in planning, running, and evaluating such programs.

Table 1. Ethnographic and medical sources

Africa

Buganda	Billington, et al. 1963; Roscoe 1911
Chaga	Raum 1940
Ghana (Accra)	Goodman 1951
Nigeria (Ile-Ife)	Long 1964; Turtell 1965
Sudan	Kendall 1953
South Africa (Alexandra Township)	Stein and Susser 1959
General	Gelfand 1964

Asia

China	Lamson 1934
Iban	Jensen 1967
India	Briggs 1920; Fuchs 1939; Ghosh 1968; Gideon 1962; Gordon, Gideon, and Wyon 1964, 1965; Minturn and Hitchcock 1963; Mistry 1952; Sarker, Choudhuri, and Ray 1955; Singh 1947; Stevenson 1920
Japan	Standlee 1959
Philippines	Ewing 1960; Frake 1957; Hart 1965; Nydegger and Nydegger 1963; Rubel, et al. 1971
Thailand	Wales 1933; Anuman Rajadhon 1965
Vietnam	Coughlin 1965

Europe

Greece	Blum and Blum 1965

North America
American Indian

Arikara	Gilmore 1930
Cherokee	Oldbrechts 1931
Navajo	Leighton and Kluckhohn 1947; Lockett 1939
Ojibwa	Landes 1937, 1938
Zuñi	Leighton and Adair 1963
Appalachia	Osgood, Hochstrasser, and Deuschle 1966
Hutterites	Eaton 1958
Rural South	Mongeau, Smith, and Maney 1960

Latin America

Guatemala	Bunzel 1959; Cosminsky 1972; Rodríguez Rouanet 1970; Reina 1966
Mexico	Beals 1946; Foster 1948; Gerdel 1949; Kelly 1965; Lewis 1960; Madsen 1965; McKay 1933; Redfield and Villa Rojas 1934; Romney and Romney 1963; Schendel 1968
Peru	Wellin 1956

Oceania

New Guinea	van Amelsvoort 1964

REFERENCES

ANUMAN RAJADHON, P.
1965   "Customs connected with birth and the rearing of children," in *Southeast Asian birth customs*. Edited by D. Hart. New Haven: Human Relations Area Files Press.
BEALS, R.
1946   *Cheran: a Sierra Tarascan village.* Smithsonian Institution, Institute of Social Anthropology, Publication 2.
BILLINGTON, W. R., H. F. WELBOURN, K. C. WANDERA
1963   Custom and child health in Buganda; III: Pregnancy and childbirth. *Tropical and Geographic Medicine* 15:134–137.

BLUM, R., E. BLUM
    1965   *Health and healing in rural Greece.* Stanford: Stanford University
           Press.
BRIGGS, G.
    1920   *The Chamars: the religious life of India.* Calcutta: Association
           Press.
BUNZEL, R.
    1959   *Chichicastenango: a Guatemalan village.* Seattle: University of
           Washington Press.
COSMINSKY, S.
    1972   "Decision-making and medical care in a Guatemalan Indian com-
           munity." Unpublished Ph.D. dissertation, Brandeis University.
COUGHLIN, R.
    1965   "Pregnancy and birth in Vietnam," in *Southeast Asian birth
           customs.* Edited by D. Hart. New Haven: Human Relations Area
           Files Press.
EATON, J.
    1958   "Folk obstetrics and pediatrics meet the M.D.," in *Patients, phy-
           sicians, and illness.* Edited by G. Jaco, 207–221. Glencoe: Free
           Press.
EWING, J.
    1960   Birth customs of the Tawsug. *Anthropological Quarterly* 33:129–
           132.
FORBES, T. R.
    1966   *The midwife and the witch.* New Haven: Yale University Press.
FORD, C.
    1945   *A comparative study of human reproduction.* Yale University
           Publications in Anthropology 32. New Haven: Yale University
           Press.
    1964   *Field guide to the study of human reproduction.* New Haven:
           Human Relations Area Files Press.
FOSTER, G. M.
    1948   *Empire's children: the people of Tzintzuntzan.* Mexico City:
           Nuevo Mundo.
FRAKE, C.
    1957   Post-natal care among the eastern Subanun. *Silliman Journal*
           4:207–215.
FUCHS, S.
    1939   Birth and childhood among the Balahis. *Primitive Man* 12:71–84.
GELFAND, M.
    1964   *Medicine and custom in Africa.* London: E. and S. Livingston.
GERDEL, F.
    1949   A case of delayed afterbirth among the Tzeltal. *American An-
           thropologist* 51:158–159.
GHOSH, B. N.
    1968   An exploratory study on midwifery practice of the local indige-
           nous dais in Pondicherry and utilization of domiciliary midwifery
           services of a health centre by a semi-urban slum community.
           Indian Journal of Public Health 12:159–164.

246   SHEILA COSMINSKY

GIDEON, H.
1962   A baby is born in the Punjab. *American Anthropologist* 64:1220–1234.
GILMORE, M.
1930   Notes on gynecology and obstetrics of the Arikara tribe of Indians. *Papers of the Michigan Academy of Science, Arts, and Letters* 24:71–82.
GOODMAN, L.
1951   Obstetrics in a primitive African community. *American Journal of Public Health* 41:56–64.
GORDON, J., H. GIDEON, J. WYON
1964   Childbirth in rural Punjab. *American Journal of Medical Science* 247:344–357.
1965   Midwifery practices in rural Punjab. *American Journal of Obstetrics and Gynecology* 93:734–742.
HAIRE, D.
1972   The cultural warping of childbirth. *ICEA News.* International Childbirth Association.
HART, D.
1965   "From pregnancy through birth in a Bisayan Filipino village," in *Southeast Asian birth customs.* Edited by D. Hart. New Haven: Human Relations Area Files Press.
JELIFFE, D. B., F. J. BENNETT
1962   World-wide care of the mother and newborn child. *Clinical Obstetrics and Gynecology* 5:64–84.
JENSEN, E.
1967   Iban birth. *Folk* 8–9:165–178.
KELLY, I.
1956   An anthropological approach to midwifery training in Mexico. *Journal of Tropical Pediatrics* 1:200–205.
1965   *Folk practices in north Mexico.* Austin: University of Texas Press.
KENDALL, E.
1953   A short history of the training of midwives in the Sudan. *Sudan Notes and Records* 33:42–53.
KILLEN, O.
1960   Rural health centres in Kiambu. *East African Medical Journal* 37:204–215.
LAMSON, H.
1934   *Social pathology in China.* Shanghai: The Commercial Press.
LANDES, R.
1937   *Ojibwa sociology.* New York: Columbia University Press.
1938   *Ojibwa woman.* New York: Columbia University Press.
LEIGHTON, D., J. ADAIR
1963   *People of the Middle Place.* Human Relations Area Files.
LEIGHTON, D., C. KLUCKHOHN
1947   *Children of the people.* Cambridge: Harvard University Press.
LEWIS, O.
1960   *Tepoztlán: village in Mexico.* New York: Holt, Rinehart and Winston.

LOCKETT, C.
1939   Midwives and childbirth among the Navajo. *Plateau* 12:15–17.

LONG, L. D.
1964   Sociocultural practices relating to obstetrics and gynecology in a community of West Africa. *American Journal of Obstetrics and Gynecology* 89:470–475.

MADSEN, C.
1965   *A study of change in Mexican folk medicine.* Middle American Research Institute, Publication 25.

MC KAY, K.
1933   "Mayan midwifery," in *The peninsula of Yucatan.* Edited by G. Shattuck, 64–65. Carnegie Institute of Washington, Publication 431.

MEAD, M., N. NEWTON
1967   "Cultural patterning of perinatal behavior in childbearing — its social and psychological aspects," in *Childbearing — its social and psychological aspects.* Edited by S. Richardson and A. Gutmacher. New York: Williams and Wilkens.

MINTURN, L., J. HITCHCOCK
1963   *The Rajputs of Khalapur, India.* New York: John Wiley.

MISTRY, J. E.
1952   "Indigenous midwifery," in *The economic development of India.* Edited by V. Anstey, Appendix A. London: Longmans Green.

MONGEAU, G., H. SMITH, A. MANEY
1960   The "granny" midwife: changing role and functions of a folk practitioner. *American Journal of Sociology* 66:497–505.

NYDEGGER, W., C. NYDEGGER
1963   *Tarong: an Ilocos barrio in the Philippines.* New York: John Wiley.

OLDBRECHTS, F. M.
1931   Cherokee belief and practice with regard to childbirth. *Anthropos* 26:17–33.

OSGOOD, K., D. HOCHSTRASSER, K. DEUSCHLE
1966   Lay midwifery in southern Appalachia. *Archives of Environmental Health* 12:759–770.

Prevention
1972   Mister midwife of San Diego. *Prevention.*

RAUM, O.
1940   *Chaga childhood.* London: Oxford University Press.

REDFIELD, R., A. VILLA ROJAS
1934   *Chan Kom.* Chicago: University of Chicago Press.

REINA, R.
1966   *The law of the Saints.* New York: Bobbs-Merrill.

ROBERTS, J.
1960   Rural health projects in North Nyanza. *East African Medical Journal* 37:186–203.

RODRÍGUEZ ROUANET, F.
1970   Prácticas médicas tradicionales de los indígenas de Guatemala. *Guatemala Indígena* 4:52–86.

ROMNEY, K., R. ROMNEY
1963   *The Mixtecans of Juxtlahuaca*, Mexico. New York: John Wiley.
ROSCOE, J.
1911   *The Baganda*. London: Macmillan.
RUBEL, A., W. LIU, M. TROSDAL, V. PATO
1971   "The traditional birth attendant in metropolitan Cebu, the Philippines," in *Culture and population*. Edited by S. Polgar, 176–186. Chapel Hill: Carolina Population Center.
SARKER, A., N. CHOUDHURI, G. S. RAY
1955   Birth and pregnancy rites among the Oraons. *Man in India* 35: 46–51.
SCHENDEL, G.
1968   *Medicine in Mexico*. Austin: University of Texas Press.
SINGH, M.
1947   *The depressed classes: their economic and social condition*. Bombay: Hind Kitab.
SOLIEN DE GONZÁLEZ, N.
1963   Some aspects of child-bearing and child-rearing in a Guatemalan ladino community. *Southwestern J. of Anthropology* 19:411–423.
SOLIEN DE GONZÁLEZ, N., M. BÉHAR
1966   Child-rearing practicies, nutrition, and health status. *Milbank Memorial Fund Quarterly* 44:77–96.
STANDLEE, M.
1959   *The great pulse: Japanese midwifery and obstetrics through the ages*. Rutland, Vermont: Charles Tuttle.
STEIN, A., M. SUSSER
1959   A study of obstetric results in an under-developed community. *Journal of Obstetrics and Gynecology of the British Empire* 65: 763–773; 66: 62–74.
STERN, C. A.
1972   Midwives, male-midwives, and nurse-midwives: an epitome of relationships and roles. *Obstetrics and Gynecology* 39:308–311.
STEVENSON, M.
1920   *The rites of the twice-born*. London: Oxford University Press.
TURTELL, B. M.
1965   Midwifery and midwife training in Nigeria. *Nursing Times* 61: 1664–1665.
VAN AMELSVOORT, V.
1964   *Culture, stone age and modern medicine*. Assen: Van Gorcum.
WALES, H. G.
1933   Siamese theory and ritual connected with pregnancy, birth, and infancy. *Journal of the Royal Anthropological Institute of Great Britain and Ireland* 63:441–451.
WELLIN, E.
1956   Pregnancy, childbirth, and midwifery in the valley of Ica, Peru. *Health Information Digest for Hot Countries* 3.
WORLD HEALTH ORGANIZATION
1966   *The midwife in maternity care. Report of a WHO expert committee*. WHO Technical Report Series 33.

Cerro Sechin: Medical Anthropology's Inauguration in Peru?

FRANCIS X. GROLLIG, S.J.

In Peru there are many well-known archaelogical zones. Travel ads have popularized, for example, Machu Picchu, the fabulous "Lost City of the Incas." And, near to it, Cuzco is sometimes referred to as the "Archaelogical Capital of the New World." The fortress of Paramonga, perhaps a hundred yards east of the Pan-American Highway, like many other ruins, has been featured on Peruvian postage stamps. But Cerro Sechin has enjoyed none of this popularity.

Cerro Sechin is an ancient but comparatively small set of ruins. It is not a whole complex like the northern Chimu's capital, Chan-Chan; nor is it a great city, like Cajamarquilla, just outside of Lima; nor is it even a vast ceremonial site, like Pachacamac on the Pacific coast south of Lima. In fact, Cerro Sechin is like a diamond: little but beautiful. The main unit of this set of ruins that has been excavated to date is one marvelous little foundation. And of this, only three sides have been cleared. The southern façade is still buried deeply under the debris of, perhaps, thirty-five centuries.

On the way to Cerro Sechin, after leaving Lima, you pass through a veritable museum some 350 kilometers long. The cemetery of Chancay, the fortress of Paramonga, and the more recently cleared ruins of Manchan — to name just a few of the sites — are within viewing distance from the Pan-American Highway North. About eight kilometers south of Casma, the ruins of Cerro Sechin are located approximately one kilometer east of the highway. An access road leads right to the ruins. The two rivers, Moxeke and Sechin, which join to become the Río Casma just a short distance to the west of Cerro Sechin are but little trickles in the dry season (when I visited the area in 1971, 1972, and

1973), but they are veritable torrents in the wet season (Tello 1956: 21).

The ruins of Cerro Sechin were discovered by J.C. Tello and T. Mejía Xesspe on 1 July, 1937, when a lad fifteen years old, who had been hired by Tello as a day laborer, led them to "the stone with the 'Indio Bravo' engraved on it." And this was the first time that they saw such an engraved stone *in situ* on the coast (Kaufmann-Doig 1969: 263). In that season some two months of excavating uncovered ninety-eight such engraved stones: the walls (eastern, northern, and western) of the building that Tello (1956: 84–252) describes as the Cerro Sechin Temple.

After such an illustrious beginning, Cerro Sechin was ignored for nearly thirty years. A guard was appointed in 1965 by the Patronato Nacional de Arqueología, but funds failed, and the appointment was not renewed. Then, in 1969, Arturo Jiménez Borja with two associates began to reopen the excavations and probe further into the mysteries of Cerro Sechin (Reynaldo Trinidad 1972: 23). When we visited Cerro Sechin for the first time, 9 August, 1971, we met Lorenzo Samaniego Román, one of the associates of Jiménez Borja. Dr. Samaniego verbally dated the ruins at 1500 B.C. (Grollig 1971) — a date that corresponds closely to the "1600 a.n.e." B.C. Bueno Mendoza and Samaniego assigned in their article (1970: 31).

CERRO SECHIN: CHAVIN OR NOT CHAVIN?

In connection with the assigning of a date for Cerro Sechin, it is interesting to note that Tello simply considered these ruins as one of the many coastal manifestations of the Chavin culture (1960: 31), with a typical distribution of large and small monoliths (1960: 33). Moreover, Tello calls it a Chavin temple when he speaks of the helmeted heads and the hand-held axes and darts on the "fantastic series encountered in the relief carvings on the monoliths which adorn *el templo Chavin de Cerro Sechin*" (1960: 36). But Kaufmann-Doig (1969: 266) indicates that although Tello held that these are of Chavin parentage, "others think that these [relief] carvings do not manifest Chavin ancestry, but rather Cerro Sechin is truly *sui generis* and probably earlier than the classical phases of Chavin de Huantar."

Later del Busto Duthurburu adverted to Kaufmann-Doig's "*aloctonista*" theory for the origin of Peruvian culture (1970: 21), but labeled a photograph of Cerro Sechin's monolith G' (XXIII) "*Cultura Chavin: estela de piedra de Cerro Sechin que representa un guerrero vencido*"

(1970: 31), even though Lumbreras (1969: 112) had used exactly the same monolith in his text and had noted that the Cerro Sechin culture could have been before Chavin. Finally, on this point, Bennett and Bird, speaking of the monoliths of Cerro Sechin, insist: "This carving style is unique in Peru. The designs are based on the human figure, and there is no suggestion of the Chavin feline," a position with which we agree. Commenting on the antiquity of these carvings, the text goes on: "If, as present evidence suggests, this construction belongs in the Cultist Period, it must antedate the spread of the Chavin horizon" (1964: 100).

Needless to add, it is no doubt an oversimplification, but to a visitor who has seen both sites and carefully examined photographs and drawings of Chavin — as, for example, those given in Lumbreras' guide to Chavin (1970) — the contrasts seem greater than the comparisons. The feline-toothed figures, the stone-paved steps, the complicated carvings, etc. — all of these Chavin traits are missing at Cerro Sechin. Perhaps it is also significant when Rowe (1967: 73) is speaking about temples "in the Chavin style," he does mention "other famous shrines at Mojeque and Pallca in the Casma Valley," but Cerro Sechin is NOT noted.

Without attempting to dispute the function of the central structure of Cerro Sechin (Tello's "Temple"), we can take a look at it and read the hand-cutting on the wall. We agree 100 percent with the description given by Jiménez Borja (1970: 39), who says the "style of Sechin is figurative. It leaves nothing to the imagination."[1] Perhaps our approach is descriptive rather than analytical: we say what we see and, for the most part, we prescind from what it may mean.

Approaching the "Temple" of Cerro Sechin, the main (and only) entrance is on the north side of the structure. The clay stairway in the center of the north façade has survived centuries of earthquakes and is in remarkably good condition (Reynaldo Trinidad 1972: 23). The north façade ends with a rounded corner and now (1973) both the east and west façades are known to end in rounded corners, where they join the (as yet unexcavated) south wall.[2] The article *"Sobre el descubrimiento*

---

[1] This quotation and others from Spanish sources are translated from the original authors' Spanish by the author of this paper.
[2] The hope of finding yet more valuable materials has been intensified by the current excavations. In the notes (Grollig 1973b) from the visit to Cerro Sechin some references include the following remarks:
a. Test pits have gone into the wall of the building east of the main temple. One pit was covered. It was north of the north wall line and opened at ground level.
b. The south wall is still completely buried. Bits of pottery have been reported

de la cultura Chavin en el Perú" by Tello, which first appeared in *American Antiquity* (9[1], July 1943) and was reprinted by Ravines (1970: 69–110), is a splendid synopsis of the earliest information on Cerro Sechin. It gives the length of the north façade as fifty-two meters and describes the distributions of the large (*mayor*) and small (*menor*) monoliths.

Much more, of course, could be said by way of introduction. But let this suffice: all around the three excavated sides of the "Temple" there is a façade of monoliths, with a regular pattern of alternation between large and small monoliths (Lumbreras 1969: 111). In general, they are also in matched pairs — similar motifs are balanced to the east and to the west of the central stairs, etc.

Admitting that we do not know WHO produced Cerro Sechin, we must also admit that we do not know HOW it was produced. Buse (1957: 96) notes briefly that some technique of wearing off (*desgaste*) or friction (*frotación*) was used in such a way that no tool marks are visible. The style of the engraving of all of the stones is identical: Tello even said, "It is uniform in all of them. There are no fundamental differences. They were all produced by one artist, or by a group of artists trained in the same school" (Ravines 1970: 93). And Kaufmann-Doig (1963: 82) agrees with Tello. Admitting the antiquity, we prescind from the cultural affinity of the creators of Cerro Sechin and turn our attention to the individual blocks produced.

CERRO SECHIN: ANATOMY IN STONE

It would be an exaggerated claim to say that the Cerro Sechin archaeological zone includes the foundation of the first medical school in the New World. Nor are these the first medical textbooks—written in stone! But the fine, clear-cut monoliths of Cerro Sechin certainly do provide us, uncontestably, with a reflection of a knowledge of human anatomy which did exist in Peru as early as 1500 B.C.

With hardly 100 stones in the inventory (Table 1), it might seem like an exaggerated claim to say that we have here a complete course on human anatomy. But the details are certainly revealing. The human fig-

---

found. Most of them belong to a later date than the original culture. Most of the older fragments are but small pieces. Little more of the colored (interior) walls have been found to date.

They expect to continue the excavation until the complete temple area is uncovered. The whole north façade is reconstructed — using the fallen pieces. But a section of the east wall is still original.

Table 1.　Monoliths of Cerro Sechin

I	X4	XXVI	h'l	LI	F'	LXXV	a
II	X7	XXVII	i'	LII	f'2	LXXVI	al
III	X3	XXVIII	E	LIII	E'	LXXVII	g
IV	Xl	XXIX	g'	LIV	f'l	LXXVIII	gl
V	X2	XXX	j2	LV	g'l	LXXIX	fl
VI	X5	XXXI	m'l	LVI	e'l	LXXX	h
VII	D	XXXII	ll'	LVII	d'l	LXXXI	hl
VIII	A	XXXIII	k'	LVIII	D'	LXXXII	el
IX	I'	XXXIV	K'	LIX	B'	LXXXIII	j'l
X	J'	XXXV	G	LX	a'l	LXXXIV	k
XI	N'	XXXVI	?	LXI	f'	LXXXV	L
XII	X6	XXXVII	g2	LXII	e'	LXXXVI	ll
XIII	L'	XXXVIII	jl	LXIII	d'	LXXXVII	l
XIV	F	XXXIX	kl	LXIV	d'2	LXXXVIII	M
XV	H	XL	f	LXV	c'	LXXXIX	ml
XVI	J	XLI	c	LXVI	c'l	XC	m
XVII	K	XLII	C	LXVII	I	XCI	N
XVIII	i'l	XLIII	b	LXVIII	d	XCII	nl
XIX	h'	XLIV	bl	LXIX	M'	XCIII	n
XX	h'l	XLV	cl	LXX	il	XCIV	Ñ
XXI	H'	XLVI	j	LXXI	a'	XCV	ñ
XXII	B	XLVII	e	LXXII	A'	XCVI	O
XXIII	G'	XLVIII	?	LXXIII	b'l	XCVII	ol
XXIV	d'	XLIX	i	LXXIV	b'	XCVIII	m'
XXV	i'2	L	j'				

Based on inventory listing by Tello (1956: 146–228). Listed in the order in which the monoliths were discovered. Capital letters are used for major monoliths, small letters for minor ones. The major monoliths A to K are at the left of the north façade, A' to K' at the right of the steps.

In the east wall only thirteen monoliths — L, ll, l, M, ml, m, N, nl, n, Ñ, ñ, O, and ol — were discovered in the first excavations (Tello 1956: 216). In the 1937 excavations along the west wall, Tello says the digging proceeded only about six meters and they encountered only seven monoliths (L', M', N', k', l', m', and m'l).

ures (all males?) represent the range from dwarf to giants. Some are complete. Some are cut in half. Numerous isolated heads decorate the walls. The anatomical inventory includes: hair, eyes, tongue, teeth, lips, arms, legs, heels, fingernails, vertebrae, stomach, and intestines.

Although practically all of the stones — with such notable exceptions as the "Banner" stones, designated by Tello as A (VIII) and A' (LXXII) (1956: 146, 176) — and practically all of the monoliths of Cerro Sechin have anatomical details, it will not be necessary to recount them one by one.[3] Rather, therefore, a selection will be made of some of the anatomical features portrayed.

[3] According to information received at Cerro Sechin, Lorenzo Samaniego, the archaeologist in charge of the site (and the whole Peruvian coastal area near Sechin), is about to release a publication on the ruins that will be a guide to the zone.

Heads

The first feature which we will consider is a number of heads that are represented on the monoliths. These heads are severed from their bodies; they are heads, not skulls. It is perhaps a contrived coincidence that we begin with the stone which Tello (1956: 226) numbers "I" in his series. It is a head (X4) which Tello describes as having been discovered on 1 July, 1937, — the day of the discovery of Cerro Sechin. The stone itself is very irregular, and Tello speculates that perhaps this is a fragment from another large monolith. Benson (1972: 74) refers to Tello's work and illustrates this head from Tello (1956: 226, Figure 100). The representation of the human head here is of the simplest form. The full face is done with the usual single simple line, and the details of the face are also done, each with a simple line, for the mouth, the nose, and the eyes (closed). "The Dwarf" (Figure 1) is the only example of a "full frontal face" given in this paper.[4]

This kind of head is the same type as is seen on the large (*mayor*)

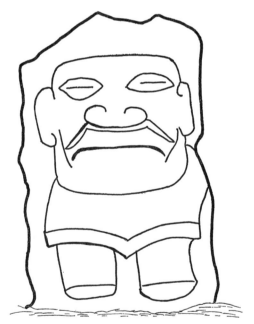

Figure 1.   The Dwarf (3058)

[4]   All of these figures were adapted from original color slides made by the author at Cerro Sechin, 1972. The slide number is given in parentheses after the title of the figure.

monoliths D (VII) and D' (LVIII) which have, on each one of them, twelve identical heads. These are portrayed in Tello (1956: 151, 183). On the two large monoliths there are two vertical columns each having six identical heads — a total of twelve heads on each monolith.

It is, perhaps, appropriate that we should begin with a discussion of the heads, because they are so numerous. There are probably more than fifty of the small (*menor*) monoliths that have one or two heads engraved upon them (Figures 2, 3, 4). In the southwestern corner of the foundation, for example, there are eight such monoliths with a total of nine heads on them — one has two heads (Figure 4).

The orientation of the heads is a bit difficult to understand; they face in all directions. Some are full-front views of faces; some are profile views. The profile-cut monoliths have the front (nose) of the face in all directions — up, down, and to either side (Figures 2, 3). In general, by contrast, the so-called warrior monoliths (Figure 5) and the other major monoliths seem to form a procession toward the central stairs.

We cannot agree with Tello (1956: 237), when he suggests that these heads "cannot be considered as perfectly human, since they are feline-like [*felinoide*]." More details on these several heads will be given in the next few paragraphs as we discuss some of the particular features of the head.

Hair

Considering the small number of possibilities, we find it interesting to note that the hair appears in several distinctively different styles. In some cases the hair comes out of the top of the head and is parted in the middle. This appears in a straight front view of the face; it is rare. Other than this there are several types portrayed: the hair comes out of the top of the head and goes over the front of the face (Figure 3), over the back of the head (Figure 2, bottom), or, more rarely straight up (Figure 6).

In all of these cases, the representation of the hair is simple: a few single lines define the straight, flowing locks. Generally, there are what appear to be three strands or bunches of hair. Rarely — e.g. h'1 (XX) — four hanks of hair, and a few monoliths like X1 (IV) and X2 (V) have six strands. Once again, there is no attempt at realism; only the "rope" of hair, not the individual hairs, is delineated by the engravings on the monoliths. Some of these lines coming out of the head are thought to be braids of hair by which a trophy head is carried.

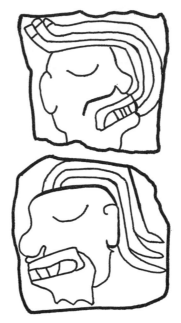

Figure 2.   Heads: (top) "Mayan" glyphs — or blood? (bottom) typical hair style (3061)

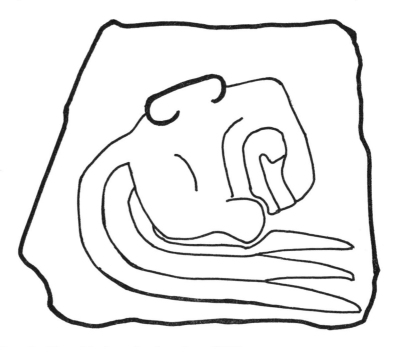

Figure 3.   Vanquished warrior, face down (3050)

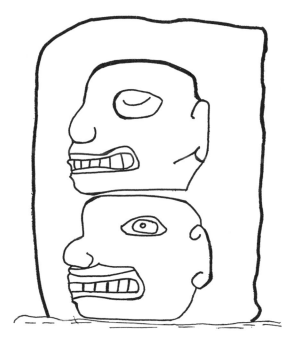

Figure 4. Monolith with two heads (3051)

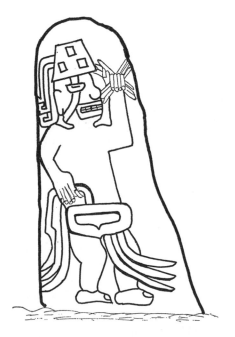

Figure 5. Warrior with darts: Tello, K (XVII) (3078)

Lips and Teeth

These two features we can deal with together. Some of the heads have the mouth closed, and then no teeth are visible (Figure 3). Others have only a line to indicate the mouth, and there is no representation even of the lips (Figure 1). But some have the lips open and then generally only the upper lip is shown.

With regard to the teeth, too, there is little variation. No attempt is made to differentiate among the different types of teeth. Thus, for example, you do NOT find exaggerated canines (as you would have if an attempt had been made to represent the feline form that is so common in Chavin sculptings). No case that we have seen presents the classic human dental formula (2–1–2–3 of incisors, canine, premolars, and molars). While a typical distribution of homodont dentition is given in monolith a′ (LXXI) as it is presented in Tello (1956: 195), where six upper and six lower teeth of the left side of the face are shown, they are all equal in width and there is no bite pattern indicated: all are flat-crowned (Figure 5). In addition to this geometric presentation of teeth, there are some mouths with only one set of teeth (not both uppers and lowers) shown (Figure 2), and some only indicate that teeth are present (Figure 7), but do not differentiate them as smaller units (Tello 1956: 241–242 and foldout).

Tongue

In the monoliths of Cerro Sechin some of the heads, e.g. j (XLVI) show the tongue extending out of the mouth. In other heads, however, the tongue is in the mouth, e.g. d′1 (LVII). Of this latter Tello (1956: 201) indicates that the line above the teeth is the tongue, and above this we find the upper lip.

In the interpretation of the monoliths of Cerro Sechin we noted that some of the figures have lines coming out of the mouth and proposed "this is reminiscent of Mayan carvings — but about 2,000 years older!" (Grollig 1973b). The monolith h′ (XIX) is an example of this, and Tello (1956: 210) says maybe the ends of the cords give the impression "of heads of serpents or tips of feathers" (Figure 2, top). This, of course, would strengthen the resemblance to the Mayan carvings at a site like Chichén Itzá — a point that Tello probably would not push too far. Later in this paper we suggest that perhaps these lines represent blood.

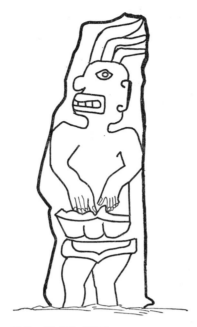

Figure 6.   Vivisection: Tello, J' (X) (3072)

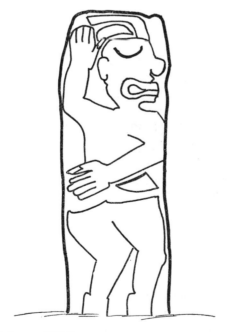

Figure 7.   Divided dancer (3081)

Another suggestion has also been made: these are cords coming out of the mouth similar to the cords with which the lips of the Jívaro trophy heads are tied shut (presumably to keep in the spirits) in the Amazon-Marañón basin. This, of course, fits with the Tello thesis for the origin of the culture traits that came from the jungle and coalesced in the civilization of Chavin. This, for him, was the matrix of all the Peruvian "high cultures."

Finally, we note that in at least one case, j (XLVI), Tello (1956: 174) was doubtful whether the lines represented the upper lip or perhaps the tongue.

Ears

Practically all of the heads on the monoliths have ears represented. Moreover, in practically all of these cases, the ears extend out from the head and the external vertical borders are flat. Curved hooks mark the top and bottom of each ear. This is consistent with the simple style of representation so familiar at Cerro Sechin.

In some of the figures — said to be warriors — the ears are prominent (Figure 5). The same is equally true of those called dancers (Figures 7 and 8). Del Busto Duthurburu (1970: 24) speaks of warriors when he says, "In the bas-reliefs of Cerro Sechin can be read the story of a great war, and victor and vanquished are personified in stone." In these cases the evidence of the victor is shown generally by the item held in the hands — a club, an axe, or darts, e.g. K (XVII), E' (LIII), or H' (XXI). The eyes are generally open. In the case of the vanquished, the eyes are generally closed, but there are some notable exceptions. For the dancers, Kaufmann-Doig (1969: 266) points out the similarity between these figures and the (perhaps) better-known figures of the dancers of Monte Albán in Mexico. He even illustrates his text with a juxtaposition of a Sechin figure and a Monte Albán dancer.

The two monoliths, D (VII) and D' (LVIII) each have two stacks of six heads and on each of these heads the ears are visible.

Eyes

All of the heads at Cerro Sechin have eyes; some are open, some closed. Other eyes are represented merely by a curved or straight line. Two monoliths, however, deserve special attention with regard to the use of

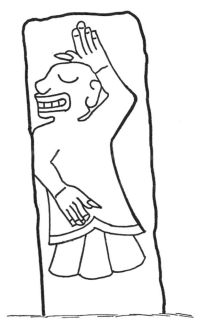

Figure 8. Bottomless dancer: Tello, G' (XXIII) (3071)

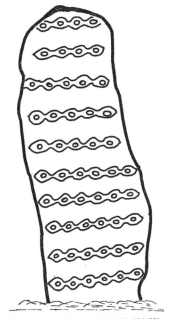

Figure 9. Eyes of Cerro Sechin: Tello, F (XIV) (3063)

eye motif, F (XIV) and F' (LI). In his description and discussion of these two moonliths, Tello (1956: 154, 187) uses three different Spanish words: *ojuelos* (little eyes), *discos pupilares* (eye pupils), or *anillos* (rings). These two monoliths show series of eyes apparently strung together (Figure 9). This, of course, could represent the horrendous practice of blinding captives. Later, we shall return to a captive (?) head which apparently has been given this treatment. Tello, in his text (1956: 162–163), discusses more fully the different types of eyes that are found on the monoliths of Cerro Sechin. Kaufmann-Doig (1963: 82) thinks the heads with closed eyes may be trophy heads (Figure 3).

Arms, Hands, Fingers, and Fingernails

The association of these different anatomical features is quite natural because the same stones which present one also present the others (Figure 10). We leave it a moot question: do the representations of the arms present cases of amputation or are they the result of the vindictive executioner's axe? The presence, for example, of the tip of the humerus extending from the severed arm (not shown here) may well indicate a surgical procedure. Tello considers X5 (VI) an example of an amputation (1956: 237). But, on the other hand, the whole context — when on the same monolith you have the carvings of two arms and two legs severed with no torso to attach them to — suggests the vindictive executioner's axe.

We do not know if it is significant or not, but the fact is that to date we have not seen a single case in which a hand is shown severed from an arm.

Some of the fingers are straight. And in this case you can see the middle finger is longer than the others (Figures 5 and 8). This type of realism is not unfamiliar on the stones of Cerro Sechin. In other cases, the fingers are bent, and there is a well-developed thumb with proximal phalanges (Figure 10). It is notable that the thumbnail is given extreme prominence in some of the figures — warriors, K (XVII) (Figure 5) and dancers, G' (XXIII) (Figure 8) alike. Curiously enough (though we have seen no reference to this in the literature), the dancer seems to have two left hands, each with a fine set of fingernails and an especially well-worked thumbnail.

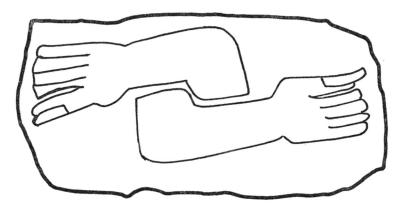

Figure 10. Arms, hands, fingers, and fingernails: Tello, f'2 (LII) (3070)

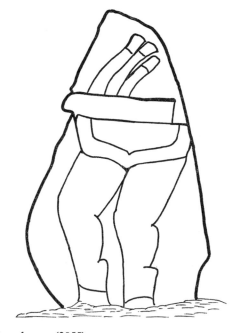

Figure 11. Topless dancer (3055)

Torso

Because the specific details of the parts of the torso are dealt with elsewhere in this article, here we will confine our remarks to noting that some cases, e.g. a monolith discovered after Tello, represent decapitated persons. From the way in which the neck terminates, it is possible that two strokes were used to sever the head from the shoulders.

In other cases, e.g. G (XXXV) and G′ (XXIII), you have just the top half of the torso represented (Figure 8). Another figure, el (LXXXII), shows just the bottom half (Figure 11) of the torso. Others such as J (XVI), J′ (X), and c′1 (LXVI), show a single person cut into two parts (Figures 6 and 7) at the belt line (Tello 1956: 235). Some of these will be further described when we discuss the intestines.

Blood

Perhaps we have in the monoliths of Cerro Sechin representations of blood. We believe this can be said of many of the monoliths. Again, we have not seen this discussed anywhere in the literature, but one can look at the monoliths and see a distinctly different type of symbol from that which is used to represent the hair. The difference lies in the distal end of the unit — if we may use that expression. The HAIR symbol ends in a point; the blood symbol ends in a squared unit almost like the fingernails. Such a representation as the "blood" symbol can be seen for example in monolith a (LXXV) where the blood comes out of the top of the head. The three strands do not terminate in the familiar pointed end, as hair representations do, e.g. monolith a1 (LXXVI). The contrast is noted in d′1 (LVII) where the hair symbol goes out the top of the head and what we are calling the blood symbol goes out of the bottom of the head, which in this case is cut off just below the chin. This monolith suggested the distinction between the two symbols. As a matter of fact, Tello (1956: 162–163, 203) gives some excellent representations of this comparison.

Our interpretation will allow an entirely different presentation for the monolith G′ (XXIX) than the one given by Tello, who says that the eye of this head is triangular and from it "come three hanks of hair" (1956: 208). We would say, rather, that this represents the excision of the left eye and the three lines are three streams of blood because the three units coming from the eye do not terminate in the usual pointed ends, to which we restrict the hair symbol (compare Figures 2, top, and 11 with others — Figures 2, bottom, and 6).

It is interesting to note that this same blood symbol is on two, XCVI and XCVII, of the last three monoliths discovered by Tello. He designated them as O and o1. He correctly guessed (1956: 220) when he said, "Later we discovered another monolith, probably a major one O (XCVI). . . ." But, apparently, these were never completely excavated by Tello.

Legs, Heels, and Toes

Essentially, all that we have to add in this category is the notation that a parallel to the presentation of the upper limbs exists in the picture of the lower limbs; just as the anatomical parts (arms, hands, fingers, and fingernails) are presented joined, so also, the lower parts are seen as a unit (legs, heels, and toes).

Although we refrain for the most part from discussing the interpretations of the monoliths of Cerro Sechin, we may make just one remark on the presentation of those who are called "the dancers": by their feet you shall know them (Figures 7 and 11)!

Vertebrae

Because the stones of Cerro Sechin, as was already remarked, "leave nothing to the imagination," when we discuss the vertebrae we find more excellently presented osteology — considering the times and the medium (stone) chosen. Tello (1956: 236) in speaking of these vertebrae says, "las cuatro facctas articulares marcados por medio de rectángulos." Here we have the presentation not merely of the spinal column, but of details, the articular facets of the spine (Figure 12). This is certainly intriguing for a presentation some 3,500 years old.

The major monoliths C (XLII), I (LXVII), I' (IX), and M (LXXXVIII) are examples of these. One (discussed below) has one of the vertebrae with some internal organs.

Stomach and Intestines

In some of the representations, the stomach and the intestines are presented as a part of a body. However, in one major monolith (unknown to Tello) is the delightful presentation of the internal organs, (stomach and intestines) without a body (Figure 13). These are shown below the (superior?) view of a vertebra with the clearly represented spinal foramen and three sections of heart valves. In this monolith the intestine has a fine loop. Because this monolith in the east wall lies to the south of ol (XCVII), we assume that Tello never saw it, and are, therefore, indebted to the recent excavations for a look at this new page in medical illustration. This is also true of several other of the monoliths illustrating the intestinal tract. One monolith shows a victim, still alive — his eyes

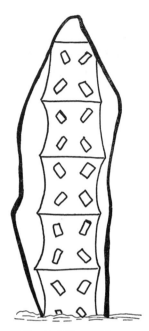

Figure 12.   Spinal column: Tello, I' (IX) (3072)

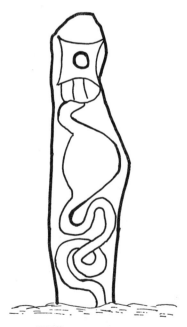

Figure 13.   Alimentary tract (3083)

are open — clutching at his stomach and intestines as they flow out where his lower torso has been cut off. Just to the north of this monolith there is another, which portrays a section of the intestines, including several loops of the same. Because the bottom (top?) of this monolith is buried by the present ground level, it is difficult to say whether there is a stomach on this monolith.

We do not claim to have found the first medical school in the New World, nor even to have found the first textbooks in stone. But the evidence seems to be clear enough: these people, 3,500 years ago, did have an accurate knowledge of human anatomy. Information like this, especially from the western hemisphere will be most welcome. Perhaps out of this eventually will come the history of the beginnings of medical anthropology.

REFERENCES

BENNETT, WENDELL C., JUNIUS B. BIRD
    1964   *Andean culture history* (second, revised edition). Garden City, New York: The Natural History Press.
BENSON, ELIZABETH, editor
    1972   *The culture of the feline.* Washington: Dumbarton Oaks Research Library and Collections.
BUENO MENDOZA, ALBERTO, LORENZO SAMANIEGO ROMÁN
    1970   Sechin: una nueva perspectiva. *Amaru: Revista de Artes y Ciencias UNI* 11.
BUSE, H.
    1957   *Huaras Chavin.* Lima: Juan Mejía Baca and P. L. Villanueva.
DEL BUSTO DUTHURBURU, JOSÉ ANTONIO
    1970   *Historia general del Perú — el Perú antiguo.* Lima: Librería Studium.
GROLLIG, S. J., FRANCIS X.
    1971   "Notes from Peru." Unpublished manuscript.
    1972   "Notes from Peru." Unpublished manuscript.
    1973a "Notes from Peru." Unpublished manuscript.
    1973b "Cerro Sechin monoliths: Casma, Peru." Unpublished manuscript.
JIMÉNEZ BORJA, ARTURO
    1970   El estilo Sechin. *Amaru: Revista de Artes y Ciencias UNI* 11.
KAUFMANN-DOIG, FEDERICO
    1963   *La cultura Chavin.* Lima: Peruano Suiza.
    1969   *Arqueología peruana.* Lima: Iberia.
KOSOK, PAUL
    1965   *Life, land, and water in ancient Peru.* Long Island, New York: Long Island University Press.
LUMBRERAS, LUIS G.
    1969   *Antiguo Perú.* Lima: Francisco Moncloa.
    1970   *Los templos de Chavin.* Lima: Proyecto Chavin.

RAVINES, ROGGER, *editor*
1970   *100 años de arquelogía en el Perú.* Lima: Instituto de Estudios
    Peruanos.
REYNALDO TRINIDAD, LEONCIO
1972   Sechin, 3500 años A.C. *Gente* 161.
ROWE, JOHN H., DOROTHY MENZEL
1967   *Peruvian archeology.* Palo Alto, California: Peek Publications.
TELLO, JULIO C.
1956   *Arqueología del valle de Casma.* Lima: San Marcos.
1960   *Chavin cultura: matriz del la civilización andina.* Lima: Imprenta
    de la Universidad de San Marcos.

The Use of Argillaceous Earth as Medicament

B. RÖMER

> If these pages should have the good fortune to attract the attention of a biochemist and physiologist and to stimulate them to a fresh investigation of the problems involved, I should feel amply rewarded for the trouble and time.
>
> BERTHOLD LAUFER [1]

Clay is formed in the breakdown of volcanic stone: basalt, granite, trachyte, and others. Aluminum silicate is found in the composition of these rocks along with aluminum, sodium, and silicon oxides. Water, containing dissolved carbon dioxide, dissolves the sodium silicate and the potassium silicate, leaving behind aluminum hydrosilicate (Supek 1971: 328).

The physical and chemical characteristics of argillaceous earths are dependent upon the nature of the hydrosilicates and their general relationship. In nature, however, argillaceous earths are never pure hydrosilicates of aluminum.

In the event that argillaceous earth is located at the place where it was formed in the decomposition of the volcanic rock, it is spoken of as argillaceous earth from the primary source and is then more or less whitish or greyish in color. Should the argillaceous earth have been removed from the original location by earthquake, water, or other physical factors, it is spoken of as argillaceous earth "of secondary source." Earths of these kinds contain various other elements which give them other colorations. The additions may be compounds of iron, calcium, or magnesium, as well as sand, carbon particles, remnants of

---

[1] In: "Geophagy," page 108.

vegetation, etc. The carbon particles may dye the earths blue or black; iron compounds may dye it yellow, greenish, or reddish.

Argillaceous earth is hygroscopic and absorbs much water, along with the various compounds dissolved in the water. In pharmacology argillaceous earth is termed bolus.

In this report the activated property of argillaceous earth is to be emphasized and shall therefore be discussed in greater depth. "Activated" is the term applied to those argillaceous earths which show a large adsorptive capacity. Such earths consist of very small particles (diameter = 0.1–1 micron). Every argillaceous earth contains a larger or smaller amount of such particles having this greater adsorptive capacity. In water these particles form a unique suspension, termed a colloidal suspension. The particles "hover" in the water. Clay particles present in a colloidal suspension have an enormous specific surface and for this reason an enormous specific surface energy as well and are, therefore, "active," i.e. they show a large adsorptive capacity (Lupibereza 1951: 59).

In ethnology the application of clay for curative purposes is frequently identified with geophagy, the eating of earth. Since argillaceous earth is applied externally as well, we will forgo a discussion of geophagy with respect to satisfying hunger, consumption as a delicacy, etc. Use of clay earths for curative purposes is well known in folk medicine throughout the world. It has its origins most probably in prehistoric times and is mentioned in the literature of classic antiquity, e.g. Hippocrates. Travel literature and ethnological writings were occupied with the problem of geophagy until the end of the last century, after which interest in this phenomenon waned. In the course of time various magic elements were attached to geophagy and, when the interest in magic in ethnology slackened, geophagy was shunted to the periphery of ethnology. Thus it was a large (and pleasant) surprise in professional circles when there appeared three excellent monographs: "Geophagy" (Laufer 1930), "Die Geophagie" (Stahl 1932) and "Geophagical customs" (Arnell and Lagercrantz 1958). In ninety printed pages Laufer worked over a voluminous mass of material which was arranged by continent. He recommended the materials to some future chemist, who, stimulated by Laufer's efforts, might arrive at scientific substantiations. Stahl characterizes his monograph with the subtitle: "Mit besonderer Berücksichtigung von Sudamerika"; he does not neglect to present the corresponding material from other regions along with the South American phenomena. Arnell and Lagercrantz provide instructive maps.

Geophagy is encountered most frequently among pregnant women in all parts of the world. The explanations for this phenomenon are extremely varied and often contradictory. It is stated, for example, that geophagy alleviates pregnancy-related nausea or that it stimulates nausea; fantastic and superstitious explanations are presented as well. In *Über die roten Erden* . . . (Ehrenberg 1868: 51) a rational explanation is attempted, namely that pregnant women eat clay so that the fetus will receive less nourishment making the delivery easier.

Modigliani (1892: 123) is of the opinion that geophagy relieves pregnancy-related nausea. Laufer (1930: 109) subscribes to the same opinion. Stahl (1932: 354) is prepared to draw a parallel between geophagy and the calcium preparations of modern birth aids; calcium preparations are prescribed for pregnant women as an aid in the skeletal development of the fetus. This may only be assumed for those clays which contain calcium compounds.

Pregnancy is not the only condition for which clay is eaten. Diarrhea, constipation, and syphilis, among others, are cured by clay; external application is made, for the most part, on wounds. Hippocrates maintained that clay possesses curative powers and recommended it as a purgative: "*Terram nigram samiam in aqua tritam, tali magnitudine praebeto*" (Hippocrates 1737). The medical ethnologists of the preceding century had already considered the possibility of the curative abilities of clay, e.g. Ploss, *Das Weib in der Natur- und Völkerkunde* (1897: 653), but this remained only a supposition; thus we are still able to read in Tischner's *Völkerkunde* (1959: 265) that "until now it has not been explained whether in geophagy it is a matter of consumption for pleasure or as a delicacy or whether it is practiced for medicinal reasons."

Almost ten years after Tischner's book appeared, the Rumanian doctor Alexandru Ispasescu published his treatise on geophagy, "Présence de la géophagie en Roumaine" (1968). Ispasescu is the first in ethnological literature to state without reservation the curative benefits of clay. He bases his opinion upon medical arguments. For Ispasescu, geophagy is an empirical treatment of illness by virtue of the aluminum silicates which are efficacious in absorbing and neutralizing secretions of pepsin and hydrochloric acid.

Ispasescu's conclusions are noteworthy and one is compelled to accept them, since, in contemporary medical practice of gastro-enterological therapy, other aluminum compounds are available as medicine. At the same time we want to emphasize that we would not yet attempt thus to explain the effectiveness of clay, as stated by Ispasescu, in the treatment of flatulence, infectious intestinal disorders, diarrhea, constipation, and poisonings, among others, and even less so for the external applications of clay. The strikingly frequent appearance of geophagy among pregnant women compels us to investigate whether clay is actually beneficial to them, how this is manifested, and which components of the clay possess the curative properties. The answers to these questions would perhaps also answer the question of the curative efficacy of clay in general. This is the question for whose answer ethnologists have searched for the last two hundred years.

Heringa in "Eetbare aarde van Sumatra" (1874: 186, 189) analyzed in Batavia a sizable number of clay types, which are effective against diarrhea, and has determined that the earths contain neither curative nor nourishing components. In South Australia Joseph Kearney, active for more than twenty years as a missionary, informed us that among the tribes of the Walmadjeri and the Sodadja it was customary to sprinkle wounds with clay, a custom superseded by antibiotics. Less Steward of the Wokaya tribe made it possible for us to examine the clay which is eaten for medicinal purposes and used in the treatment of wounds. Steward and other natives have assured us that this material is eaten not only by the pregnant women but by the men as well in treatment of abdominal distress.

This information led us to believe that here it was a matter of antibiotics, since modern medicine knows of a series of antibiotics which have been discovered in the earth: streptomycin, chloramphenicol, canamycin, etc. Negative results, however, from the investigation of clays from Australia with regard to antibiotic properties along with the spread of geophagy among pregnant women in the entire world (which could not be ascribed to antibiotic properties) compelled us to give up the idea of the antibiotics properties of clay.

An indication of where the answer to the question of the curative powers of clay could be found was given us by the great physician of antiquity – Hippocrates. Hippocrates states that pregnant women eat clay and charcoal (*Liber de superfoetatione*):

Si qua praegnans mulier terram edere concupiscat, aut carbones, eaque edit, in capite pueri, ubi natus fuerit, signum a talibus apparet.

He refers here to wood charcoal which was generally known at that time. Let us set aside Hippocrates' subjective opinion on the consequences of this custom and analyze the question of why exactly "clay and charcoal" appear together and what they have in common.

Let us first observe the characteristics of charcoal. It is generally known that charcoal (wood or animal charcoal) is used as a medicine in abdominal disorders, digestive disturbances, poisoning, etc. and that activated charcoal has a characteristic adsorptive effect. It is not difficult to establish a parallel between activated charcoal and clay when one considers the activated characteristic of clay, as explained earlier. However, this would provide a solution in and of itself only for cases of diarrhea and similar illnesses of the digestive organs, but not for geophagy among pregnant women, the most widespread instance in the literature of ethnology.

As is generally known, pregnant women suffer very often from flatulence, i.e. from a build-up of gases in the intestines, which results in cramps and other discomfort. This results from the displacement of the normal position of the intestines because of the increase in size of the womb and other hormonal causes. Without entering into the strictly medical area, we may assert that the activated argillaceous earth functions adsorptively, i.e. the intestines are relaxed and pressure on the stomach is reduced which results in some relief of nausea. It is interesting to note that some authors in the past had already observed that the adsorptive effect of clay possesses special qualities. This decisive characteristic of clay was, however, only mentioned, without being investigated more closely. In the nineteenth century the adsorptive nature of clay is mentioned in *Eetbare aardsoorten en geophagie* (Altheer 1857: 96).

Employing the adsorptive effect of clay, one might explain geophagy among pregnant women and those suffering from abdominal illness as well as the application of clay to seeping wounds, for which one must find substantiation outside of ethnology, in the literatures of medicine, pharmacology, and chemistry. From research in the literature we have established that, although ethnological interest in geophagy has already reached its nadir, in various pharmacopoeias clay has affirmed itself as a medicine, either *per os*, as an enema, or applied externally. The *Drogistenlexikon* (Irion 1955: 61), under the heading, "Germ free white clay, Bolus alba sterilisata," states:

Germ free white clay ('Merck') is at 100° sterilized white clay D.A.B.6. of special fineness and of particularly good adsorptive effect . . . . Internal use: 2 teaspoons and more mixed with water in infections abdominal illness with acidic characteristics; also as an enema, and externally as drying agent undiluted on seeping wounds and catarrhs of the mucous membranes.

We inquired at the firm of E. Merck in Darmstadt to learn why and how the plant had decided on the production of this preparation. The firm informed us that:

This preparation had already been withdrawn from trade at least thirty years ago. It had been introduced about the turn of the century; from this time came in any case the first publications. . . . The introduction had come about as the result of the stimulus of Prof. J. Stumpf, Würzburg.

Thus, this is similar to Kearney's information that clay had been replaced by antibiotics in the treatment of wounds in Australia.

Professor Stumpf explains the bactericidal property of clay as follows:

The curative properties of clay are founded in its special physical character-istics, above all in the distribution of its minute particles. Individual clay particles are smaller than many bacteria. If infected mucous membranes are more or less flooded with clay, the bacteria are completely sur-rounded by clay particles and are thus separated from their source of nourishment and become imbedded in the inorganic material. Growth and the survivability of the bacteria are thus halted almost instantaneously, and from this is explained the strikingly speedy abatement of the symptoms of infection and/or symptoms of poisoning in acute infectious diseases of the alimentary canal (Stumpf 1916: 19).

In *Lehrbuch der Pharmakologie,* Poulsson (1928: 447) explains the effectiveness of clay drawing upon the principles of colloidal chemistry:

If a suspension of finely distributed particles, e.g., bolus, talc, or charcoal, is mixed with solutions of salts, dyes, alkaloids, colloids, or with other fine suspensions, there exists on the surfaces of all of the small particles a bound-ary layer, where the concentration is greater than that of the surrounding medium. This physical fixing, which is termed according to Du Bois-Reymond as adsorption, is a surface effect and for this reason particularly large, if the surface is very large (and conversely, the particles extremely small).

In bacteriology it is assumed that bacteria are finely suspended in the host; the toxins, however, are colloidal suspensions. In order to prove our assertions with a practical example, a melancholy possibility was chosen from the past, the occasion being the cholera epidemic of approximately sixty years ago in 1913 in Serbia. The German staff doctor Aumann and the Russian military doctor Rabin fought against the epidemic in a friendly, cooperative undertaking. From Dr. Aumann's report (1913: 590ff.) we quote the following:

As another prophylactic I should wish to recommend the bolus alba, by virtue of our findings relative to acute nausea attacks and, above all, to advanced diarrhea. . . . For other reasons we had been compelled to set up along side of the barracks for the cholera patients a division for receiving soldiers stricken with attacks of diarrhea accompanied by vomiting. For all of these cases the bolus alba — 100 grams given once daily in 200 grams of water — served us well. The attacks were inhibited after a few hours, the patients were again fit for duty on the next day. In an experiment carried out on myself in treating a severe intestinal catarrh, I was able to convince myself of how quickly and of how beneficial is the effect of bolus alba. The cramps and painful peristaltic intestinal reflexes subsided shortly after the administration of 100 grams of bolus alba; there was no subsequent appearance of diarrhea; within a few hours I felt completely restored.

We want to especially emphasize a sentence found later in Aumann's text: "Since it is absolutely not recommended to use sterilized bolus, the medicine is prepared rather cheaply." Thus we have here an authentic geophagy from folk medicine!

Having read the report by Dr. Aumann we were indeed sorry that clay had been supplanted by antibiotics, having investigated its source in folk medicine. After further research in pharmaceutical writings, we encountered, however, a pleasant surprise in that we discovered that clay has reentered recent pharmaceutical practice. The Hungarian medicinal manufacturer EGYT introduced two new preparations based upon clay, namely "Bolus laxans" tablets (indication: constipation, flatulence, etc.) and "Bolus adstringens" tablets (indication: acute intestinal infections, infectious processes in the bowels, among others). The advantage of the bolus preparations, as reported to us by the firm, is that it does not color the contents of the intestines, as charcoal preparations do, so that possible hemorrhage in the stomach or the small intestines is not disguised.

Ethnologists have sought for a long time for an answer to the question of the curative property of clay. It is most probable that the only doctor who did research in ethnology was Professor Julius Stumpf of the University of Würzburg. Following his successful external application of clay he resolved upon its internal use, having learned of geophagy of the Otomaks. Professor Stumpf writes of this as follows (1906: 19):

I openly admit here that actually for years, already with my first experiments with bolus, the idea of a possible internal application of clay had occurred, always in a larger, albeit somewhat indistinct form, after I had read, somewhere around the year 1887, of "earth-eating wild peoples" in Alexander von Humboldt's *Ansichten der Natur.* . . .

In contemporary science, researchers follow two paths. Medicine has not made any claim on geophagy, and ethnology does not take into account the chemical and pharmaceutical literature at all. It was our task to reduce these two streams to a common denominator, at perhaps the last moment, when geophagy is confronted today by the relentless advance of antibiotics. The primary curative property of argillaceous earth lies in the adsorptive effect of its colloidal form. This does not exclude other possible curative properties of clay, which require further biochemical investigations. If an application of clay is found in the cure of syphilis as well, it will be necessary to examine clays compounded with arsenic, bismuth, and/or mercury, and possibly other elements too, which medicine has not yet employed in the cure of this disease. This no longer belongs to the sphere of ethnology. Geophagy has offered a contribution to medicine and to pharmacology in the same way as creosote, aspirin, and most recently a medicine with kava-kava as a base have benefited from ethnological research in the past.

REFERENCES

ALTHEER
1857   *Eetbare aardsoorten en geophagie.*
ARNELL, B., S. LAGERCRANTZ
1958   Geophagical customs. *Studia Ethnographica Upsaliensia* 17:1–81.
AUMANN
1913   Über die Massnahmen bei der Bekämpfung der Cholera in Serbien. *Berliner Klinische Wochenschrift* 13:590ff.
EHRENBERG, C. G.
1868   *Über die roten Erden als Speise der Guinea-Neger.* Berlin.
HERINGA, JOD
1874   Eetbare aarde van Sumatra. *Natuurkundig Tijdschrift voor Nederlandsch Indie* 34:185–189.
HIPPOCRATES
1737   *De natura mulierum,* volume two, section eighty-one.
1737   *Liber de superfoetatione,* volume ninety-three.
IRION, HANS
1955   *Drogistenlexikon,* volume two. Berlin.
ISPASESCU, ALEXANDRU
1968   Présence de la géophagie en Roumaine. Déductions etnoiatriques sur la géophagie. *Etnoiatria* 2:29–33.
LAUFER, BERTHOLD
1930   Geophagy. *Field Museum of Natural History, Anthropological Series* 18:101–193.
LUPIBEREZA, TODOR
1951   *Glina.* Beograd.

MODIGLIANI, ELIO
1892   Fra i Batacchi indipendenti. Rome.
PLOSS, H.
1897   Das Weib in der Natur- und Völkerkunde. Leipzig.
POULSSON, E.
1928   Lehrbuch der Pharmakologie. Leipzig-Oslo.
STAHL, GÜNTHER
1932   Die Geophagie. Zeitschrift für Ethnologie 63:347–374.
STUMPF, JULIUS
1906   Über ein zuverlässiges Heilverfahren bei der asiatischen Cholera
       sowie bei schweren infektiösen Brechdurchfällen. Würzburg.
1916   Bolus für medizinische Anwendung. Darmstadt.
SUPEK, ZVONIMIR
1971   Tehnologija s poznavanjem robe. Zagreb.
TISCHNER, H.
1959   Völkerkunde. Frankfurt.

Interaction of Traditional and Western Medical Practices

Introduction

HAROLD B. HALEY

We had an hour-and-a-half session on the interaction between native practices and Western medicine. Certainly, in much of the world, cultural change and health care change are most visible in the medical anthropological area. We essentially discussed four issues. I will outline these briefly and make some reference to some individual authors. I will comment on what seemed to be our four main subjects. The ideas came from papers.

To begin with, our discussion was opened by Dr. Vijay Kochar, Ph.D. (India), now temporarily at Johns Hopkins, who raised the questions: What are the boundaries of medical anthropology? Can we define it? What is medical anthropology? He expressed it in this way. He felt that any contribution to the field had to answer positively to two questions: (a) How much does the specific contribution relate to medicine and public health? And, (b) How do these contributions relate to anthropology? Fr. Grollig had written a letter to me in February of 1973 as we were working on the organization of the session, and he had taken a quotation from Dr. Horacio Fabrega's monograph on medical anthropology that essentially says the same thing. This was the basis on which we had attempted to organize this conference and this section.

The second subject was raised first with the very innocent-sounding question from Miss Luisa Urdaneta, a nurse from Cali, Colombia, now working for a doctorate at Southern Methodist University. Doing fieldwork in relationship to American physicians in Austin, Texas, she raised the question: How can we teach medical students and ultimately how can we teach physicians to look at patients, illness, and disease from an anthropological viewpoint? A very interesting, a very quiet, a very sweet

question. I kept notes: twelve people discussed it! Miss Sheila Cosminsky agreed that this should be done and indicated that she thought that
this should be done quite early in education before patterns are too solid-
ly established. At that time, a medical student who was present in the
meeting spoke up. Having had four years of part-time work in an ad-
dict clinic in Chicago, he thought we needed more consumer education: too many of the patients they were dealing with were not sufficiently health-conscious. His overall feeling was that the doctors needed education and so did the patients — certainly not original, but unfortunately, still true. Dr. Dale Ritter, a practicing physician, made the point
that the physician, in caring for his patient, has as his first goal the desire to do what is right and what is best for the patient. He will change
his orientation but he has got to be convinced at the pragmatic level that
another approach — such as an anthropological approach — will
improve patient care. Dr. Richard Kessler, Associate Dean at Northwestern University's medical school, contributed very actively to the discussion and to this particular point he gave two comments. The medical student, while he is in school, is primarily disease-oriented. This is
partially the education he is being given, but is also partially what some
of his primary motivation is in entering medicine. We have to recognize
that if you try to teach anthropology to these people, you are teaching
a group for whom the rest of what they are doing is disease-oriented;
therefore, some special arrangements — none of which he suggested —
would be needed to shift to the more people- or culture-orientation of
anthropology. Dr. Kessler then shifted to the physician's side of the
equation and talked about the fact that physicians are like other people:
they resist change. Change in viewpoint, change in thought, change in
process cannot be imposed from the outside. He again followed the
same thought Dr. Ritter did: the M.D. must WANT to change in order
to be able to see that he can care for his patients better. At this time,
Dr. William Stablein made an interesting shift in viewpoint when he said
that the work that he had done in Nepal in setting up the medical clinic
for Tibetan refugees wasn't so much to change the system but rather to
accommodate it. He thought the accommodation was better than change.
That brought an immediate response from Dr. Kessler; he agreed that
this was just as true in Chicago as it was in Nepal.

From that point we developed three definitions which seem rather
important. Dr. Kessler raised for discussion the difference between
medical care and health care. These are two different things. After a rather brief discussion of this, Miss Urdaneta went into another definition
(related but different), when she said that we must define the differ-

ence between what IS and what SHOULD BE. Dr. M. Gracia, a Cuban physician who is now the director of a state mental hospital in Montana, has a tremendous medical and anthropological interest in the North American Indian people in Montana. He pointed out the importance of cultural definitions in diseases; that the physician starts from the point of diagnosis; and, if you make your diagnosis wrong on a cultural — or any other — basis, you are in trouble. He gave a beautiful example of the American Indian who, as a patient in a hospital, is a very silent person. Under some circumstances, some individuals have interpreted the silence as being a manifestation of schizophrenic catatonia, when actually it is a reflection of silence in the Indian's culture. Here, understanding the cultural basis is necessary for understanding the case history in order for a proper and appropriate medical diagnosis to be made.

The third subject we discussed was the relationship between health and culture change. Then we moved into the factors that are the bases for consumer or patient utilization of various health services. One of the papers, by Clyde Woods, Ph. D., and Theodore Graves, Ph. D., is a superb study of cultural change in the Guatemalan Atitlán Lake district of San Lucas Tolimán. I enjoyed that paper because in it they talked about a clinic they were involved with and the care that was given. They mentioned the clinic and a papal volunteer from the United States coming at periodic intervals and seeing patients. Actually, that was on Saturday mornings. In 1967 I did have the experience of spending one day in the San Lucas Tolimán clinic and I do have in my records that there were twenty-two patients that I helped with care on the particular day: it was a bit of a homecoming for me to read their paper. One of their themes was that the availability of modern Western medical care was an instrument in causing changes in belief systems much wider and broader than medical care. This was a catalytic function. They didn't use that terminology: I do.

This led to discussion with Dr. Antonio Quintanilla, a Peruvian physician who was originally a sociologist and who is now a specialist in internal medicine and nephrology on the faculty of Northwestern University and the Veterans' Research Hospital in Chicago. He has worked with, and his paper is related to, the highland Indians of Peru, the Quechua and the Aymara. When they migrate to the cities, particularly Lima, what happens? He makes a very interesting chronological sequence. The mountain Indian coming into the city adapts very quickly and easily to technology. That is the first and the easiest change made; second is adaptation to differences in foods. But the last and the most difficult change is the change in health beliefs; people do not change their health beliefs without major disruption in their other belief systems. There is an interesting contrast between Drs. Woods' and Graves' paper on the one hand and Dr. Quintanilla's on the other. Dr. Quintanilla says that in a medical school in Peru they were taught Western science and disease and not given the opportunity to participate in transcultural exchange with any of their patients. He made the point that transcultural exchange is something that has to be lived and is quite difficult to teach. And I think we are having that same situation in the United States.

From this discussion we got into the fourth issue: how the patient or the consumer chooses his medical care. To begin with, one of the speakers made the point that you have to go with a situation when you have no options, and there are many areas in developing countries where alternatives do not exist. Where they do exist, then different bases develop. One theme, repeated by Dr. Kochar and Miss Cosminsky, and a number of others, was that, when various traditional and Western healers are available, there tends to be use of the Western healer for acute diseases and the native healer for more chronic diseases. Miss Sheila Cosminsky said that was pretty much true in Guatemala, but that in Guatemala with the Indians all disease was considered supernatural and there tended to be an early use of Western medicine; if and when that failed, recourse to the healer was invoked. Dr. William Stablein and his work in Nepal give us details of work with three different groups using different medical sources. One thread that went through the thought of a majority of these people when they talked and is in their papers is the presence of what we would call "non-Western diseases." It was interesting to hear Miss Belcove talking about Taos, New Mexico, and Dr. Quintanilla talking about Peru, and each of them in their papers talking about *susto* and conditions of this kind. There are these well-defined, intracultural diseases for which we do not have a Western counterpart. Then Miss Urdaneta pointed out that in Austin, Texas, 18 percent of the people are Mexican and, as she put it, "there's a *curandero* in every block." She thought in given situations that the higher the educational and socioeconomic level, the more use of Western healing; the lower the level, the more the use of the *curanderos*.

Those are the four main concepts; I think that the thoughts that these individual authors and discussants presented relate to and are the bases for the issues we present in this section.

Editor's Note: This, then, gives the Pre-Congress Conference context in which five of the eight papers in this section of the volume were discussed. In addition to the papers of Drs. Gracia, Kochar, Quintanilla, Stablein, and the co-authors Woods and Graves, we have included the contributions to the Congress of Vinigi Grottanelli, Ph.D. (University of Rome), "Witchcraft: an allegory?"; Dr. Haley's own paper, "Endemic goiter, salt, and local customs in Central America: prevention of a preventable disease"; and the brief communication to the Congress of Dr. Kamuti Kiteme on "Traditional African medicine."

Human Factors in the Regulation of Parasitic Infections: Cultural Ecology of Hookworm Populations in Rural West Bengal

V. K. KOCHAR, G. A. SCHAD, A. B. CHOWDHURY,
C. G. DEAN, and T. NAWALINSKI

The literature on parasitic diseases[1] is replete with explicit statements or implicit assumptions about the significance of human factors in disease ecology (for examples, see Audy 1972; Bisseru 1967; Cockburn 1967; Cort 1942; Fox 1966; Garlick and Keay 1970; Gordon 1966; Gray 1965; Lariche and Milner 1971; May 1959; Nelson 1972). The great variety of factors[2] is treated with varying degrees of sophis-

Field studies and subsequent work were conducted under the sponsorship of the Johns Hopkins Center for Medical Research and Training in Calcutta and Baltimore and were supported by PHS grant 5 R07 TW00141–05CIC, NIH grant R07–AI–10048–12–13 and foreign research grant 01–027–01 (PL 480 grant 6x4327 from the Government of India). The project was supervised by Dr. G. A. Schad, Department of Pathobiology, School of Hygiene and Public Health, Johns Hopkins University, and Dr. A. B. Chowdhury, Chairman, Division of Parasitology, and Director, Calcutta School of Tropical Medicine, Calcutta.

The principal author is a social anthropologist responsible for presenting the anthropological aspects of this inquiry to the anthropological audience. All other collaborators, except Mr. C. G. Dean (a nematode ecologist), are parasitologists. Anthropological field investigations were assisted by Messrs. Amitava Basu, Basudeb Laha, Biren Ghosh and Gopinath Basu. Mr. Jacob Thomas, statistician, Johns Hopkins Center for Medical Research and Training, Calcutta, provided enormous help in analysis of the data presented here. Generous help and guidance of Dr. Dwain W. Parrack, Department of Pathobiology, School of Hygiene and Public Health, to the principal author in preparation of this paper are gratefully acknowledged. Comments by, or discussions with, Dr. R. I. Anderson, Dr. Paul E. White, Dr. Tom Sasaki and Dr. Neville Dyson-Hudson have helped in clearer formulation of some ideas.

[1] Although at times used in a broad sense, the term "parasitic" in this paper is generally used in the context of helminth infections in general and hookworm infection in particular.

[2] The variety of human factors mentioned in the more important sources on hookworm infection, to which the search was confined, is indeed amazing. Chand-

tication.[3] Some careful attempts have been made to develop a systematic body of information on human factors;[4] however, it is generally recognized that even the key human factors in the ecology of the most important parasitic diseases have not received careful attention.[5] Although repeated assertions have been made about the significance of human factors in disease ecology, a tremendous gap exists between these assertions and effort directed towards increasing the actual state of knowledge about such factors.

Great progress has taken place in medical anthropology, particularly in the social epidemiology of chronic diseases and in the social processes within (or in relation to) modern medical institutions. However, there have been few studies by anthropologists on the ecology of parasitic diseases.[6]

---

ler (1929) alone mentions about seventy-five different human-factor categories in the discussion of the epidemiology and ecology of hookworm disease.

[3] Nelson (1972) provides an overview of the kind of behavioral and social information that is usually sought by biomedical scientists about parasitic diseases. In contrast, other papers in the same volume illustrate the level of information sought about behavior of other animals involved in parasitism.

[4] Fabrega (1972) has reviewed disease studies from evolutionary perspective and epidemiological studies in primitive communities. Further examples could be mentioned. Audy (1965) gives a résumé of human influences on the natural foci of diseases. Chandler (1926–1927) in his hookworm studies in the different parts of India gives detailed descriptions of settlement patterns and defecation habits.

Cort (1926) made an extensive study of the traditional system of composing night soil for use as fertilizer in China. Dunn (1972) in his recent study provided partial validation of his earlier hypothesis about the ecological complexity and degree of parasitism on the basis of field investigations among the different cultural ecological groups in Malaya.

Ford (1970, 1971) did an extensive study of land use in Africa from historical perspective in relation to the ecology of the vectors of trypanosomiases in man and cattle. Duggan's (1970) historical note on the African trypanosomiases is also on the same theme. Giglioli (1963) studied changes in human and cattle populations leading to eruption of malaria in a previously eradicated region.

Husting (1968) in his yet unpublished dissertation studied social factors in the epidemiology of schistosomiases (cited by Nelson 1972). Imperato (1972) has produced yet another very interesting account of the nomadic habits of pastoralists in Mali in order to develop a suitable vaccination program in the region. Wright (1970) has summarized his own studies and those of others that indicate the role of human factors in the ecology of schistosomiasis.

[5] See Stewart's (1972: 370) comment on the status of knowledge about human factors in the epidemiology of venereal diseases; Wright's (1970: 77) and Nelson's (1972) comments on the knowledge of human factors in the ecology of schistosomiasis; Fox's (1966: 99) comments on the ecology of viral diseases. See also Fabrega's comments (1972: 205, 206).

[6] In contrast to the previous reviews, Fabrega (1972) for the first time devotes a section on disease ecology and cites biomedical studies of parasitic diseases. He also discusses the growing possibility of using the approach of population biology in medical anthropology.

Biomedical studies do not provide anthropologically interesting and useful information, nor do the anthropological studies provide appropriate information on medically relevant social aspects. A kind of no man's land exists between biomedical and social sciences, as if each were held back by the unavoidable intricacies of the other. Conceptual and methodological problems of satisfactorily exploring the "social" domain for understanding phenomena in the "biological" domain, or *vice versa*, are forbidding.

As pointed out by Scotch (1963:65) and others, the two domains need to be theoretically integrated. This is more acute in social sciences if the involvement in medicine and public health is to extend beyond "the most transient consultative relationships" (Rapoport 1962: 190). While some would question the "tendency to define anthropology's role in this field essentially as an academic discipline" (Hochstrasser and Tapp 1970: 248), there is no escape from the fact that the pursuit of academic or professional priorities that anthropologists may want to seek from such interdisciplinary involvement (Polgar 1970: 264) is probably the best chance to make substantive contributions to the "science of man" despite the so-called management bias.

It would seem that with strong biological, historical, and ecological orientations, the anthropological tradition, emphasizing a natural-history approach, has great potential in this context. However, the reviews (Polgar 1962; Scotch 1963; Fabrega 1972) indicate that these traditional strong points constitute undercurrents rather than the main currents. With more and more social scientists and biomedical scientists learning each other's trades, at times working together, and a few crossing boundaries and exploring from the other side, new strategies of research and theoretical integration in this interdisciplinary domain are taking shape.

AN EMERGING STRATEGY

Some recent advances have paved the way for what might be called a cultural-ecological approach in medical anthropology. Research from many different directions is converging on this approach. The following description is a crude distillate of ideas dormant in the writings of some anthropologists and socioecologically oriented biomedical scientists.[7]

[7] Some of the ideas developed here are indirectly expressed in the writings of anthropologists (Alland 1966, 1969, 1970; Dunn 1968, 1972; Cassel 1960; Fabrega

The knowledge of the etiologic organism, its life cycle, and its ecology is the basis of an inquiry into the interconnections between social factors and the natural history of a disease. The reference points of this approach are not the disease symptoms in an individual but the complex chain of events and processes involved in the disease cycle (see Figure 1). The life history or the natural history of the parasite population is the key process in the disease cycle.

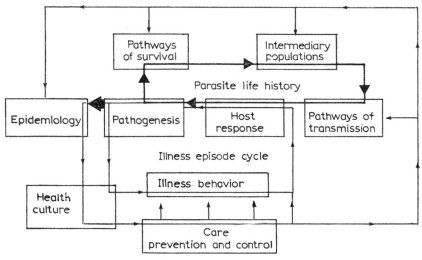

Figure 1.   The disease cycle
Life history of the parasite leads to the cycle of pathogenesis in the human body. Illness leads to the cycle of illness behavior and treatment. Cumulation of illness in a population leads to the cycle of care, prevention, and control leading to a new pattern of disease in the population and a new level of parasite life history

The life history can be conceived as a varied and complex chain of events, situations, and pathways through which populations of a given parasite pass in order to complete individual life cycles. The life cycle is one, but life histories are numerous for a parasite population. The life histories of human parasites may involve a great variety of intermediary populations such as alternative hosts, intermediate hosts, paratonic hosts, vectors, reservoirs, etc. (Sprent 1969: appendices).

These interacting and interdependent populations involved in a disease cycle constitute a complex ecological network. A certain structure of these populations and certain pattern of interactions among these populations are intrinsic to a given pattern of disease in a hu-

1972; Gray 1965; Polgar 1964) and in the general writings of biomedical scientists (Audy 1958, 1965; Cockburn 1971; Burnet and White 1972; Fox 1966; Gajdusek 1970; May 1954, 1959; Schofield 1970; Sprent 1969; Wright 1970).

man population. It is an ecological system, a sequence of "interlocking cause-effect pathways" (Watt 1966: 2). In this system, complex factors from many dimensions play a role (social, genetic, biological, environmental, etc.).

Instead of thinking in terms of causality (of a disease) or in terms of strength of association between a set of variables and a final cause (the disease), an alternative perspective is to think in terms of regulation; not regulation of the disease in an individual, but the regulation of populations, and of interactions among populations at specific points in the natural history of the parasite population. As shown later, some human factors may act positively for the parasite populations and some negatively.

Persistent patterns of interaction between populations constitute the basis of the host-parasite relationships. These relationships evolve through time; that is, these are based upon adaptations occurring in repeated life histories of the parasite and host populations. Disease in a human population at a particular time is an expression of a particular state of equilibrium between ever-persistent and ever-changing biological, ecological, and cultural phenomena.

In areas where the landscape is shaped by the agricultural or other activities of human population, the structure of the biotic community is directly or indirectly subject to human choices and social usages. Furthermore, biological entities, including those involved in the disease cycle, are integrated into a culture, i.c. these become a part of the complex sociocultural relationships and belief system of a people. Infection or parasitization can thus be viewed as an expression of the culture-parasite relationships.

Different specialists study the different aspects of the disease cycle using different techniques and conceptual frameworks. Such multidimensional approaches are complementary even though these may in fact emphasize only one dimension. From the anthropological perspective, disease is a dimension of culture; it is an "anthropological phenomenon" (May 1959: v) amenable to anthropological theory and methods. A disease is a part of situations and processes inherent in the relationships of persons in a community (1) to each other, (2) to the flora, fauna, and other ecological entities, and (3) to the cultural entities affecting their health.

The anthropological goal implicit in this approach is twofold. First, the goal is to explore the underlying function of specific behavior patterns and social usages in the regulation of disease cycle. Second, it is to relate these patterns to various other aspects of a culture that are involved in the regulation of diseases. The regulation can be studied in relation to any one or more facets of the disease cycle. In this paper only the free-living phases in the life cycle of a parasite are considered.

Man becomes involved in helminth zoonoses when his activities impinge upon the overall life history of a potential parasite, i.e. during any part of the biological period comprising development from one sexual generation to another (Sprent 1969: 340).

The life cycle provides the starting point and a basic frame for organizing field inquiries. Depending upon the available information it is possible to identify ecological, biological, and human factors that are known to be or are deemed to be involved in the disease ecology (see Figure 2). It is also necessary to know how these factors bear upon the parasite population.

For a parasite population, the natural history can be considered in terms of multiple natural foci and multiple pathways to and from these foci, through which the parasite populations are channeled in a given environment. The different pathways have different degrees of significance for the parasite populations in survival, development, and contact with the host populations.

Having identified the main pathways and the human factors, anthropological investigations can then be planned to provide precise information on these factors. It is useful to conceptualize variables as specific behavior patterns that directly relate to the known bioecological factors. These patterns can be then related to the other sociocultural factors at successively higher levels of abstraction and cultural integration (see Figure 2).

HOOKWORM INFECTION IN RURAL BENGAL: THE PROBLEM

The life cycle of the human hookworm may be summarized as follows. The adult worms of two species of human hookworm reside in the small intestine of man. A female worm releases five to twenty thousand eggs per day. These eggs enter the external environment with the feces. Under favorable conditions the eggs hatch in less than twenty-four hours, releasing first-stage free-living larvae which feed and grow; these molt after about two days and develop into second-stage larvae which again molt after about five days into the infective third-stage larvae.

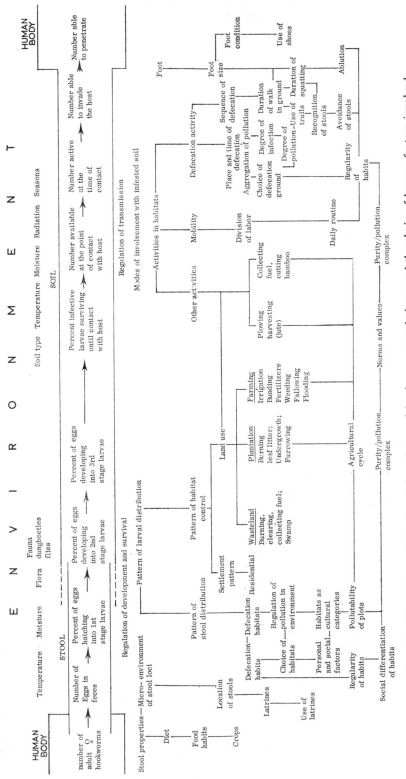

Figure 2. Life history of the free-living phases of hookworm populations and the chain of human factors involved

No further development takes place until these are able to penetrate the skin of the human host. In the host the larvae migrate via the bloodstream and reach the lungs where they undergo the fourth molt. These reach the intestine via the trachea and esophagus. The larvae undergo the final molt in the intestine and develop into adult worms.

In the human population studied, an adult male villager passes on the average about one million eggs per day in his stools, whereas the female villagers pass about half this number. Mortality of eggs and larvae is very high even under favorable environmental conditions. Only about 2 to 3 percent are known to survive in the infective stage in silt loam plots (*Johns Hopkins Report* 1965–1966: 47–48).

The intensity of infection is measured by counting the number of hookworm eggs in a sample of stool and is expressed as eggs per gram (EPG) of feces. Egg count is an indirect indication of the number of hookworms in the intestine. Hookworm disease is attributed largely to the loss of blood due to the feeding activity of adult hookworms in the intestine and therefore it depends upon the number of worms harbored. Roche and Layrisse (1966:1034, 1092) found that children and adult females with egg counts of 2,000 EPG and adult males with the egg counts of 5,000 EPG begin to show a significant decline in hemoglobin levels. Intensity of infection below 3,000 EPG is taken here to represent a light infection.

High prevalence of hookworm is usually associated with a high intensity of infection, a situation found to exist in many areas of the world where hookworm is endemic (World Health Organization 1964:13). In rural West Bengal, however, it has been known since the twenties and has been confirmed recently (Chowdhury and Schiller 1968:308) that despite almost universal prevalence, the average villager carries a light hookworm infection. The overall prevalence of infection in the study population was found to be 90 percent and the mean intensity or level of infection in the sample population about 2,500. Of the egg counts 73 percent were below 3,000 EPG and only 4.4 percent of the egg counts were above 10,000 EPG (Schad, et al. n.d.).

Because no treatment program was operating in the study area, low intensities of infection in the face of high prevalence of infection pose an interesting problem. It suggests that some natural mechanisms must be regulating the hookworm populations. For the anthropological inquiries it was hypothesized that in this traditional rural society, where hookworm infection is believed to have a long history, the behavior patterns of the host population might be playing a role in regulating the hookworm population and thereby limiting the level of infection.

Chandler's statement (1929:195) that "the majority of the worms are acquired from defecation areas during the act of defecation," identifies defecation behavior as the key element in the regulatory process.

In the following discussion, the importance of various aspects of defecation behavior is assessed in two ways: (1) how such factors affect the survival, development, and distribution of the free-living populations of hookworm; and (2) how the patterns of defecation affect the chances of larval contact with the human population. These two ways of assessment are used below as qualitative measures of the role of function of specific human habits.

This study was a part of an interdisciplinary project concerning the ecology of interacting populations of hookworm and man in rural West Bengal. The field study was conducted in Bandipur *anchal* of Hooghly district, West Bengal, from October 1968 to December 1970. A population from twelve contiguous villages (6,268 people) was chosen for the study. A random sample of 100 households, made up of 750 people, was selected for an epidemiological survey. All 100 households were included in a general social survey. Additionally, a subsample of fifty households was drawn from these for detailed anthropological investigations.

The following kinds of field records have been used for the discussion below: (1) interrogations of all subsample household members once every month, for fifteen months, about the time and place of defecation, (2) identifications of one stool of one subject from each subsample household every month for observations around the "identified stools" (including simulation of time periods involved in various activities associated with defecation), (3) observations of the actual sequence of defecation behavior of unidentified subjects in the different habitats, (4) land-use maps and stool-distribution maps in three study villages, and (5) ethnographic and socioanthropologic records.

Only selected material with regard to the defecation activity will be presented here.

CHOICE OF HABITAT AND TIME OF DEFECATION

Studies show that hookworm larvae have a very limited ability to migrate beyond the area occupied by a stool *(Johns Hopkins Report 1965–1966: 42).* Because the choice of where to pass a stool lies with the people, larval populations can only exist and abound where human habits foster them. The pattern of distribution and aggregation of free-living larval populations thus is largely a question of where people prefer to pass their stools.

Human Behavior

People in different villages pass stools in various habitats in the environment (see Table 1). On the average about 50 percent of the

Table 1.   Local variation in the deposition of stools in different habitats (in percent)

Villages	Fields	Bamboo groves	Banana garden	River bank	Pond bank	Tree grove	Bushes	Residential	Other*
Laltejol	82.6	4.8	1.9	0	0	0.2	0	3.2	7.4
Beleputa	78.4	0	0	0	8.0	0	0	7.8	7.8
Jadabbati	71.1	10.3	0.4	0	0	0	0.4	7.7	8.3
Nabason	64.7	20.8	0.5	0	0	0	0	8.2	5.8
Khanarber	42.0	29.8	0	0.8	5.4	0.3	5.1	13.2	3.9
Lalpur	40.0	10.8	13.3	13.5	1.6	1.5	0	11.2	8.2
Hasimpur	38.3	18.4	0.3	11.1	2.3	0	7.4	11.0	11.1
Bhimpur	35.9	0	2.6	0	28.6	0	0	17.9	13.5
Choalpara	32.3	19.5	4.0	4.6	7.0	0.5	6.6	14.5	9.5
Khankhanpur	27.9	12.4	5.5	0	13.8	8.9	14.7	10.1	6.9
Mohalla	16.8	25.9	18.1	0.4	1.3	0	15.1	15.5	6.9
Bandipur	3.4	75.9	4.1	0	0	0.4	0.4	11.8	4.1
All villages	42.6	22.4	4.1	3.6	3.8	1.0	4.1	10.7	6.9

* Includes stools deposited in latrines or stools for which subjects provided ambiguous location.

stools are passed in the fields[8] and other sparsely shaded habitats. Laltejol and Bandipur villages present polar contrasts in the use of fields and bamboo groves — the two typical defecation habitats of the study population. People seasonally change their defecation habitats from fields to bamboo groves and *vice versa* (see Figure 3). The time of defection activity shows a marked peak in the morning and a suggestion of a smaller peak in the afternoon (see Figure 4).

[8] In the context of soil pollution, fields are generally unshaded habitats, except fields under jute crop for about one and one-half months when sufficient shade exists on the soil surface.

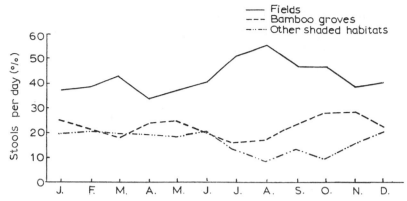

Figure 3.   Seasonal variation in the percentage of stools passed in fields, bamboo groves and other shaded habitats by the sample population

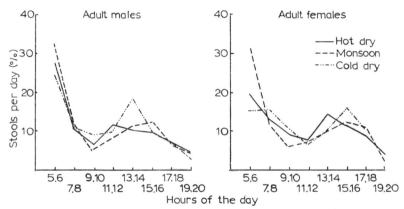

Figure 4.   Diurnal and seasonal variation in defecation time of the adult males and adult females

Bioecology

Free-living hookworm larvae are extremely susceptible to desiccation and, hence, during the long dry season between October or November to June, transmission ceases (Chandler 1935; Schad, et al. 1973). From the beginning of the monsoon season in June until October or November, depending upon the year, soil moisture is adequate for larval development and survival. However, daytime temperatures are high and in stools ovicidal temperatures are often attained at about midday (*Johns Hopkins Report* 1969–1970: 9).

Chandler (1929:147) and Beaver (1953) have noted that alternate wetting and drying are deleterious for the larvae. Added stresses of solar radiation and temperature have the potential of affecting the activity and longevity of the larvae, thereby changing their infectivity and accumulation in the unshaded habitats. Under adverse conditions the infective larvae are known to become inactive for prolonged durations.

Implications of Human Behavior

Whether stools are passed in shaded or unshaded habitats will not materially alter hookworm development and survival between November and May. Between June and October, however, whether or not people choose to pass stools in shaded habitats has an important bearing on the probability that the eggs will survive to contribute to the transmission. The shifts in the habits and choices of the human adults during this period result in the deposition of 56 percent to 65 percent of the stools in fields and other sparsely shaded habitats. This will result in elimination of a substantial proportion of larval populations from the unshaded habitats in contrast to the shaded habitats.

Similarly, the environment of the villages (such as Bandipur) where people predominantly use bamboo groves and other shaded habitats for defecation will foster greater larval populations than the environments of villages (such as Laltejol and Beleputa) where unshaded habitats are predominantly used for defecation. This does not necessarily mean that infection levels in the former villages will be higher, because, as shown below, other factors also affect the chances of transmission.

In general, persons who regularly pass stools in early morning are more likely to contact active larval populations on the soil surface than those who regularly defecate during the midday when soil surface conditions are unfavorable for hookworm larvae.

The stools passed in the afternoon in unshaded habitats will not be exposed to temperatures lethal for hookworm eggs until after about twenty hours. By this time the eggs may have hatched. As noted above, men pass about twice as many hookworm eggs in their stools as women. However, since more women than men tend to defecate in the afternoon, the hookworm eggs in their stools are more likely to hatch and contribute to the transmission. Such factors are important in judging the relative importance of age-sex groups in maintaining the high endemicity; the egg output data alone are not sufficient.

Human Behavior and Culture

Land-use maps of three villages were prepared to study how people structure their environment. Marked differences between villages, *para* [hamlets], and houses were noticed. Table 2 gives land use and stool distribution in three villages. Land use sets the limits to the choice of defecation habitats, but within limits various factors govern the villager's choice for a defecation ground.

Table 2. Percentage of area under different habitats in three villages and the percentage of stools in those habitats

Village	Fields area	stools	Bamboo groves area	stools	Bushes area	stools	Banana garden area	stools	Residential area	stools
Bandipur	25.2	3.4	8.5	75.9	16.5	0.8	9.3	4.1	16.2	11.8
Jadabbati	55.1	71.1	6.5	10.3	3.7	0.4	1.9	0.4	13.2	7.7
Khanarber	56.6	42.0	4.2	29.8	19.1	10.8	0	0	14.1	13.2

Among the reasons given for their choice, the more important are: proximity to their homes; proximity to a pond; social acceptability of using the place or plot for such purpose; agriculture or plantation within the plot; the amount of ground cover, flooding and insect population in the ground; degree of fecal pollution in the plot; ownership of the plot; relationship of the family or neighborhood with the owner of the plot; defecation as a group activity (for children and females); privacy and shame among women in using a place visible to or frequented by males; avoidance, by males, of a defecation area where certain female kin might be present; state of health; weather and time of defecation; idiosyncrasies.

Normative and attitudinal factors are also involved in this behavior in regard to defecation. It is considered ideal to pass stools first thing in the morning. The ritual norms of daily routine emphasize the importance of regularity and discipline with regard to defecation, and elders often rebuke their children when they fail to conform.

A popular text in Bengali on the daily routine for Hindu households notes that omission of these acts is sinful. The first act, after arising and chanting the first morning prayer, is defecation. The book even mentions the places which should be avoided (Bhattacharya n.d.: 11), namely, paths, heaps of ash, pastures, plowed fields, water, cremation grounds, hills, ruined temples, ant hills, pits, and river banks. The book also recommends that while defecating in the morning one should face north and in the evening face south.

The agricultural cycle is a social timetable influencing everything in the life of villagers, including the defecation activity. It is an important consideration for changes in the time and place of defecation. Some fields may remain fallow for months and continue to be used as a place for defecation (called *hegomath*). Others are plowed and sown soon after rain or irrigation, which prohibits the use of a field for defecation. The caste of the owner, suitability of its location, and the cropping pattern on the plot are important considerations in the formation of a *hegomath*.

AGGREGATION OF FECAL POLLUTION

Bioecology

If the stools and hence the larval populations are highly aggregated in an infested focus, where some regular activity is carried out by man, then obviously the probability of host-parasite contact will be high in that area. Further, assuming that defecation is the only regular activity in the infested foci, the probability of contact with the parasite population will be determined by the frequency and duration of human contact with the infested stool points during defecation. This will depend upon the number and the pattern of distribution of stools in the infested foci in relation to the pattern of defecation activity. Repeated use of the same focus for defecation will increase the probability of contact, while recognition and avoidance of stool points during walking or squatting will reduce the probability of contact.

Human Behavior

The location of all stools in three study villages was plotted on enlarged land-use maps upon which a grid, marking 10 square-foot units, was superimposed. Polluted units (with one or more stools) accounted for only 1.0 to 2.6 percent of the total area of the village settlements. Fecal pollution is thus highly localized within small areas of the environment. More than 60 percent of the defecations reported by the sample population occurred in socially recognized defecation grounds. About 40 percent of the subjects reported using the same habitat in at least 85 percent of their responses over fifteen monthly interrogations. Stools are not uniformly distributed WITHIN the defecation grounds. Some areas of the grounds are free of stools, some areas have heavy aggregations of stools, and some areas are lightly polluted by occasional use. Further observations revealed that these patterns of aggregation changed with time. Another important observation was that although there were few, if any, stools on the trails within the defecation grounds, areas along the trails usually developed aggregations. In fields where trails did not exist, aggregations developed linearly along the bunds, narrow dikes partitioning individual plots, which are used as paths. In some fields, particularly *hegomaths*, stools were distributed evenly, reaching up to fifty stools per 100 square feet in some grounds in the dry months.

With reference to defecation activity only, the frequency of interaction with infested foci is equal to the number of stools passed — about 1.7 per day per person. Table 3 shows the density of fecal pollution around the identified stools. Stool points are recognizable up to five to seven days, even in the rainy season. Table 3 indicates that 48 percent of the identified stools in the fields were found to lie within a fecal pollution density of less than five stools per 100 square feet. Only about 21 percent of the identified stools in bamboo groves, in contrast to fields, were located within such low pollution density.

Table 3.   Percentage of stools identified in different habitats and percentage of fecal densities within 100 square feet

Location of identified stools	Number of square feet from identified stools							
	5	5–9	10–14	15–19	20–24	25–34	35–39	≥ 40
Fields	47.5	19.2	8.3	7.5	3.3	3.3	9.2	0.8
Bamboo groves	21.1	21.1	23.1	17.3	5.8	7.7	3.8	0
All habitats	34.2	19.4	15.1	11.9	6.8	6.8	5.8	1.0

Implications of Human Behavior

These observations support Chandler's remark that people repeatedly use the same areas for defecation (Chandler 1929:195). This pattern ensures the repeated contacts of the hosts with the earlier stool points and hence provides a favorable setting for the parasite populations.

Lower densities of pollution are encountered by the subjects defecating in the fields. The populations of hookworm larvae generated in fields are generally less likely to be contacted by the host in the course of defecation than are the larval populations generated in the bamboo groves.

Chandler thought that most people preferred to use an individual spot repeatedly and that therefore they reinfected themselves from the larvae generated in their own stools. Despite repeated inquiries only a small number of people were found to do so, particularly the sick and aged persons.

Human Behavior and Culture

On interrogation people generally reported that they do not like to defecate where other stools are present. Their professed avoidance of polluted areas, their acute recognition of old stool points, and the cultural norms of pollution and purity suggest that people would naturally avoid other stools while walking around or in the selection of a defecation spot. This, however, is not the case.

People using a defecation ground would start polluting a particular corner of the ground that seemed suitable. For the same reasons more people use the same area of the ground and gradually pollution increases to such a level that users start moving to another cleaner area within the same ground, forming new trails and new foci of pollution. Some move to another ground. Those most fastidious perhaps move first. Some persons, particularly the aged, would linger on and continue to use the old focus for some time. In bamboo groves, the system was to periodically use a focus and then abandon it. In the fields such shifts of the defecation grounds were much more frequent because of periodic changes in agricultural activity. This accounts for lower stool densities (in fields) in general (except the *hegomath*).

The concept of the avoidance of polluted foci (within the defecation grounds) operates at various thresholds of individual sensitivity. A great variety of social and cultural factors, mentioned earlier, result in a highly localized stool distribution within small areas of the environment which are repeatedly visited for defecation.

THE SEQUENCE OF DEFECATION BEHAVIOR

Bioecology

Besides entering a habitat (focus or nidus) man has to behave in a manner which is conducive to infection. In helminth anthropozoonoses the behavioral (ethological) factors are just as influential as the ecological factors. Even within the habitat, actual infection will depend upon such behavior factors . . . (Sprent 1969: 340).

Similarly, aspects of defecation behavior in hookworm infection need to be examined in more detail to elucidate the exact situation. Most important is the behavior that affects the duration and frequency of contact with the stool points.

Human Behavior

Less than 1 percent of the people were observed wearing shoes while going to defecate and only 4 percent used latrines regularly. Thus two most important deterrents to hookworm infection do not exist in the population.

About 95 percent of the subjects for whom stools were identified selected a defecation spot within a walking time of three minutes from their homes. Of the subjects (observed) 82 percent spent less than two minutes in walking within the defecation ground exploring for a suitable place to squat. This exploratory walk was partly along the trails. The location of the identified stools of 94 percent of the subjects was (on simulation) found to lie within fifteen seconds' walk from the trails and, hence, represents but a few footsteps.

Once a suitable spot for defecation was chosen, the subjects squatted for less than five minutes (see Table 4). Despite verbal statements by the people about avoidance of fecal pollution and despite their ability to recognize "traces" of stool (stool points turned into soil but still recognizable), about 75 percent of the stools identified had one or more recognizable stool points within three feet. Subjects were more prone to squat close to a trace than to a fresh or partially turned stool (41 percent vs. 26 percent). About 15 percent of the individuals squatted sufficiently close to a trace of old stool, i.e. within one foot, to suggest that their feet could have been in contact with the infective larvae.

People in the villages studied customarily ablute, i.e. wash the perianal skin, after defecation by entering a pond or other body of water found close to the defecation ground. In actual behavior, the time lapse between finishing defecation and entering water was less than one minute for 41 percent of the subjects, less than four minutes for 83 percent, and less than five minutes for 90 percent of the subjects (see Table 4).

Table 4.   Frequency distribution for the time spent in each activity associated with defecation (based on direct observation)

Time spent at each activity (in minutes)	Subjects timed at any one activity (in percent)			
	Total time within defecation ground (entry to exit)	Walking time in the defecation ground	Squatting time	Time lapse from end of squatting to entry into water source
<1	2.7	62.8	16.7	41.5
1–<2	9.1	19.2	17.6	13.2
2–<3	14.5	7.7	22.5	13.2
3–<4	24.5	6.4	14.7	15.1
4–<5	12.7	1.3	7.8	7.5
5–<6	15.5	0	9.8	0
6–<7	5.5	0	5.9	3.8
7–<8	7.3	0	4.9	1.0
8–<9	2.7	0	0	0
9–<10	3.6	1.3	0	0
10–<11	1.8	0	0	0
11–<12	0	0	0	3.8
12–<13	0	1.3	0	0
13–<14	0	0	0	0
Totals (in percent)	99.9	100.0	99.9	100.0
Number of individuals observed per activity	110	78	102	53

Implications of Human Behavior

Most transmission would be confined to defecation habitats available within a limited distance from the houses (within about 300 yards). Walking on trails, avoidance of trails for defecation, and the short duration of walking within the infested areas of the ground (particularly off trails), have a twofold effect. This behavior, on the one hand, increases aggregation of stools in small areas along the trials within the defecation grounds, and thus ensures repeated contact with the larvae. On the other hand, these patterns of behavior limit the duration of exposure to the infested soil.

The duration of squatting is particularly important. This is the time when the villagers remain stationary and when the infective larvae have the best chance to invade humans. The above estimates that 15 percent of the stools are found within one foot of a trace is an underestimate because of completely unrecognizable old stool points where hookworm larvae might still be present. If we assume that the position of the stool points coincided with the position of the feet only half the time, roughly 15 to 20 percent of the squattings are likely to be in direct contact with the stool points.

The interval between defecation and ablution ($<$ five minutes) is also very important. Unless the larvae that adhere to feet during the defecation activity are able to penetrate within such short durations, they are likely to be washed away in the ablution process. Experimental infections by two colleagues indicate that even after exposures lasting fifteen to thirty minutes under favorable experimental conditions about 60 percent of the larvae failed to penetrate the forearm skin.

Human Behavior and Culture

As in the instances discussed before, the equivocal attitude of people toward fecal pollution is an important element in selection of a defecation spot. The exploratory walk within the defecation ground was at first thought (by us) to be a search for a pollution-free spot.

However, fecal pollution found around identified stools led to further inquiries which revealed that the search is not only for such a spot but also for a number of other choices such as: lack of visibility from the main path; avoidance of others already squatting; avoidance of spots known to be used frequently by the opposite sex; absence of ground cover; a vantage point allowing a view of others entering the ground; and direction of the wind and foul smell.

These criteria seemed to override the ritual considerations of fecal pollution. Ambivalence rather than conformity is the key to their behavior.

When outside defecation grounds people showed concern for fecal pollution within the ground, but when within the ground they did not appear to be very much concerned about other stools around them. Defecation *per se* is a ritually polluting activity irrespective of the ritual pollution attributed to entering a defecation ground or to stepping over feces. The presence of other stools close to the squatting spot is therefore unimportant ritually.

For some high castes, simply entering a bamboo grove is itself a kind of pollution, requiring washing of feet and changing of clothes whether or not the person defecates. Adults would not want to enter a bamboo grove when they are "clean." Avoidance of "stools" voiced by the people is more with reference to the sight and odor of stools. Frequent spitting during the defecation activity was described to be a "natural" response to unpleasant sight and smell.

Other defecation grounds such as fields or tree groves do not connote the same degree of taboo as do bamboo groves. Bamboo groves receive all kinds of "filth" and impurities besides stools (such as useless brooms and pots, clay pots used in offerings to ancestor spirits or in cremation, menstrual pads, the placenta of domestic animals, etc.). In folklore, bamboo groves are also associated with ghosts and witches (at night). On the other hand, fields are "good" and "clean." Stools in fallow fields are a kind of manure, not merely "filth." Many farmers do not like to plow a *hegomath* and hire a low-caste agricultural laborer to do the job. Pollution of fields under jute crop, extensively planted in recent years, is permissible after weeding has been finished. No food crop is pollutable.

Ablution, followed by rubbing hands with soil (taken from or around a pond), is a necessary ritual after defecation. This habit is sanctioned by norms as a purificatory act. Termination of defilement is symbolized by taking a mouthful of water and spitting it out. Many people also prefer to take a bath as a continuation of this ritual. In any case, the clothing worn during defecation is changed. Many people change their "clean" clothes or even shoes before going for defecation. The high castes are required to tie their sacred thread around their right ear (as a sign of desecration) until after they have purified themselves. Only the left hand must be used for rubbing the anus during the ablution. Rural Bengalis do not use the left hand for holding any food material while eating or serving because it is defiling.

The high castes tend to conform to these norms more often than do the low castes. Similar differences exist in socialization of children for appropriate defecation habits. These suggest that differences in the pollution levels should be looked for along these lines.

DISEASE ECOLOGY, HUMAN BEHAVIOR, AND CULTURE

With further study it is possible to replace the qualitative statements about the implications of the behavior with quantitative statements. These can then be used like other population data to develop life tables for the parasite populations (Hairston 1962; MacDonald 1965). Another perspective for epidemiological analysis is to investigate the relationship of some key behavioral/social factors of situations to the levels of hookworm infection.

The qualitative statements are indicative of the direction in which these behavior patterns impinge upon the life history of the parasite. The question central to the anthropological interest is: what overall relationship between culture and disease can be deduced from such an analysis of the function of a set of human factors in regulating the natural history of the hookworm in rural Bengal? This would involve questions such as why people do what they do and how varied behavior patterns relate to other aspects of sociocultural life. As illustrated in the examples given, a consideration of these questions provides numerous points of interconnection between simple behavior patterns and culture.

Burnet defines an endemic disease as "an infectious disease present in a community in which the social circumstances do not offer any effective barrier to its spread" (Burnet and White 1972:202). In contrast to the often emphasized notion that diseases are "manmade" maladies (Gordon 1966: 344; Audy 1972: 79), Burnet recognizes the fact that some human factors act as effective barriers to the spread of disease. In any culture, factors that both promote and restrict diseases are simultaneously present. The pattern of parasitic diseases in a human population can thus be viewed as the net result of these opposite and complementary effects of human factors acting at specific points in the disease cycle.

The various facets of defecation behavior discussed above may be similarly classified as those favoring or limiting the hookworm populations in the study area.

1. Cultural factors that favor the parasite:

a. The habit of fecal pollution of the soil;

b. The habit of going barefoot for defecation;

c. Habits leading to the aggregation of fecal pollution in highly localized and socially recognized foci regularly visited by the population for defecation;

d. Habits and choices of time and place (habitats) which increase the probability of development and survival of hookworm larvae and of contact with active larval populations.

2. Cultural factors which protect man and limit the parasite populations:

a. Habits and choices that restrict contact with the stool points;

b. Choices restricting the duration of exposure and transmission;

c. Habits restricting involvement with the regular defecation grounds and habits restricting deposition of stools in areas (other than defecation grounds) where involvement is much more likely;

d. Habits and choices of time and place (habitats) which decrease the probability of development and survival of hookworm larvae and of transmission.

The first set of factors ensures the continued survival of the parasite population and the second ensures protection of the human population from excessive parasitization. It has been shown above how the different aspects of defecation behavior and habits depend upon traditionally established culture patterns. The two focal trends are complementary effects of the same cultural setting — a combination of complex cultural factors regulating the traditional pattern of defecation habits and behavior. The key elements in this setting are land use, agricultural cycle, cropping pattern, purity/pollution idiom, ambivalent attitude to fecal pollution, conformity to the norms of defecation and ablution, and regularity of habits.

Given the fact that we are dealing with a disease pattern that seems to be naturally regulated by human factors, the above discussion may be summed up under the following general propositions for further examination:

1.   Conformity to the traditional social setting identified above is an effective cultural mechanism regulating the hookworm infection in rural West Bengal (compare Cort 1926: 390; Scott 1937: 525).

2.   Social change altering the key elements of this social setting will upset the traditionally established culture-parasite relationship in the study population (cf. hookworm disease in plantation areas, immigrant and unsettled populations).

REFERENCES

ALLAND, A.
  1966   Medical anthropology and the study of biological and cultural adaptations. *American Anthropologist* 68:40–51.
  1969   "Ecology and adaptation to parasitic diseases," in *Environment and cultural behavior*. Edited by A. P. Vayda, 80–89. New York: Natural History Press.
  1970   *Adaptation in cultural evolution: an approach to medical anthropology*. New York: Columbia University Press.
AUDY, J. R.
  1958   The localization of disease with special reference to the zoonoses. *Transactions of the Royal Society of Tropical Medicine and Hygiene* 52:308–334.
  1965   "Types of human influence on natural foci of disease," in *Theoretical questions of natural foci of diseases*, 83–88. Symposia Československá Věd. Prague: Czechoslovakian Academy of Sciences.

1972 "Aspects of human behavior interfering with vector control," in *Vector control and the recrudescence of vector borne diseases*, 67–84. World Health Organization. Washington: Pan American Organization.

BEAVER, P. C.
1953 Persistence of hookworm larvae in soil. *American Journal of Tropical Medicine and Hygiene* 2:102–108.

BHATTACHARYA, T.
n.d. *Nityakarma Padhdhati* [Procedures for daily rituals]. Calcutta: Orient Library. (In Bengali.)

BISSERU, B.
1967 *Diseases of man acquired from his pets*. London: Heineman.

BUCK, A. A., R. I. ANDERSON, T. T. SASAKI, K. KAWATA
1970 *Health and disease in Chad: epidemiology, culture and environment in five villages*. Baltimore: Johns Hopkins Press.

BURNET, M., D. O. WHITE
1972 *Natural history of infectious disease* (fourth edition). Cambridge: Cambridge University Press. (Originally published 1966 by M. Burnet.)

CASSEL, J. R., *et al.*
1960 Epidemiological analysis of health implications of culture change: a conceptual model. *Annals of New York Academy of Sciences* 84(17):938–949.

CHANDLER, A. C.
1926–1927 The prevalence and epidemiology of hookworm and other helminthic infections in India (in twelve parts). *Indian Journal of Medical Research* 14:185 to 15:695.
1929 *Hookworm disease*. New York: Macmillan.
1935 A review of recent work on the rate of acquisition and loss of hookworms. *American Journal of Tropical Medicine* 15:357–370.

CHOWDHURY, A. B., E. SCHILLER
1968 A survey of parasitic infections in a rural community near Calcutta. *American Journal of Epidemiology* 87(2):299–317.

COCKBURN, A.
1971 Infectious disease in ancient populations. *Current Anthropology* 12(1):45–62.

COCKBURN, A., *editor*
1967 *Infectious diseases: their evolution and eradication*. Springfield, Illinois: Thomas.

CORT, W. W.
1942 Human factors in parasite ecology. *American Naturalist* 76:113–128.

CORT, W. W., *editor*
1926 *Researches on hookworm in China*. American Journal of Hygiene Monograph 7. Baltimore.

DUGGAN, A. J.
1970 "Historical introduction," in *The African trypanosomiases*. Edited by H. W. Mulligan. London: Allen and Unwin.

310   V. K. KOCHAR, G. A. SCHAD, A. B. CHOWDHURY, C. G. DEAN, T. NAWALINSKI

DUNN, F.
1968   "Epidemiological factors: health and disease in hunter-gatherers,"
       in *Man the hunter*. Edited by R. B. Lee and I. DeVore, 221–228.
       Chicago: Aldine.
1972   Intestinal parasitism in Malayan aborigines (Orang Asli). *Bulletin
       of the World Health Organization* 46:99–113.
FABREGA, H.
1972   "Medical anthropology," in *Biennial review of anthropology*.
       Edited by B. J. Siegel, 167–229. Stanford: Stanford University
       Press.
FORD, J.
1970   "Interactions between human societies and various trypanosome-
       tsetse wild fauna complexes," in *Human ecology in the tropics*.
       Edited by J. P. Garlick and R. W. J. Keay, 91–95. New York:
       Pergamon.
1971   *The role of the trypanosomiases in African ecology: a study of
       the tsetse-fly problem*. Oxford: Clarendon.
FOX, J. P.
1966   The environment and the virus. *Archives of Environmental Health*
       12:91–100.
GAJDUSEK, C. D.
1970   Isolated and migratory population groups: health problems and
       epidemiological studies. *American Journal of Tropical Medicine
       and Hygiene* 19(1):127–28.
GARLICK, J. P., R. W. J. KEAY, editors
1970   *Human ecology in the tropics*. New York: Pergamon.
GIGLIOLI, G.
1963   Ecological change as a factor in renewed malaria transmission in
       an eradicated area. *Bulletin of the World Health Organization*
       29:131–145.
GORDON, J.
1966   Ecologic interplay of man, environment and health. *American
       Journal of Medical Sciences* 252:341–356.
GRAY, R. F.
1965   "Medical research: some anthropological aspects," in *The African
       world: a survey of social research*. Edited by R. A. Lystad,
       352–370.
HAIRSTON, N. G.
1962   "Population ecology and epidemiological problems," in *Bilharziasis*.
       Edited by G. E. W. Wolkstenholme and M. O'Conner, 36-62.
       Boston: Little, Brown.
HOCHSTRASSER, D. L., J. W. TAPP, JR.
1970   "Social medicine and public health," in *Anthropology and the
       behavioral and health sciences*. Edited by Otto von Mering and
       L. Kasdan, 242–271. Pittsburgh: University of Pittsburgh Press.
HUNTER, J. M.
1966   River blindness in Nangodi, northern Ghana: a cyclical advance
       and retreat. *Geographical Review* 56:398.

HUSTING, E. L.
1968   "A biological and sociological study of the epidemiology of bilharziasis." Unpublished doctoral dissertation, University of London.

IMPERATO, P. J.
1972   Nomads of the Niger. *Natural History Magazine* 81(10):61.

Johns Hopkins Report
1965–1966   *Johns Hopkins Center for Medical Research and Training Report.* Calcutta.
1967–1968   *Johns Hopkins Center for Medical Research and Training Report.* Calcutta.
1969–1970   *Johns Hopkins Center for Medical Research and Training Report.* Calcutta.

LARICHE, W. H., J. MILNER
1971   *Epidemiology as medical ecology.* Edinburgh: Churchill, Livingston.

MAC DONALD, GEORGE
1965   The dynamics of helminth infections, with special reference to schistosomes. *Transactions of the Royal Society for Tropical Medicine and Hygiene* 59(5):489–506.

MAY, J. M.
1954   The cultural aspects of tropical medicine. *American Journal of Tropical Medicine and Hygiene* 3(3):424–429.
1959   *The ecology of human disease.* New York: M.D. Publications.

NELSON, G. S.
1972   "Human behavior in the transmission of parasitic diseases," in *Behavioral aspects of parasite transmission.* Edited by E. V. Canning and C. A. Wright, 109–122. New York: Academic Press.

POLGAR, S.
1962   Health and human behavior: areas of interest common to the social and medical sciences. *Current Anthropology* 3(2):159–205.
1964   "Evolution and the ills of mankind," in *Horizons of anthropology.* Edited by Sol Tax. Chicago: Aldine.
1970   "Commentary," in *Anthropology and the behavioral and health sciences.* Edited by Otto von Mering and L. Kasdan, 263–266. Pittsburgh: University of Pittsburgh Press.

RAPOPORT, R. N.
1962   Comments. *Current Anthropology* 3(2):190.

RAPPAPORT, R. A.
1967   Ritual regulation of environmental relations among a New Guinea people. *Ethnology* 6(1):17–30.

ROCHE M., M. LAYRISSE
1966   The nature and causes of hookworm anemia. *American Journal of Tropical Medicine and Hygiene* 15:1031–1102.

SCHAD, G. A., *et al.*
n.d.   "The ecology of interacting populations of man and hookworm in rural West Bengal." Unpublished manuscript.
1973   Arrested development in human hookworm infection: an adapta-

tion to a seasonally unfavourable external environment. *Science* 180:502–504.

SCHOFIELD, F. D.
1970   Some relations between social isolation and specific communicable disease. *American Journal of Tropical Medicine and Hygiene* 19: 167–169.

SCOTCH, N. A.
1963   "Medical anthropology," in *Biennial review of anthropology*. Edited by B. J. Siegel, 30–68. Stanford: Stanford University Press.

SCOTT, J. A.
1937   Observations on the transmission of hookworm infection in Egypt. *American Journal of Hygiene* 26:506–526.

SPRENT, J. F. A.
1969   Helminth "zoonoses": an analysis. *Helminthological Abstracts* 38(3):333–351.

STEWART, G. T.
1972   "Communicable diseases," in *Trends in epidemiology*. Edited by G. T. Stewart, 346–393. Springfield, Illinois: Charles Thomas.

WATT, K. E. F.
1966   "The nature of systems analysis," in *Systems analysis in ecology*. Edited by K. E. F. Watt, 1–14. New York: Academic Press.

WORLD HEALTH ORGANIZATION
1964   *Soil transmitted helminths*. World Health Organization Technical Report 277. Geneva.

WRIGHT, C. A.
1970   "The ecology of African schistosomiasis," in *Human ecology in the tropics*. Edited by J. P. Garlick and R. W. J. Keay, 67–80. New York: Pergamon.

Analysis of Incidence of Excessive Alcohol Intake by the Indian Population in Montana

M. F. GRACIA

This study is based on 1970 admission information on the Indian patients in the Alcoholic Treatment and Rehabilitation Program at Montana State Hospital, the only state psychiatric hospital in Montana. Statistics on sex, age, reservation of origin, with or without tribal background, as well as information on those Indians who came from outside the reservation or particular Indian area will be presented.

It should be noted that some Indian patients were not admitted into the treatment program because of lack of motivation or because excessive alcohol intake was not the main problem of the individual or because the medical staff felt the individual was not a good candidate for the program.

We will review age, sex, place of origin (reservation and tribal background) and discuss the ratio of admissions in relation to particular groups, reasons offered by the different groups for acceptance or non-acceptance of treatment and identify factors influencing individual decisions based on past clinical experience as well as anthropological and ethnographic factors that might explain or influence the data obtained.

According to Table 1, 183 males were admitted and 129 (seventy percent) accepted the alcoholic treatment offered. Of the 34 females admitted to the hospital, 18 (fifty-three percent) accepted treatment. Drinking is a male social activity and the amount and strength of the liquor consumed denote one's manliness. "Sissies" do not drink. Females are not accepted into this purely male social activity. As in the old tribal days, the female's role is a secondary one, i.e. to be at home and take care of family needs and socialize with her own female peer group.

Of the reasons given for females not accepting treatment, the need to

Table 1. Hospital admission according to tribal group

| Reservation and area | Tribe | Population | Reservation acreage | Male | | Female | | Total admitted |
				Admitted	Accepted treatment	Admitted	Accepted treatment	
Crow	Crow	3,126	1,598,067	55	42	5	4	60
Fort Peck	Assiniboine Sioux	3,000	998,755	30	27	7	4	37
Blackfeet	Blackfeet	4,850	983,128	46	32	8	4	54
Fort Belknap	Assiniboine Gros Ventre	1,344	626,959	11	6	2	1	13
Flathead	Selish Kutenai	2,212	625,986	8	6	3	2	11
Rocky Boy	Chippewa Cree	915	107,511	3	1	1	0	4
Yellowstone County (possibly Crow)				6	1	1	0	7
Areas other than reservations (counties)				24	14	7	3	31
Totals				183	129	34	18	217

be at home and care for the rest of the family was the most genuine and the most frequently given excuse, while denial of a drinking problem was the second most frequently given excuse. As far as the need to be at home was concerned, marital status made no difference. It is more acceptable for men to be alcoholics than women, not only from their viewpoint, but also from that of family and friends. With Alcoholics Anonymous groups being established on some of the reservations and the fact that there is an increased interest in the female role in other societies, we expect to see more acknowledgment of female alcoholism and more acceptance of treatment programs.

Table 2. Hospital admission according to age and sex groups

	0 to 20 years		21 to 35 years		36 years and older	
Reservation and area	Male	Female	Male	Female	Male	Female
Crow	1	0	23	2	31	3
Fort Peck	0	0	11	5	19	2
Blackfeet	4	0	14	4	28	4
Fort Belknap	0	0	2	0	9	2
Flathead	0	1	5	0	3	2
Rocky Boy	0	0	1	1	2	0
Yellowstone County (possibly Crow)	0	0	4	1	2	0
Areas other than reservations (counties)	1	0	13	4	10	3
Total	6	1	73	17	104	16

As noted in Table 2, there was little difference in the age ratios of admitted male and female patients. Three percent of both sexes were in the younger age group; 50 percent of the females and 40 percent of the males were in the 21 to 35 age group; 47 percent of the females and 57 percent of the males were 36 years and older. Although statistically there is little difference between admitted females in the middle and older age groups, we felt that there were more acknowledgment and acceptance in the younger females of alcoholism being a problem than in the older females. Because the older females had been on the reservation longer, had less education and less chance for education and because their duties in the home have decreased and activity outside the home is not acceptable to them, frustration becomes a more dominant part of living. Alcohol may help relieve this frustration, but is not an acceptable outlet for either the woman or those around her.

As noted in Table 3, from the four largest reservations, the highest incidence of admissions per population base was found, namely the

Table 3.   Ratio of admissions per reservation population

Reservation	Number of admissions	Population	Ratio per population
Crow	60	3,126	1:52
Fort Peck	37	3,000	1:81
Blackfeet	54	4,850	1:90
Fort Belknap	13	1,344	1:100
Flathead	11	2,212	1:200
Rocky Boy	4	915	1:229

Crow with 60 admissions (1:52), Fort Peck (Assiniboine and Sioux tribes) with 37 admissions (1:81), the Blackfeet with 54 admissions (1:90) and Fort Belknap (Assiniboine and Gros Ventre tribes) with 13 admissions (1:100). There was little difference in the ratios per population of admissions from the Flathead and Rocky Boy (Chippewas and Crees) reservations, 1:200 vs. 1:229. Indians were hospitalized from two other regions. From Yellowstone County, one of the most densely populated areas in Montana with good economic stability, the lowest ratio of Indians was admitted. Known for its mixed population, Yellowstone County has a predominance of Crow Indians who have intermingled with Caucasians, ethnic groups such as those with Spanish and Indian backgrounds, and a small number of blacks. The remaining patients were from various counties in Montana and many of these Indians originally came from reservations.

With the highest ratio of admissions and from the largest and most geographically isolated reservation, the Crow once lived in earth lodges, grew corn and tobacco (for ceremonial purposes only), and made pottery. Because of pressure from other Siouan-speaking Indians, they migrated from the Great Lakes area through North Dakota into Montana and became nomadic hunters. Originally, they divided into the River and Mountain Crow and their organized clans are even now in existence as social organizations.

While the Crow had the highest ratio of admissions, the Indians housed at Flathead and Rocky Boy reservations had the lowest. With 1:200 admissions, the Flatheads (or Selish as they prefer to be called) and the Kutenai tribes were once buffalo hunters and fishermen and ate plant foods such as roots, berries, and nuts. Selish, the Flathead tribal language, is spoken by many tribes from Montana to Puget Sound while their brother tribe, the Kutenai, speak a language which is unique and has no connection with any other. Sun dances and winter spirit ceremonies were a part of the religions of the Kutenai, while their neighbors, the Flatheads, sought guardian spirits in the mountains. Native American Indians, the Flatheads were the first tribe housed on a Montana reservation. Preferring Bitterroot Valley because of its climate, they are still resentful of the fact that they were housed at Mission Valley in 1872.

With the lowest ratio of admissions, 1:229, Rocky Boy reservation houses the Chippewa and Cree tribes. The Chippewas speak Algonquin, while the Cree's language is a mixture of French, Chippewa, and Cree. Culturally, the Crees, a mixture of Mongolian, Caucasian, and French, are rejected by other Indian and ethnic groups as not culturally Indian. Nomadic warriors, these landless Canadian Indians were settled on public land at Rocky Boy by an Act of Congress in 1910. Long ago they accepted the Christian religion. Little is left of their Indian heritage.

In comparing the tribes with the highest and lowest number of admissions, it was found that the Crows are geographically isolated from the hospital and other Indians and as an isolated group tend to drink more. With ex-alcoholics on the reservations having formed Alcoholics Anonymous groups, there are more awareness and referral to the hospital treatment program. The Flatheads are near the hospital and come more on their own, while the Crows come in groups. A more mobile tribe, the Crows have mixed more with other groups and have little knowledge of their heritage and tradition; the Flatheads are more insular, tend to marry their own, and are more united and proud of their tribe and its heritage. The Crows have a very poor economy, while the Flatheads have a strong economy and are more independent. Being one of the last groups of Indians to enter Montana, the Crows have not been able to establish as strong a tribal identity in and outside the reservation as have the Flatheads, who came to Montana over 100 years ago and are still resentful about their relocation. The Flatheads have strong control over members of the younger generation, while the Crows have little control over this group.

The Indians housed at Rocky Boy are isolated from other Indians and fewer come to the Hospital. Even the name of their reservation refers to a geographical area and denotes their non-Indian status as far as other groups are concerned.

The second greatest number of admissions came from Fort Peck reservation which houses the Assiniboine and Sioux tribes. Thirty-seven Indians or 1:81 were admitted. The largest number of admissions, 21, came from the older age group, while the middle age group had 16 admissions. There were none from the under 20 years of age group. Originally from North Dakota, the Assiniboine were settled at Fort Peck in 1888, while the Sioux migrated from Canada later. Both of these nomadic tribes were expert horsemen and warriors. Formerly buffalo hunters, too, the Assiniboine speak Sioux. Enemies of the Blackfeet tribe, the seven councils of the Dakota Confederacy still govern many aspects of their daily life.

The Blackfeet tribe had 54 admissions or a ratio of 1:81. For all age groups, this tribe had the second greatest number of admissions of all reservation tribes and the largest number of admissions, 4, in the age 20 and under group. The Blackfeet were the second group of Indians to settle on a Montana reservation in 1874. Migrating from Canada south and west, the Blackfeet were buffalo hunters and fishermen and lived off plant foods. A military society, they requested spiritual help in love, war, gambling, and healing. Their language was Algonquin.

The fourth largest reservation, Fort Belknap, housed the Assiniboine and Gros Ventre tribes. The Assiniboine tribe has been previously discussed since part of this group is housed at Fort Peck. Fort Belknap had 13 admissions or a ratio of 1:100 and almost all of the admissions were Indians from the older age group. The Gros Ventre migrated from French Canada west through North Dakota to Montana. A part of the Algonquin Confederacy, the largest confederacy of Indian tribes on the continent, the Gros Ventre speak Algonquin. They used to make pottery and do some hunting.

After examining the above data, it was found that the tribes who came from a more cohesive and organized society with a more intact tradition and a better economic situation were less willing to come to the hospital for treatment than the individuals who came from a more loose society with less of a traditional background and less identification with any particular group. The groups who were exposed to more mixing and less identity were more interested in coming for treatment. We can speculate that with the lack of tradition and the frustration faced by individuals no longer interested in tradition as well as the loss of identity with the past, these Indians used their alcoholism to escape from guilt, suffering, frustration, or a lack of sense of importance and purpose.

From our knowledge of their heritage, it is apparent that the loss of old rituals created a spiritual crisis and that exposure to a different culture and their difficulty in making a compromise, substitution, or accommodation to new values as well as the fading of old traditions and the indifference of the younger generation to old ideas and values made them confused and frustrated. Progress and evolution of new ideas were replacing the meaningful old rituals which in the early days helped to take care of the task of daily living for the individual, the group, and the tribe. Alcohol became a substitute and modified this painful reality and made it a more acceptable way to live despite the legal, social, economic and other complications of chronic alcoholism.

In some instances we found that a lack of communication between individual Indians and staff members could impair the possibility of acceptance or nonacceptance of the treatment offered. For example, silence is important in Indian culture and is a part of their daily life, but was seen by many staff people as a manifestation of resentment, hostility, or a negative attitude. It was only a reflection of their heritage and a defense mechanism against a new experience, such as the hospital environment.

A knowledge of Indian folklore and an anthropological background will give individuals working with Indians and their problems a better understanding of their frustrations and their individual needs and goals.

Finally, it should be noted that in recent years, the younger generation of Indians has developed an intense interest and pride in their past, their rituals and tradition, and we feel that this might be one of the ways of saving this rich folkloric life and might be a source of personal strength and support for these tribes and become a foundation for the formation of new goals and ideals. Not only for the Indians, but for others as well, these myths and legends might play an important part in explaining the role of man on earth and, from a historical point of view, help many individuals understand themselves and others as well as the environment in which they live.

REFERENCES

ABBOT, C. N.
1964   *Montana in the making* (thirteenth edition). Billings: Gazette.
ALFONSO, E.
1957   *La Atlantida y América*. Madrid: Cultura Clásica.
AMABILIS, M.
1963   *Los Atlantes en Yucatán*. Mexico: Orion.
DONNELLY, I.
1949   *Atlantis: the antediluvian world* (second edition). New York: Harper.
DORSON, R. M.
1950   *America begins*. Greenwich: Fawcett.
EGGAN, F., *et al.*
1947   *Social anthropology of North American tribes*. Chicago: University of Chicago Press.
ELIADE, M.
1964   *Myth and reality*. London: Allen and Unwin.
FREUD, S., D. E. OPPENHEIM
1958   *Dreams in folklore*. New York: International Universities.

HOFF, E. C.
1963   *Aspects of alcoholism.* Philadelphia: Lippincott.
JOSEPHY, A. M., JR.
1961   *The American Heritage book of Indians.* New York: American Heritage.
JUNG, C. G.
1958   *Psyche and symbol.* New York: Bollingen.
1964   *Man and his symbols.* London: Aldus.
Larousse
1959   *Larousse encyclopedia of mythology.* New York: Prometheus.
Montana
1958   *The Montana almanac, 1959-1960.* Missoula: Montana State University.
NORTENSEN, A. R.
1964   *The American West.* Salt Lake City: University of Utah Press.
STAFFORD, H. E.
1959   *The early inhabitants of the Americas.* New York: Vantage.
VETTER, G. B.
1958   *Magic and religion.* New York: Philosophical Library.
VILLASENOR, D. V.
1963   *Tapestries in sand, the spirit of Indian sandpainting.* Healdsburg: Naturegraph.

Witchcraft: An Allegory?

VINIGI L. GROTTANELLI

A field of research in which contemporary anthropologists have remained staunchly entrenched in their Western ethnocentrism is the study of witchcraft. Well aware of the fact that one society after another, in many parts of the world, asserts a firm belief in the actual existence of witchcraft phenomena, they have unanimously taken for granted that such beliefs are illusory. Even to raise the possibility that the societies in question might after all be right in affirming the reality of witchcraft and the anthropologists wrong in denying it has apparently been deemed unworthy of serious scholarship.

I am using the term "witchcraft" in the usually accepted sense of "a mystical and innate power, which can be used by its possessor to harm other people" (Middleton and Winter 1963: 3), and I am not here concerned with the still largely unsolved question of the partial overlapping of this concept with the concepts of sorcery, evil medicine, and magical powers in general. Inasmuch as my main frame of reference is Africa, for the clarity of the argument I shall begin by summarizing the essential traits of the belief in witchcraft among the Nzema, the southern Akan society with which I am most directly acquainted.

Witchcraft (*ayɛne*) is an inborn spirit (*sunsum*) already present in some babies of either sex when they are in their mother's womb and which remains with them throughout their lives. It can occasionally be thrust upon adults, transmitted by succession, or "sold," but even in such cases it is acquired unwittingly. A person possessing *ayɛne* cannot take it into the nether world; before dying, he must pass it on either to another human being or to some domesticated animal, or wrap it up into a bundle, from which *ayene* will later emerge to "embrace" one of the witch's heirs.

Though in rare cases used for good purposes, *ayene* normally corrupts human nature; it causes its bearers to damage other people's property or to destroy their lives. Witches feast jointly on human flesh, each one of a group in turn providing a victim who is killed and devoured in the course of nocturnal banquets. The victim must be a close kinsman of the witch acting as host, usually (but not necessarily) a member of his or her segmented matrilineage. Witches perform most of their deeds at night, and their usual way of locomotion is flight; while the body lies in apparent sleep, the witchcraft spirit flies about, flapping its wings like a bat; its cry, resembling that of some night bird, can be heard up in the air. A witch is gifted with second sight: he or she can see things in complete darkness as clearly as in the daytime or watch things happening far away, and can also see gods, ghosts, or other preternatural beings who are invisible to common mortals. Witches can instantly transform themselves into snakes, bats, hogs, millipedes, or any other animals of their choice. They can work all sorts of wonders (such as, for example, tying together two palm fronds from distant places to make an aerial bridge on which they then run at fantastic speeds, or pulling out a person's eye and using it to replace a lorry's damaged headlight, etc.).

In its essential traits, this pattern corresponds to witchcraft beliefs known from other parts of west Africa, and to some extent also from different societies in other areas. In other terms, the Akan (or, more generally, the African) commoner will accept the fact that witches of this sort DO exist and that the actions and prodigies ascribed to them, while unachievable by common mortals, do actually take place in everyday life — in a word, are REAL. To the average European of the twentieth century, on the other hand, this whole set of beliefs is bound to appear unacceptable, objectively "impossible," UNREAL.[1]

Faced with the alternative between these two positions, antithetical and at first sight irreconcilable, anthropologists have either openly sided with the latter view, or they have ignored the issue altogether, in both cases shifting their analysis to a different level — the sociocultural and functional explanation of that illusion, witchcraft.

In his epoch-making monograph on Zande witchcraft, oracles, and magic, Evans-Pritchard chose the first of the two attitudes mentioned.

---

[1]   The refusal to admit the reality of witchcraft (as opposed to sorcery) antedates by at least ten centuries the rise of anthropological science. Among the authorities who in the Middle Ages held that *strigae* [witches] were no more than a fiction of popular superstition and did not exist in reality are St. Agobardus, Archbishop of Lyons between 816 and 840, Regino of Prüm, Abbot of the famous Prüm Monastery in Eifel between 892 and 899, and Burckhard, Bishop of Worms in the first quarter of the eleventh century.

"Witchcraft is imaginary," he wrote, "and a man CANNOT POSSIBLY be a witch." In a following chapter, he fleetingly referred to the Azande's own attitude not toward witchcraft *per se*, but toward the "deception" and "inefficiency" of witch doctors:

... as in many other of their customs, we find a mingling of common sense and mystical thought, and we may ask why common sense does not triumph over superstition. ... Their idiom is so much of a mystical order that criticism of one belief can only be made in terms of another that equally LACKS FOUNDATION IN FACT (Evans-Pritchard 1937: 119, 193–194; emphasis added).

The obvious implication is that, in the author's mind, Zande "mystical thought" is equated with "superstition," both being contrary to "common sense" — the latter embodying the prevalent opinion of twentieth-century Westerners shared by the author.[2]

The same position was taken years later by Gunther Wagner in his synopsis of Luyia ("Kavirondo") culture: "The charges levelled against [the witch] may be so fantastic that THEY COULD NOT POSSIBLY HAVE A FACTUAL BASIS" (Wagner 1954: 40; emphasis added).[3]

Whether overtly declared, as in these instances, or — as more frequently is the case — tacitly taken for granted, the assumption that witchcraft is inadmissible runs as a red thread throughout the literature. This applies to the authors of general treatises who in recent decades have leaned more or less heavily on Evans-Pritchard's authority (e.g. Radin 1953: 144ff.; Parrinder 1954: 122ff.; Hoebel 1954: 266ff.; Howells 1962: 104–124; Lienhardt 1964: 149–158; Douglas 1967), as well as to social anthropologists who in postwar years have conducted field research on African witchcraft or have edited new studies on the subject (Middleton and Winter 1963; Marwick 1965; Harwood 1970). The issue in question is indeed hardly touched upon in the scholarly little book in which Lucy Mair has recently epitomized all relevant theories on the subject (Mair 1969). By and large, modern anthropologists appear to have concentrated mostly on the attempt to analyze the role of the witchcraft complex in given social contexts: its significance in relation to local frictions and tensions, especially in the framework of the various kinship and political systems and the like. I am contending not that this approach has not led to some fruitful hypotheses, but that it is too narrow. The issues involved are not merely social; they are moral and metaphysical and can be properly understood only in this broader framework.

[2] Some authors go as far so to lament overtly the persistence of this class of beliefs. Nadel (1951: 52) writes: "... no one would dream of defending the perpetuation of a state of ignorance and superstition, of beliefs in witchcraft ...."
[3] But for a more prudent evaluation, see Wagner (1949: I, 112).

Interpreted and "explained" in their mere social setting, native witch-craft beliefs lose some of their apparent absurdity, so contrary to our common sense. But it has strangely never occurred to anthropologists — with the laudable exception of Robin Horton[4] — that "common sense" is hardly an adequate criterion for the scientific assessment of the alleged phenomena concerned; that our duty is not only to verify the object of judgment (i.e. the authenticity of magic powers), but also, and first of all, to verify the validity of the *categoria iudicans* 'the category being evaluated' itself (i.e. of the concept of reality). For this is the very crux of the problem: once I have ascertained that the members of the African society I am studying are convinced, say, that certain persons called witches fly at night, and since in my own society such an action is reputed to be impossible, am I justified as a scientist in assuming at the outset that the African's mind must be blinded by ignorance and superstition, while my own conviction is founded on objective truth? What is "reality" to him, and what is it to me? Am I justified in holding that the only method of assessing or rejecting the authenticity of psychic and behavioral phenomena is the experimental one accepted in our Western sciences?

Questions such as these were propounded and discussed a quarter of a century ago in a book by E. De Martino that has regularly been overlook-ed in anthropological literature abroad, but nonetheless remains a sig-nificant contribution to methodology. In his attempt to analyze the problem of magical powers, De Martino does not directly discuss witch-craft as such, his examples being taken from the cognate fields of clair-voyance, shamanism, fire walking, and precognition, instances of which are quoted from both ethnological and parapsychological sources. His basic criticism, nevertheless, applies equally well to our present topic:

The very possibility of paranormal phenomena is intimately repugnant to the inner history of modern scientific trends .... [It] represents for science a real "sign of contradiction," a "scandal" .... The analysis of the problem of magical powers in the history of ethnology provides us ... with a further opportunity of realizing this: that we take for theoretical evaluation of the magic world what really is only practical expediency, and that we mistake for understanding what in fact is still polemic negation, emotional attitude. But once we have acknowl-edged this situation, by this very fact we have attained a higher historiographic perspective, we are laying the foundations for a worthier humanism .... The comprehension of the magic world is only possible in so far as we extend and deepen our criticism of realistic dogmatism (De Martino 1948: 69, 256–257; my translation).

---

[4]   One could now add the name of M. G. Marwick (1973), whose article came to my notice after the present paper had been written.

Unimpeachable as De Martino's position is at the epistemological level, one must admit that his conclusions are only indirectly constructive for the furthering of anthropological research. True, the inadequacy of what he calls the "naturalistic method," the "experimental science of nature," to solve the problems raised by paranormal phenomena is blatant. True, more specifically, the general omission of any systematic attempt to check the factual foundations (if any) of alleged wizardry phenomena is largely due to the researchers' *a priori* skepticism. But of course this is not the only obstacle: the fact that the very societies which profess belief in witchcraft (as in other paranormal phenomena) enshrine this belief in what we call a "mystical aura" discourages empirical investigation. The gap in *Weltanschauung* is simply too wide.

So, while De Martino's appeal for a "higher" or more comprehensive approach on the part of the anthropologist remains essential, I suggest there is another way by which we should attempt to bridge the intercultural chasm: by a more thorough effort to evaluate the real nature of beliefs at the other end.

Scarce attention has hitherto been given to the ascertainment, along psychological and statistical lines, of the actual degree of faith in witchcraft among the societies concerned. Though the general pattern of belief certainly follows the blueprint accepted in each society and is rooted as such in the minds of most men and women of that society, its nature — to put it in Shirokogoroff's terms — is that of a "hypothesis" (a culture-sanctioned hypothesis), as contrasted with "positive knowledge." The belief may (and, among the Akan of whom I am cognizant, does) find varying degrees of acceptance in the minds of different individuals. Prevalent consensus does not imply totalitarian faith by the whole society, nor a lifetime's unwavering belief at the individual level.

A rare opportunity for a control of this type, apart from direct investigation in the field, is provided by a recent pamphlet on witchcraft written by an educated Nzema in his own language (Aboagye 1969), which I have elsewhere translated and commented upon (Grottanelli 1973), and which may be taken to reflect the opinion of today's literate, urbanized section of the Akan on the subject.

The author describes at such length and with such wealth and precision of details the faculties and deeds of witches, some of which are summarized at the beginning of the present paper, that readers are left with no doubt as to his firm belief in the reality of witchcraft. Yet a recurrent expression, which he untiringly uses in relating those alleged "facts," sheds a significant light on the nature of his belief. According to Aboagye, witches actually DO the perfidious or miraculous things he reports, but they do them "in ayɛne way." Here are a few examples from his text (my translation, emphasis added):

The exchange of meals among *ayɛne* people is done eating human beings.... When the time comes, one of them takes a relative, son or daughter, father or mother ... [and] kills this person at once IN AYƐNE WAY, or hangs him till he is fat before killing him (§ 18).... When they eat meals IN AYƐNE WAY they become well satisfied (§ 19).... If your *ayɛne* friends tell you it is your turn [to provide a human victim for the common meals], and you refuse, all together they will attack you and fight you IN AYƐNE WAY (§ 20).... If one of his relatives owns a lorry to transport passengers, the witch may sell it IN AYƐNE WAY ... and keep the money for himself (§ 22).... A witch may invent an aeroplane, a steamer, a motorcar, a train, IN AYƐNE WAY (§ 95).

The contents and style of the booklet make it plain that Kweis Aboagye did not write it for the sake of scholarship, but in order to provide his fellow countrymen with "factual" information as to the real nature and behavior of witches and with advice as to the practical means to defend themselves against them. At the same time, however, he stresses the fact that the nefarious deeds of witches are performed on a plane of reality conceived as distinct from that of profane, everyday life. This, I believe, is a way of suggesting — in terms comprehensible to the average Akan reader — that the whole witchcraft complex must be understood as a body of symbols,[5] a compromise, as it were, between naive popular belief and Western-inspired skepticism.

If this interpretation is correct, it would point to a possible rapprochement of the two antithetical positions mentioned above. A symbolical explanation of witchcraft, and more generally of magic, is by no means a novelty for Western scholars (cf. Beattie 1966: 202–212); if we are prepared to accept such an explanation, a major obstacle to our understanding of witchcraft beliefs is no doubt removed.

To illustrate the point with one more example from Aboagye's pamphlet: if we are asked to believe that a certain female witch actually transforms her unsuspecting husband into a horse at night in order to ride him, we refuse to do so. Such a metamorphosis is in patent conflict with our "scientific" mentality, so we declare it to be "impossible." But if the same prodigy is submitted to us as having a metaphorical meaning, implying that some domineering wife is constantly ordering her weak husband about, thus reducing him to mental and even physical exhaustion, then we are inclined to accept the fact as likely or even true, because we know from experience that such situations do in fact exist in almost every

[5]   Another Akan writer, a Francophone Anyi from the Ivory Coast, refers to witches' alleged cannibalism as "symbolic meals" (Amon D'Aby 1960: 58, Note 1).

society. In Italy, indeed, this prepotent sort of wife may be referred to jocularly as a *strega* — 'a witch'.

To what extent the average illiterate African accepts and interprets such a metaphorical conception of witchcraft is of course a relevant question. When an Akan says that a witch has "stolen" such and such a man's brain, or has "cut off his head," he KNOWS very well that the victim's head is still visible — we would say objectively — on his neck. When another informant tells us that a witch "flies away" at night, he is well aware that the witch's body is still in its place, asleep in bed, as anyone can see; he means it is only the unfathomable spiritual essence that flies away.[6] In other terms, he is referring to a "symbolic" flight; but in his mind the culture-sanctioned image of *ayɛne* surpasses ordinary human nature so greatly in power, knowledge, and harmfulness,[7] that the symbol overshadows profane experience and is more "real" than everyday reality. In some cases, no doubt, symbolism escapes simpler minds altogether, so that the beliefs are accepted in their literal, vulgar sense. But then we should not forget that the same is true in all societies, including Western ones. It is only a minority of the initiates that perceives the subtleties of symbolical expression in religion, art, and other sectors of culture.

Regardless of the degree of awareness of this symbolism, to the Akan the idea of witchcraft remains essentially the translation into culturally significant terms of an everlasting existential problem, the unavoidable presence of evil — more precisely, of that quintessence of evil brought into this world by the destructive hatred and envy lurking in the heart of close kinsfolk. Inasmuch as another essential trait of this particular kind of evil is its SUBVERSIVE nature (in the literal and etymological meaning of the adjective; see Grottanelli 1973), the witchcraft complex could be defined as AN ALLEGORY OF SOCIAL AND MORAL SUBVERSION.

Here again, I suggest that this definition of witchcraft can be translated in terms compatible with our own conception of this category of evil. That

---

[6] Both opinions are alternatively held by African peoples: that witches fly out IN SPIRIT at night to do their nefarious work and that they go out IN THE FLESH. According to Junod and to Stayt, the Thonga and Venda of southeastern Africa accept the former theory, while according to Schapera the latter prevails among the Kxatla (Schapera 1934: 294). Further inquiries along quantitative lines might help to ascertain how exclusive these two contrasting conceptions are among the peoples concerned.

[7] Carlos Castaneda's studies of Yaqui magic (1971), a recent edition of which was translated into French in 1973 under the telling title *Voir*, have lately called our attention to the fundamental relevance of paragnomic versus "natural" ways of seeing. Exactly like the Copper Eskimo shaman (cf. Rasmussen 1932: 27), the Nzema (Akan) witch is described as "one who has eyes": hence his immense superiority over common mortals.

our own psychic balance, our vitality, and our very physical health are constantly being impaired and undermined ("devoured") by calamities and adversities whose final causes are often inscrutable, and particularly by the avowed or unavowed hostility of our neighbors, is an existential truth that few people in the modern "civilized" world would question. And that hostility and ill-feeling are all the more painful and destructive of our well-being and peace of mind when we detect them in our nearest kinspeople is equally undoubted. Now it is very much the same social and psychological truth that Africans try to assert when they attribute misfortune, illness and death to *aysne* or similar entities, just as our own ancestors did, and indeed as some of our Western contemporaries continue to do.

If we are prepared to accept "the allegory that is witchcraft" as a formulation of existential risks to which our own society is no less exposed than are African ones, expressed in a symbolical phrasing that by its very nature eludes the requirements of experimental control, we will have gone a step further towards solving the age-old dilemma of the "reality" of witchcraft.

REFERENCES

ABOAGYE, P. A. K.
   1969   *Aysne*. Accra.
AMON D'ABY, F. J.
   1960   *Croyances religieuses et coutumes juridiques des Agni de la Côte d'Ivoire*. Paris: Larousse.
BEATTIE, J.
   1966   *Other cultures*. London: Cohen and West.
CASTANEDA, C.
   1971   *A separate reality*. New York: Simon and Schuster.
DE MARTINO, E.
   1948   *Il mondo magico*. Torino: Einaudi.
DOUGLAS, M.
   1967   Witch beliefs in central Africa. *Africa* 37: 72–80.
EVANS-PRITCHARD, E. E.
   1937   *Witchcraft, oracles and magic among the Azande*. Oxford: Clarendon Press.
GROTTANELLI, V. L.
   1973   "La stregoneria Akan vista da un autore indigeno," in *Demologia e folklore: Scritti in memoria di G. Cocchiara*. Palermo.
HARWOOD, A.
   1970   *Witchcraft, sorcery and social categories among the Safwa*. London: Oxford University Press.

HOEBEL, E. A.
1954 *The law of primitive man.* Cambridge, Massachusetts: Harvard University Press.
HORTON, R.
1967 African traditional thought and Western science. *Africa* 37:50–71, 155–187.
HOWELLS, W.
1962 *The heathens: primitive man and his religions.* Garden City, New York: Doubleday.
LIENHARDT, G.
1964 *Social anthropology.* London: Oxford University Press.
MAIR, L.
1969 *Witchcraft.* London: Weidenfeld and Nicolson.
MARWICK, M. G.
1965 *Sorcery in its social setting.* Manchester: Manchester University Press.
1973 How real is the charmed circle in African and Western thought? *Africa* 43:59–70.
MIDDLETON, J., E. H. WINTER, editors
1963 *Witchcraft and sorcery in East Africa.* London: Routledge and Kegan Paul.
NADEL, S. F.
1951 *The foundations of social anthropology.* London: Routledge and Kegan Paul.
PARRINDER, E. G.
1954 *African traditional religion.* London: Hutchinson's University Library.
RADIN, P.
1953 *The world of primitive man.* New York: H. Schuman.
RASMUSSEN, K.
1932 *The intellectual culture of the Copper Eskimos.* Copenhagen: Gyldendale.
SCHAPERA, I.
1934 "Oral sorcery among the natives of Bechuanaland," in *Essays presented to C. G. Seligman.* Edited by E. E. Evans-Pritchard, R. Firth, B. Malinowski, and I. Schapera. London: Kegan Paul, Trench, Trubner.
SHIROKOGOROFF, S. M.
1935 *Psychomental complex of the Tungus.* London: Kegan Paul, Trench, Trubner.
WAGNER, G.
1949 *The Bantu of north Kavirondo,* volume one. London: Oxford University Press.
1954 "The Abaluyia of Kavirondo (Kenya)," in *African worlds.* Edited by D. Forde. London: International African Institute.

The Process of Medical Change in a Highland Guatemalan Town

CLYDE M. WOODS and THEODORE D. GRAVES

THE RESEARCH SETTING

The research upon which this report is based was conducted in San Lucas Tolimán, the *cabecera* [head town] of one of the thirteen *municipios* (geographic and political subdivisions of Guatemala's twenty-two Departments) which surround Lake Atitlán in the southwestern highlands of Guatemala (Tax 1937: 169; Woods 1968; Nash 1969). The population is composed of 3,214 people who consider themselves Indians (81 percent) and 761 people who consider themselves Ladinos (19 percent). While this biethnic distinction implies one population of Spanish-European ancestry (Ladinos) and another whose forebears in the New World predate the Spanish Conquest (Indians), considerable interbreeding has occurred and the contemporary distinction is based less on biological than sociocultural factors. As Richard Adams states the case, the Ladinos and Indians ". . . represent what we can best call sociocultural groups which have historical and racial parallels" (Adams 1957: 267).

Generally speaking, Ladinos speak Spanish, wear Western style

The field research on which this report is based was conducted in 1965–1966 and was sponsored by the Stanford program in Medicine and the Behavioral Sciences, under the directorship of Benjamin D. Paul, with funds from a Public Health Service Grant (No. ES 0068 01) awarded to Dr. Rolf Eliason, Department of Civil Engineering, Stanford University. Supplementary funds were supplied by the Russell Sage Foundation. The present analysis and write-up were facilitated by a Faculty Research Support grant from UCLA to Woods and an NIMH Special Fellowship (1-F03-MH-43,794-01) to Graves. Abelino Celada, a local Ladino, and Genaro Lec, a bilingual San Lucas Indian, provided invaluable aid throughout the field period in their capacity as research assistants.

clothing, practice nominal Catholicism, tend towards nonagricultural occupations, are better educated, economically better disposed, and maintain superior housing, sanitation facilities, diet, and health than do Indians. Conversely, Indians retain their native dialect, distinctive costume, and traditional world view (Tax 1941), engage primarily in subsistence agriculture (maize, beans, and squash cultivated with a primitive technology), and maintain the social, political, and religious life of their communities through sharing service in a series of rotating offices in the civil-religious hierarchy (Carrasco 1961; Nash 1958b). In Guatemalan Indian communities the religious component of this hierarchy consists of a number of ranked and interrelated religious fraternities (*cofradías*), each of which has the responsibility for the veneration and care of a particular saint.

A dynamic environment of change, however, tends to blur many of these sociocultural distinctions in contemporary San Lucas. Phlegmatic in the past, a continuing process of transculturation, whereby traits are lost from the Indian tradition (de-Indianization) and acquired from the Ladino or modern tradition (Ladinization), has taken on a more dynamic aspect in recent years. This can be traced in part to increased Ladino intrusion and influence and to the imposition of external political control.[1] But perhaps more importantly, it is stimulated by an acceleration of modernizing influences, such as increased communication with the outside world (mass media, travel, roads), occupational specialization, religious proselytizing, and various educational, economic, and medical aid programs (Woods 1968, 1969, 1970).

As used here, "Ladinization" and "modernization" refer to similar but not identical change processes. Although local Ladinos provide the Indians with a first-hand model of the more "modern" way of life, their rural expression of national Ladino culture does not exhibit the entire range of modern traits manifested by their urban counterparts. Hence, they too are subject to similar modernization influences. Aid programs, for example, are directed to both populations. Modernization, therefore, ". . . the process by which individuals change from a traditional way of life to a more complex, technologically advanced and rapidly changing life style" (Rogers 1969: 14), should be taken as the more inclusive phenomenon with Ladinization as one manifestation of this process at the local level.

---

[1] Ladinos began their intrusion into the remote highland Indian areas coincident with the coffee boom in the late nineteenth and early twentieth centuries. Political reorganization at local and national levels following the "revolution" (1944) resulted in the loss of considerable local political autonomy in most Indian communities.

Numerous scholars have discussed Ladinization in Guatemalan communities (Siegel 1941; Wagley 1950; Gillin 1951; Tumin 1952; Adams 1957, 1960; Nash 1958a; Reina 1960), and Adams has suggested a continuum of several transitional types as change progresses in these communities. Moving from the most to the least traditional, these types are delineated as: (1) the Traditional Indian Community, (2) the Modified Indian Community, and (3) the Ladinized Indian Community. At the final point in the continuum all Indian traits have been lost, and the Indians enter the Ladino category. In this scheme San Lucas most closely approximates the Modified Indian Community where, according to Adams, a number of Indian traits become weakened or lost, and there is a crystallization of "Indianism" around another group of traits. Those lost or weakened traits include:

... the political-religious organization and the distinctive dress of the men ... all the men and many of the women become bilingual, but the Indian language is still retained as the mother tongue ... women generally retain distinctive clothing although it may not always be possible to identify one's village by the nature of the costume ... the use of the *temescal* often disappears, the Maya calendar is usually no longer functional, and the curers and diviners find considerable competition from Ladino spiritualists and other lay curers (1957: 271).

The Modified Indians, however, still retain many traits which set them aside as clearly Indian, such as:

... the women's distinctive costume, the leadership of men in religious activities ... the cooking still done between three stones on the floor ... the men still use the tumpline for carrying goods and the community retains its integrity as an Indian community. The people still manifest resistance to one of their number becoming a Ladino through the adoption of Ladino traits (1957: 272).

While this typology has obvious descriptive merits, it suffers from two shortcomings which restrict its usefulness in illuminating the actual process of Ladinization. First, along with many of the studies cited above, it lacks a systematic body of data which would allow a consideration and comparison of specific indices of change across communities. Second, by concentrating on gross differences BETWEEN communities, the typology ignores differences in degree of change WITHIN communities. This lack of a sufficient data base and disregard for variation within the society rule out, we think, any serious consideration of process. In this paper we offer an alternative to this static approach by considering specific indices of change and accounting for the degree of variability along these dimensions of change with a body of systematically collected, empirical data. It is variation WITHIN A COMMUNITY, we think, that permits a controlled investigation of the actual process of change.

THE ENVIRONMENT OF CHANGE

The climate of modernization in San Lucas is summarily outlined below in order to place the transitional nature of the community in appropriate perspective. This is necessary for the consideration of the medical and related changes which follows. A house-to-house census of the entire urban population, conducted with the aid of two local research assistants, supplied the data for this analysis. It should be apparent in the discussion of these different dimensions of behavioral modification that the direction of change is clearly away from the Indian tradition and towards the Ladino or modern tradition.

Dress and language are perhaps the most obvious of these modifications in San Lucas. In the past, the members of each of the many Indian societies in Guatemala could be identified by a distinctive homemade costume. In San Lucas, only 16 percent of the adult males retain this symbol of community identification, which consists of red and white striped knee-length trousers embroidered with animal figures, a many-colored shirt, red cloth belt, and dark blue waist-length woolen jacket. The rest have adopted the factory-made shirts and trousers used by the Ladino population. Although the majority retain the use of sandals or go barefoot, 13 percent of the Indian males age sixteen and over have acquired the Ladino practice of wearing factory-made shoes. None of the Indian women have changed to Ladino dress, although most tend toward the factory-made generalized costume found in many other towns in the Guatemalan Republic. Dress, therefore, is no longer a clear indication of community identification for the majority of the population. While the native language, Cakchiquel, a branch of the Mayan-Quiché family, remains the primary language spoken in the home, bilingualism is becoming a norm among the Indian community. Eighty-nine percent of the males and 65 percent of the females age fourteen and over claim some speaking competency in a rudimentary form of Spanish (the national language) and many of the men are fluent in this language.

Family organization and residential patterns have undergone some changes. The tendency is now away from generation-extended households grouped into joint family compounds toward nuclear units residing in separate residence plots. In 1937 Sol Tax noted that the typical pattern of Indian residence in San Lucas was in compounds (1946: 27). Seventy-one percent of all Indian households are now nuclear and only 37 percent are grouped into family compounds. Further, over half of the latter are simple two-household clusters. Although these tendencies more closely approximate Ladino patterns, Indians are still less likely to own the property on which their dwellings stand. Seventy-five percent of the Ladinos but only 40 percent of the Indians own their residence plots.

Changes in house construction and household services are less apparent, though some Indians are beginning to adopt Ladino practices here also. Generally, Indians reside in *ranchos* with a straw roof, walls of cane or a cane frame filled with mud and rocks *(bajareque)*, and dirt floor, while Ladinos occupy *casas* with a tin or tile roof, plastered wooden or rock walls, and cement floors. Presently, some 90 percent of the Indian population have left the traditional *rancho* for a Ladino-style *casa* (6 percent of the Ladinos reside in *ranchos)*. Although 95 percent of all Indian households retain the open fire between three stones on the floor for cooking *(tenemastes),* 4 percent have adopted the raised hearth *(poyo* or *plancha)* of the Ladinos and one boasts a gas stove. Again, while the majority of Ladino homes have sanitary facilities, running water, and a radio, and many have electricity and employ domestic help, only a minority of the Indians have adopted these conveniences. Seventeen percent have built outhouses, 3 percent have running water, and 9 percent have purchased radios. Ten households now use the town's electrical supply and several pay for the services of domestic help.

Another significant departure from tradition in this area is the diminishing use of the sweat bath *(temescal).* In the past this played a central role in native curing practices and the postnatal care of females, and it was also used for bathing. The majority of Indians have now adopted the Ladino practice of bathing in the lake, while new health programs have discouraged the use of the sweat bath for its other functions. Eighty-four percent of Indian households are now without sweat baths and the state of disrepair which typifies many of those still standing is further testimony to the decrease in their popularity.

A number of other changes can be summarily mentioned. School records indicate that more Indians are taking advantage of educational facilities than in the past, although they still lag well behind their Ladino counterparts. Only 15 percent of the Indian population age eighteen and over claim any education, as opposed to 92 percent of the Ladino population of the same age range. And, whereas 97 percent of the present school-age Ladinos attend school, only 22 percent of the Indians do so. An increase is apparent even though the figures remain low. Generally speaking, however, the Indians place less value on the educational process than do Ladinos. This reflects economic realities in this Indian community: along with limited opportunities for nonagricultural employment, time spent in school is time lost working in the fields. Here too, however, some change is evident. Although the majority of the Indian population remain small subsistence farmers, 14 percent of the adult males are now engaged in nonagricultural activities as their major occupational endeavor. Indians still use the tumpline for carrying heavy loads, although it is not uncommon to see the less economically privileged Ladinos utilizing this method in transporting produce from the fields. Where the terrain permits, however, Ladinos prefer a crudely fashioned wheelbarrow.

Courting is more open than in the past and marriage-by-elopement *(robo)* now offers an alternative to the traditional marriage-by-contract *(pedido)*. This has been accompanied by an increase in the incidence of marriage alliances with official civil and/or religious sanction. Twenty-one percent of the current Indian marital unions have been consummated with a civil and/or religious ceremony, as opposed to 77 percent of the Ladino unions. Lois and Benjamin Paul (1963) offer a discussion of similar changes in marriage patterns in a neighboring lake town.

Perhaps the most significant departures from tradition in San Lucas can be seen in the decline of the civil-religious hierarchy. Traditionally, the social, political, and religious life in Guatemalan Indian communities has been maintained by brotherhoods *(cofradías)* whose members share civil and ceremonial responsibility through alternating service in a series of interrelated and ranked civil and ceremonial offices (Nash 1958b; Carrasco 1961). Although this institution remains relatively intact in some communities, its importance has diminished considerably in others. The reasons are multiple and generally involve varying degrees of alienation from traditional patterns by members of the Indian population. Many — particularly those who are younger, have served in the military, and have been more exposed to the world outside their respective communities — choose to invest their time and money in an effort to improve their own financial positions rather than serving a costly one-year period of community service every three or four years. In addition, various subsidiary service and religious groups, including official Catholicism, whose doctrines commonly prohibit service in the traditional offices, compete for Indian loyalty. Once recruited by these rival groups, Indians are no longer available for ceremonial service in the religious fraternities. This increases the burden of responsibility and requires more frequent periods of service for those still willing to serve, thereby further weakening the system and making eventual dissolution more probable.[2]

In San Lucas the system is clearly on its last leg (Woods 1968). Its political functions have been almost totally usurped by the local and national Ladino power structure, and its role in the socioreligious life of the community is being effectively threatened by various social and religious groups which compete for the participation of the local population. While 81 percent of the Indian population are Catholic, 13 percent of these have switched to Reformed Catholicism as interpreted by newly resident priests and no longer serve the religious offices. Many others refuse service because of the heavy burden on their time and finances. Fifty-six of the latter have formed a subsidiary religious group which now bears responsibility for Easter Week activities. Because they retain this responsibility year after year, they no longer feel obliged to participate in regular service. Another 13 percent of the population have become ineligible for service due to their affiliation with one of the three newly formed Protestant sects in the community (6 percent claim no religion). These factors, among others, have combined to reduce the number of men available to staff the traditional offices, and Indian elders express considerable concern over the possibility of staffing even the more important positions in the next few years. On the basis of our formal analysis of the systematic data collected in San Lucas we will have more to say later about pressures leading to the dissolution of the *cofradía* system there. A summary of all these changes in the Indian way of life in San Lucas is presented in Table 1.

In conjunction with these changes there is a less obvious but significant shift in adherence to traditional beliefs. Sol Tax has described the "primitive world view" of Indians living in the western highlands of Guatemala (1941, 1953) and along with other students of Guatemalan Indian communities has noted the tenacity of this set of be-

---

[2] The various factors involved in the decline of one such system in a neighboring town are discussed by Paul (1969). For a detailed account of the Reformed Catholic movement in the Lake Atitlán region see Rojas-Lima (Tax 1969: 56–60).

Table 1.   Changes in traditional Indian practices in San Lucas Tolimán, Guatemala (in percent)

Trait	Indian With	Without	Ladino With	Without
Spanish language (males only)	89	11	100	00
Modern dress (males only)	84	16	100	00
No sweat bath	84	16	100	00
Nuclear household	71	29	77	23
Single household plot	63	37	94	06
Residence plot ownership	40	60	75	25
School population in school	22	78	97	03
Sanctioned marital union	21	79	77	23
Sanitary facilities	17	83	86	14
Nonagricultural occupation	14	86	73	27
Shoes	13	87	91	09
Radio	09	91	57	43
Ladino-style house (casa)	08	92	94	06
Raised cooking hearth	04	96	96	04
Running water	03	97	58	42
Electricity	02	98	44	56
Domestic help employed	01	99	43	57

liefs in the face of apparent changes in material culture (Siegel 1941; Tumin 1952; Adams 1957; Nash 1958a; Reina 1960; Tax and Hinshaw 1970). A questionnaire composed of a set of traditional beliefs was designed to systematically investigate the homogeneity and tenacity of belief in San Lucas. The beliefs tested were taken from a list collected by Tax in the late 1930's and subsequently supplemented by Robert Hinshaw in 1964 in conjunction with his attempt to establish homogeneity of Indian belief throughout the western highland area (Hinshaw 1966; Tax and Hinshaw 1970). The resulting set of ninety-four beliefs was pretested on a small purposive sample of Luceños. It was then added to and eventually reduced to a list of forty-eight beliefs, which this sample appeared to be commonly aware of. The resulting questionnaire was orally administered (with the use of an interpreter when necessary) to a nonrandom sample of forty non-Protestant Indian household heads, selected as representative of the lower socioeconomic strata (which account for over 75 percent of the total population). Each was asked if he were aware of the belief and whether he accepted or rejected its validity. The scores range from a low of eleven to a high of forty-six beliefs accepted as valid, with a mean score of twenty-eight and a standard deviation of eleven.

These findings clearly suggest that belief is neither homogeneous nor rigidly tenacious in San Lucas. It is also significant that many respondents were aware of beliefs which they rejected as no longer valid. Hence, commensurate with our previous findings, considerable variation within the community is manifested in belief as well as behavior. A further breakdown of these beliefs along with a discussion of the relationship between changing belief and behavior is incorporated in the analysis of the change process below.

In spite of these observed variations on traditional patterns, it would be a mistake to disregard the fact that San Lucas is still an Indian community. (See Nash 1958a; Reina 1960; and Tax and Hinshaw 1970 for parallel interpretations.) The Indian population is set apart from their Ladino neighbors by a body of custom and belief, albeit in attenuated form, and by their own identification with the community. Not only are they Indians, but Luceños, and hence consider themselves distinct from Atitecos (Indians from Santiago Atitlán), Maxeños (Indians from Santo Tomás Chichicastenango), and Pedraños (Indians from San Pedro La Laguna). Informants note that whether for economic opportunity, marriage, or other reasons, it is still a drastic step for an Indian to sever ties with his own town. Community endogamy is the rule and even marriage to local Ladinos remains a rare occurrence. Only fifteen out of 732 households in San Lucas (2 percent) contain a mixed (Indian-Ladino) marriage. While 27 percent of the local Ladinos resident in San Lucas in 1966 were born elsewhere, all but 6 percent of the Indians were born in the town.

In sum, although the Indian population in San Lucas retains its integrity as an Indian community, modifications in belief and behavior are evident. Further, the direction of change is clearly away from traditional Indianism and toward a more modern Ladino way of life. Mutually reinforcing external and internal forces operate in this process; the quest of material goods and alternative life style leads to increasing involvement in the cash economy and alienation from traditional social, political, and religious institutions. The severely handicapped and disappearing civil-religious hierarchy provides the most dramatic example of this breakdown in traditional structures. As these local institutions lose their "compulsive validity," i.e. fail to meet the needs of a significant portion of the society (Mandelbaum 1941), and cultural disorganization proceeds, the search for workable alternatives takes on an element of necessity (Keesing 1952; Broom, et al. 1954; Wallace 1962). Hence, we find in this and many similar situations an internal predisposition for external influence (Gluckman 1940: 135). One important channel for this external influence is the large and influential resident Ladino population in San Lucas which offers a clear and ever present model of a more modern way of life.

SYSTEMS OF MEDICINE

The transition from traditional to modern in San Lucas is particularly apparent in modified medical behavior. Native curers are experiencing considerable competition from other medical resources available to the community and their services are increasingly relegated to traditional etiological categories, such as evil eye, fallen fontanel, and witchcraft, which are not recognized by the practitioners of scientific medicine (Woods 1968). Similar findings elsewhere in Latin America have been reported by Adams (1952), Erasmus (1952), Simmons (1955), and Rubel (1960). Although elder informants were able to supply a list of thirty-six native curers practicing twenty-five years ago, only thirteen shamans were active in 1966, none of whom practiced his traditional role on a full-time basis. Alternative solutions to medical problems are offered to both Ladinos and Indians by Ladino pharmacists, spiritualists, practical nurses, lay curers, and university-trained doctors.

Our research in San Lucas focused on the process of medical change. More specifically, it was an attempt to locate, describe, and explain changes in medical practice and belief initiated by the interaction of three conceptually distinct and competing systems of medicine: Folk Indian, Folk Ladino, and Modern. Modern Medicine, a relatively recent import, encompasses a system of beliefs and practices from the tradition of Western scientific medicine, while Folk Indian Medicine takes its principles from indigenous Indian patterns. Folk Ladino Medicine derives primarily from the national Ladino tradition but has been influenced by both other traditions and represents something of an amalgam. Each of the various medical practitioners in San Lucas can be placed into the appropriate conceptual category according to the nature of the beliefs and practices each brings to the curing situation.

The practitioners of Folk Indian Medicine in San Lucas include shamans, midwives, and a number of lay (or occasional) curers. All are Indians and adhere primarily to the principles of curing inherited from the traditional Indian way of life. By traditional we do not imply pre-Conquest Mayan patterns, but the configuration which developed through the fusion of Spanish and Mayan elements after the Conquest but before the Ladinos became locally dominant in the late nineteenth and early twentieth centuries. Space considerations permit only a brief synopsis of this configuration as it relates specifically to medical beliefs and practices.

The system of traditional beliefs in San Lucas includes several related elements which bear directly on curing practices (Woods 1968, 1969, 1970). The most important of these concern beliefs in (1) a direct relationship between the incidence of misfortune (including illness with the possibility of death) and infractions of a stringent moral code, (2) a vaguely defined preordained lifeway, and (3) an overwhelming pantheon of supernatural agents which maintain absolute power over life and death.

The moral code prescribes that the Luceño should work hard, be patient and content with his station, provide as well as possible for his immediate family, avoid all arguments, be humble and amiable in interpersonal relationships, respect the rights and property of others, and above all, believe in and love God and show proper submission and reverence to all the supernatural powers. On the negative side he must never use evil words or have evil thoughts, talk against other people, show envy over the good fortune of others, or be belligerent with his fellows. Illness, with the possible consequence of death, is a commonly accepted sanction for violations of this code. The Indian who departs from these rigid standards is subject to direct sanction from God; he becomes open prey for a host of free-roaming malevolent spirits, and a likely candidate for witchcraft. Similarly, he can seek his own misfortune through carelessness, neglect, and minor sins.

Related to this is the Indians' belief in a form of predestination. God not only endows man with body and spirit, but with a vaguely defined preordained lifeway best explained with the concepts of *suerte* [luck] and *destino* [destiny], where *suerte* is the preordained path of one's life and *destino* the fulfillment of that journey. Jointly they account for the totality of events and activities which comprise the unique configuration of each man's mortal existence. This includes such things as his occupation, luck with the opposite sex, calamities, and, centrally important to this paper, the career of his health. The kinds of illnesses a person contracts, the frequency of their occurrence, and the cause of death are said to be marked in the *suerte* and are conceived as one's *destino* when they occur. The Luceño, therefore, finds himself in a curious bind. He is sanctioned for violations of the moral code, but these sanctions and the violations which bring them about are believed to be preordained in his *suerte* at birth.

There is, however, an element of individual responsibility in Luceño cognition. Each man is charged with the task of searching out his true *suerte* through determined effort, diligent application of his intelligence, and strict adherence to the moral code. When this element of self-mastery fails, of course, he can retreat to his belief in predestination to explain his own shortcomings and perhaps to disregard the plight of his fellows. Mortal man is, after all, powerless to interfere with the fixed course of his own *suerte* or that of his neighbors.

These comments underscore the Luceño's feeling of impotence and helplessness in the face of overwhelming supernatural odds. God, and the lesser powers which fall within His realm, must be revered in daily prayer and petitioned for forgiveness and aid in time of crisis. In addition each man must be constantly on guard against a multitude of evil spirits who share man's everyday world and are ever ready to take advantage of his mortal weakness. The Luceño's approach to these supernaturals further dramatizes his impotence. Although daily prayers at the household altar or occasional visits to the saints in the church or *cofradía* can be conducted through his own efforts, all important contacts with the supernatural world require the use of an intermediary. The shaman, witch, and lay curer are the more traditional of these mediums between mortal man and his distant deities, although the spiritualist and the priest have been recently added for some. This strong belief in the necessity of supernatural intercession in the curing process in conjunction with the fatalistic notion that illness is an unavoidable result of immoral behavior explains, in part, the Indian's reluctance to relinquish the use of traditional curers and the esoteric knowledge they possess.

The thirteen practicing shamans in San Lucas, several of whom are also considered witches, conduct their traditional divination and curing ceremonies *(costumbres)* in private homes, religious fraternities *(cofradías)*, the Catholic church, hillside caves, and several special locations in the countryside. Nonlocal shamans, who either journey to San Lucas or are visited by Luceños in their own localities, are also used. Because most Ladinos, progressive Indians, and proponents of Modern Medicine consider shamanistic practices primitive and their adherents backward, much of the shamans' activity is clandestine.

Six Indian midwives deliver the majority of the newborn in San Lucas, although a few Indians and the more affluent Ladinos resort to a nurse or a doctor for this service. Four of these women are certified by the Public Health Service, while two are uncertified novices. Midwives are also used as knowledgeable resources in the treatment of illness, especially where an infant is involved.

The Indians have no specific term for lay curers, merely noting that in some cases they seek the services of *uno que sepa* [one who knows]. In most cases these are elderly Indian women who, through years of experience, have become familiar with various symptoms, remedies, and treatment procedures. Similar to the shaman, the lay curer commonly follows a treatment procedure which includes (1) diagnosis, (2) a search for the cause of the ailment, (3) the supplication of appropriate supernatural figures, and (4) the administration of secret remedies and procedures.

Modern Medicine in San Lucas is represented by three doctors, two registered nurses, and several practical nurses. One of these doctors, a Guatemalan national employed by the Alliance for Progress, has been resident in the town for three years and is the community's major contact with the tradition of scientific medicine. Although he does not restrict his practice to San Lucas, he schedules consultations locally two days each week and is available for emergency calls most evenings. The other two doctors, one a Guatemalan national and the other a papal volunteer from the United States, make irregular visits to a public health clinic and a Catholic parish dispensary, respectively. In their absence the clinic is operated by a Guatemalan registered nurse and the dispensary by nuns from the United States. With the appearance of the resident Alliance doctor, the public health service doctor discontinued his weekly visits to San Lucas, which had reportedly begun several years earlier. The doctor at the parish has only been available for a matter of months and his visits are only temporary. Some Indians have used the hospital across the lake in time of serious illness, but this remains an infrequent practice. Several practical nurses, who reside in the community and have received the bulk of their training from formally trained medical personnel, provide additional medical resources in this category. While Modern Medicine has made rapid headway in the community, it is clear that its basic principles remain obscure to the bulk of the Indian population. Notions of preventive medicine, germ theory, and contagion through contact are still foreign ideas to most.

The local proponents of Folk Ladino Medicine include two pharmacists, two spiritualists, and several lay curers. All claim some knowledge of Western medical science and rely primarily on medicinal remedies from this tradition. Nevertheless, none have received formal training in the principles of Western medical science and some of their practices and beliefs appear more closely related to the Folk

Indian Tradition. Within this category, the pharmacists, who have been represented in the community for several decades, are by far the most important and frequently used resource. In addition to selling medicine across the counter, they make house calls and prescribe treatment for ailments diagnosed on the basis of visual or verbal symptoms. The hypodermic needle is foremost in their repertory of treatment.

Neither of the local Ladino spiritualists is considered to be particularly effective, and they are sought more for their reputed knowledge of herbal and patent remedies than their ability to communicate with the spirit world. Although an occasional séance is held, Ladinos and Indians desirous of this form of aid are more likely to seek the services of a more reputable practitioner in one of the centers of spiritualism in the larger urban areas. This low frequency of use of local spiritualists should not be taken as an indication that spiritualistic beliefs are uncommon in San Lucas. Quite the contrary. Other studies have indicated that spiritualism is an integral part of Ladino beliefs in Middle America and there is little reason to suspect otherwise in San Lucas. Although no systematic investigation of local spiritualism was conducted, interviews and informal conversations with various representatives of the Ladino population suggested that there was wide support for these ideas and many of the representatives reported regular usage for both curing and "surgical" purposes. Spiritualism is also entering into the Indian system of practice and belief. This can be attributed in part to the acceptance of superiority in Ladino traditions (informants commonly noted that the best way to counteract a strong case of shaman-induced witchcraft is to acquire the services of a competent Ladino spiritualist) and to a similarity between traditional Indian and spiritualist methods. Like the shaman, but unlike the doctor, the spiritualist claims supernatural power, serves as an intermediary between distant supernaturals and the stricken, and employs similar curing techniques. Hence, spiritualist practices and beliefs do not come into conflict with Indian traditions as does Modern Medicine. Madsen (1965) describes a parallel case in Mexico.

Lay curers in the Ladino tradition are often called upon to treat similar ailments as are their Indian counterparts. They are more likely, however, to use pharmaceutical preparations and the hypodermic needle in their procedures. Some claim the ability to communicate with the supernatural, conduct sorcery, cure alcoholism, and practice love magic.

Each medical system can be further divided conceptually into "major" and "minor" resources. As shown in Table 2, the doctor, pharmacist, and shaman are regarded as "major" curing resources while the public health service nurse, parish clinic nuns, lay curers, midwives, and spiritualists are considered "minor" resources. Minor resources are used primarily for the acquisition of free or inexpensive remedies and occasional minor treatment.

Table 2. Three medical systems in San Lucas Tolimán, Guatemala

Medical system	Major resources	Minor resources
Modern	Doctor	Nurse; nun
Folk Ladino	Pharmacist	Lay curer; spiritualist
Folk Indian	Shaman	Lay curer; midwife

Patients often have no actual first-hand contact with the resource since other family members may be sent for medicine and advice. The use of major resources involves greater financial and emotional investment. Cost is generally much higher and the patient is under the direct supervision of the practitioner for varying amounts of time, depending on the prognosis of the ailment. This is true when the doctor and pharmacist administer treatment during house calls or at their respective establishments, or when the shaman conducts ritual ceremonies and applies secret remedies. It should be mentioned also that in all three of these competing systems of medicine, minor resource personnel are predominantly women while major resource personnel are men (one female shaman practiced on an irregular basis during the period of investigation).

Two alternative responses to health complaints are not included in this conceptual scheme: self-treatment and no treatment at all. Both are high-frequency responses for the majority of Luceños, both Indian and Ladino; they may occur anywhere in a curing sequence while other resources are being used or they may constitute curing strategies in and of themselves. Ignoring symptoms, however, most commonly occurs in the early stages of an illness episode prior to the use of other curing resources.[3] Self-treatment includes the use of inexpensive patent medicines purchased at the pharmacies, home remedies such as herbs, poultices, juices, and alcoholic beverages, or quite commonly, a combination of the two.

[3] As used in this paper, a "complaint" generally refers to the patient's personal report of symptoms, although this information was sometimes supplied by family elders, particularly where children were concerned, and occasionally from one of the local curing specialists. An "illness episode" is the history of a given series of related complaints from initiation to termination, where the latter is represented by

After a brief discussion of the methodology employed for the observation of medical behavior, the differential use of these various curing alternatives by a sample of the Indian and Ladino population will be considered.

Data for the analysis of resource utilization and medical behavior which follows were collected from our basic sample of forty Indian households, already described, plus a comparison sample of fifteen lower socioeconomic Ladino households. Over a period of six months, from January through June of 1966, a running account of the medical practices of these forty Indian households (234 people) and fifteen Ladino comparison households (ninety people) were recorded. At least once each week each household was visited and members were interviewed regarding (1) symptoms or illness contracted (syndromes with a specific verbal referent), (2) the prognosis of previously reported complaints, (3) the curing alternatives being used to combat these complaints, and (4) the cost, source of reference, and reason for using these resources. When a major illness episode was in progress, households were visited more frequently, often on a daily basis.

The corpus of data obtained by these procedures was further augmented by the systematic community census, informal interviews, and formal questionnaires periodically administered to sample household heads, which provided information regarding past medical behavior, interviews with various curers, records available from local medical agencies, participant observation in a number of curing episodes, and the informal round of conversation that inevitably accompanies major illness in a small community.

During the observation period 1,008 complaints were registered by the Indian sample (an average of 4.3 per person) and 430 by the Ladino sample (an average of 4.8 per person). Table 3 shows that the Indians disregarded 32 percent of their complaints and responded with self-treatment for 41 percent while the Ladinos disregarded 35 percent of their complaints and relied on self-treatment in another 35 percent. Therefore, major and minor resources from the three systems of medicine outlined above were used to treat only 27 percent of Indian and 30 percent of Ladino complaints. The differential utiliza-

---

either discontinuation of treatment or death. Complaints are related when reported symptoms are identical or closely similar from one household visit to the next and when the patient or his spokesman believes them to be the same, rather than a new, problem. A "curing sequence" refers to the sequential use of actual curing resources to combat complaints in an illness episode. Obviously there could be an illness episode without a curing sequence, e.g. no resources used to combat complaints.

Table 3. Indian and Ladino responses to health complaints by a sample of forty Indian and fifteen Ladino households during a six-month observation period

	Indian complaints registered		Ladino complaints registered	
	Frequency	Percent	Frequency	Percent
No treatment	324	32	150	35
Self-treatment	416	41	150	35
Medical resources	268	27	130	30
Totals	1008	100	430	100

Table 4. Comparative use of medical resources by a sample of forty Indian and fifteen Ladino households in San Lucas Tolimán, Guatemala, during a six-month observation period

Resource used	Indian Frequency	Percent	Ladino Frequency	Percent
Minor				
Nurse; nun	143	53	60	46
Ladino lay; spiritualist	16	6	13	10
Indian lay; midwife	4	2	4	3
Subtotals	163	61	77	59
Major				
Doctor	54	20	44	34
Pharmacist	31	12	9	7
Shaman	20	7	0	0
Subtotals	105	39	53	41
Totals	268	100	130	100

tion of these resources is shown in Table 4. While the use of minor resources is similar for both samples, significant departures are apparent where major resources are concerned. Ladinos resort to the doctor frequently and exclude use of shamans from their curing practices. Further, although space considerations preclude inclusion of the empirical data, Ladinos incorporate the services of a doctor earlier in the curing process. Hence their illness episodes tend to be shorter than those of their Indian counterparts (Woods 1968: 177).

We can draw several generalizations about the curing behavior manifested by the Indian sample during the observation period. Initial complaints may be disregarded or countered with self-treatment or minor medical resources, or, commonly, a combination of these. No attempt at diagnosis is sought beyond the practical knowledge of immediate household members. The probability of moving to major medical resources increases where symptoms persist or become more severe. When an incapacitating ailment is involved, this move borders on certainty. At this juncture, however, Indian curing behavior is characteristically heterogeneous. The kind of resources used and the order of their appearance in the curing sequence depend on a number of interdependent factors. The history of the illness episode, past experience, economic considerations, advice from others, and diagnosis are particularly important in this regard. A number of changes between alternative resources in the search for an effective cure is commonplace, even where traditional etiological categories (with supposedly automatic traditional curing strategies) are brought to bear. During the observation period 28 percent of the Indian sample used both the doctor and the pharmacist, 10 percent used both the shaman and the doctor, and 8 percent used both the shaman and the pharmacist. In many cases these competing medical practitioners were used concurrently. In this respect, even though practitioners of Modern Medicine may be incorporated into the curing sequence, they sometimes serve to supplement rather than to replace their folk counterparts.[4]

Despite this evidence of syncretism, the extent to which modern medical practices are replacing traditional practices among these Indians, even in the brief time they have been available, is impressive. Only 30 percent of the sample Indian households employed a shaman during the six-month observation period, whereas almost 60 percent went to one of the doctors. Only one Indian household used the services of an Indian lay curer or midwife during this same period, whereas almost three-quarters used the nurses or nuns. Clearly change is proceeding apace in this domain.

This generalized description of medical behavior in San Lucas documents the existence of changing medical practices among these Indians, but offers little information about the actual process of change. Clearly, considerable variation within society manifests itself here as in other areas of behavior in the environment of change in San Lucas: some Indians retain the use of traditional curers, most have turned to modern curers, while a few use a combination of both. By focusing on this intrasociety variation within our Indian group we hope to illuminate better the process of change. We will be particularly concerned with the relationship between changing medical practices and the un-

---

[4] Similar findings have been reported by others who have studied the introduction of Modern Medicine into traditional areas (Redfield 1941; Simmons 1955; Firth 1959; Gonzáles 1964; Madsen 1965; Wolff 1965; Schwartz 1969).

derlying belief systems which support them, as these relate to intra-community differences in other areas of past and present Indian behavior.

THEORETICAL CONSIDERATIONS

Culture change theory at present is relatively unsystematic and contradictory. The few efforts at synthesis either end up as a catalogue of relatively unrelated ideas (Broom, et al. 1954; Kushner, et al. 1962) or emphasize only one of several competing viewpoints (Barnett 1953; Hagen 1962; Rogers 1962, 1969). Given this state of theoretical chaos, the present study was undertaken with no explicit guiding hypotheses. Rather, it was designed pragmatically to explore a range of alternative points of view: to see what was actually going on in San Lucas Tolimán and if this empirical evidence might help clarify some of the theoretical controversy in the field. This does not mean that the research was without theoretical guidance, however, as will become apparent below.

Culture change research can focus on the problem at several points. Three which seemed particularly pertinent to our situation were (1) characteristics of the "innovators" and "early adopters," i.e. what sorts of people are most or least receptive to new techniques and ideas, (2) characteristics of the innovations, i.e. what sorts of cultural elements are most readily adopted or modified, and (3) characteristics of the change process itself, i.e. what is the typical sequence of change, what touches it off, what types of secondary, linked reactions may be set in motion. Each of these general problem foci will receive attention here, and our conclusions will attempt to consider some of the interactions among these three areas of interest as well.[5]

The characteristics of innovators and early adopters, i.e. persons who accept novel beliefs and practices well before the majority, is a subject of both theoretical and empirical controversy. On the one hand are those who picture the innovator as a "deviant" or "marginal man," who is less committed to tradition because he is less frequently a recipient of traditional rewards. Barnett's notion that the disgruntled, maladjusted, frustrated, and incompetent are the most

---

[5] Studies of directed change may also focus on characteristics of the change agent, i.e. what sorts of people are most effective in introducing new elements; and cross-cultural comparative studies can inquire about what sorts of sociocultural settings are most conducive to or resistant to change. Neither of these problems was addressed in the present research.

likely innovators (1941, 1953) is typical, and has been echoed by others (Linton 1952; Rogers 1962; Hagen 1962). This same rationale has been used as the basis for postulating that young people are more receptive to innovations than those whose age and experience have tied them more closely to the traditional prestige and reward system. Empirical support, in addition to the case material on which these ideas were based, is substantial. For example, in Robert Maher's systematic study of culture change in New Guinea, he found that those Papuans most ready to adopt a modern way of life were younger and less wealthy in pigs, shell ornaments, and wives (1960). In contrast to this viewpoint is Everett Rogers' work, initially within the United States, but now including substantial cross-cultural material. While agreeing that innovators tend to be young, he also typically finds early adoption associated with wealth and high social status (1969: 296 ff). Because wealth and status tend to be positively associated with age, these results appear internally contradictory.[6] Our data from San Lucas Tolimán help resolve some of these apparent inconsistencies.

A second (and less controversial) set of innovator attributes centers on the EXPOSURE of a potential adopter to alternative techniques or viewpoints through literacy, the mass media, contact with change agents, travel, etc., and associated psychological characteristics of "empathy," "cosmopoliteness," and "innovativeness" (Rogers 1969). Again our Guatemalan data are relevant, linking these notions as well to a model of the change process.

The many debates concerning characteristics of those traits most susceptible to change will not be dealt with at any length here. The only matter of interest is whether health-relevant BELIEFS or health PRACTICES will change first, and how these two elements may be linked in the change process. Within anthropology there is a strong tradition which states that changes in the ideological sphere are preceded by changes in the technological sphere (Linton 1936; White 1949). By contrast, a competing theoretical viewpoint (Weber 1953; Vogt 1960; Hagen 1962) argues that ideological systems are fundamental, either inhibiting or predisposing toward change. Belief systems incompatible with modern practices, therefore, must change first, thereby setting in motion changes in social relationships and technology.

---

[6] Rogers' empirical research cross-culturally (1969) thus appears to contradict in some aspects this earlier theoretical formulation concerning the social marginality of innovators (1962). But such contradictions are frequent in the literature. McConnell (1965) has provided a useful review.

Finally, in Moore's "theory of partial autonomy" he argues that certain elements of culture, namely aesthetic forms and supernatural beliefs, are relatively autonomous and can change independently of other areas of the system. Hence, their loose connection with ordinary patterns of behavior ". . . means that relatively autonomous change might occur without a kind of 'systemic resistance' deriving from interlocking patterns" (1963: 75).

Ethnographic observations in Guatemala support the notion that native epistemologies remain largely intact and are surprisingly resistant to change. But they are less clear as to whether these beliefs are relatively autonomous, are changing in response to other nonideological changes, or constitute a fundamental factor which must be modified BEFORE substantial change can take place in other areas. For example, Sol Tax has for years reported the persistence of a "primitive world view" among Indians of the highlands (1937, 1941, 1953) and discusses the effectiveness of this tenacious set of beliefs in inhibiting the acculturation process (1941). Nash reports that while many changes followed the introduction of a textile factory into a traditional Guatemalan Indian community, belief systems remained intact (1958a); and Reina writes about another Guatemalan community where the Indians have not hesitated to add material items to their cultural inventory as long as these superficial adoptions do not conflict with their traditional world view. He concludes that extensive external change influences have not yet drastically affected the main aspects of the Indian culture, its configuration, or orientation (1960: 102). Finally, a recent restudy of Panajachel, a community across the lake from San Lucas studied by Tax from 1934 to 1941, focused on shifts in traditional world view (Hinshaw 1966). In a recent report on this work, Tax and Hinshaw (1970) note that with "economic ladinization" has come a gradual shift in traditional beliefs in the direction of the Ladino patterns. But they further suggest that the form of acculturative accommodation which is thereby occurring can be traced to a "Protestant ethic" inherent in the value orientations of the Indian population. Again, our data from San Lucas Tolimán may help resolve these controversies.

These various foci of concern find their synthesis in the study of the adoption PROCESS. Processual implications are inherent in much of the theory and empirical findings already sketched: (1) Does exposure to new ideas lead to a cosmopolitan world view and predisposition to change, or does such a predisposition lead a person to seek out contact with alien agents and ideas? (2) Do changes in beliefs follow upon technological change, or do they determine the course of that change? (3) What role does age and wealth play in this process? Again our data from San Lucas can be brought to bear. We will pay particular attention to the sequence of changes in different areas of native life while at the same time taking cognizance of Rogers' warning that modernization is a multivariate phenomenon:

The basic tenet is that the multitude of possible modernization concepts are connected in a cobweb of interdependent relationships, such that they function in a state of dynamic equilibrium. Variations in any one variable, therefore, trigger corresponding changes in numerous other concepts (Rogers 1969: 316).

OPERATIONAL PROCEDURES

Our first task is to establish adequate indices of our two major "dependent" variables: medical beliefs and practices. It is the differences among Indians in these attributes that our research hopes to explain. As in the measurement of most variables in this study, several alternative and operationally distinct indices were devised. This permits an examination of the "convergent validity" of our measurement procedures, as well as the construction of combined indices which tap the underlying concept more broadly than does any one index alone.

Medical Practice

Four scales of medical practice, representing a continuum from traditional to modern, were constructed. Three rely on the actual use of different curing resources during a six-month observation period while the fourth combines the latter with reported resource preferences and past usage.

1.   MAJOR RESOURCE USE: A scale of the use of major curing resources during a six-month observation period. Resource use was weighted from traditional to modern in the following manner: Each use of a doctor (Modern Medicine) was multiplied by two; each use of a pharmacist (Folk Ladino Medicine) was multiplied by one; and each use of a shaman (Folk Indian Medicine) was multiplied by zero. The total of these weighted scores (numerator) was then divided by the total possible score (denominator) had all resources used been modern. The resulting proportion was used for purposes of scaling with a range from 00 (all traditional) to 100 (all modern).

An example is shown in Table 5.

2.   MINOR RESOURCE USE: A scale of the use of minor curing resources

Table 5. Use of major resources

Resource used	Frequency	Weight	Numerator	Denominator
Doctor	4	2	8	8
Pharmacist	2	1	2	4
Shaman	2	0	0	4
			10	16

10/16 = .63 (scale score)

during the six-month observation period. Scale scores were computed using the same procedures outlined for major resource use, but substituting for the doctor, pharmacist, and shaman the parallel minor curing resource: nurse or nun (Modern), Ladino lay curer or spiritualist (Folk Ladino), and Indian lay curer or midwife (Folk Indian).

3. COMBINED RESOURCE USE: A scale combining the use of major and minor resources during the six-month observation period, but doubling the weight given the use of major resources. The score on the use of major resources was multiplied by two and added to the score on the use of minor resources. The resulting figure was used for scaling purposes as shown in the following example:

Major Resource Use Score .63 x 2 = 1.26
Minor Resource Use Score .32 x 1 = .32   1.58 (scale score)

4. RESOURCE PREFERENCE AND USE: A Guttman Scale (reproducibility = .92) was constructed from four measures of the preference and use of traditional and modern medical resources.
a. The informant rejects use of the shaman.
b. The informant has not used a shaman in the previous five years.
c. The informant has used a doctor at least once in the previous two years.
d. The informant does not reject use of the doctor.
Note that this scale includes elements of the other medical practice scales in that items (b) and (c) also include resource use during the six-month observation period.

The correlation between major and minor resource usage was only .19, but both correlated much more strongly with the Preference-Use Scale (.73 and .27, respectively). The Combined Resources Scale, however, correlated even more highly with this alternative measure (.76), suggesting that it is useful to include both major and minor resources. Because of this comprehensiveness of content, as well as the reliability of the six-month data collection, this Combined Resources Scale has been chosen as our key measure within this domain.

Belief

This domain was measured by means of a structured questionnaire consisting of a list of forty-eight traditional beliefs. The method for obtaining these beliefs has already been discussed. Each Indian in our sample was given the questionnaire concerning these widely ranging beliefs about the nature of the world and was asked whether he was aware of the belief and whether or not he personally accepted its validity. The subject was then given a total score based on the number of these traditional beliefs he rejected. When translated into proportions, the range is from .04 to 77 percent modern, with a median of 25 percent. In addition to this total score, three sub-scales were constructed tapping potentially distinct domains of belief:

1.   BELIEF IN EVIL SPIRITS: A sub-scale measuring the rejection of from one to sixteen items involving belief in evil spirits.

2.   MEDICAL BELIEF: A sub-scale measuring the rejection of from one to thirteen items indicating that perceived infractions of the moral, natural, or supernatural order leads to a negative change in the violator's physical or mental state.

3.   NONMEDICAL BELIEF: A sub-scale measuring the rejection of from one to nineteen items indicating that no perceived infractions are involved or that these infractions do not lead to a change in the violator's physical or mental state.

The correlations among these three sub-scales ranged from .74 to .82. These high correlations suggest that native beliefs in this area constitute a single domain, from which it is impossible to isolate "medical" from "nonmedical" elements. They also serve as an index of the high internal homogeneity (one type of "reliability") of the total scale.

Innovativeness

"Innovativeness" is defined by Rogers as "the degree to which an individual adopts new ideas relatively earlier than others in his social system" (1969: 314). Measures of this trait have been employed by many investigators as their major dependent variable, i.e. the thing they want to explain. In our research, however, we have treated innovativeness as a psychological "predisposition" to adopt a modern way of life, as seen by past behavior. It thus becomes a potential "predictor" of future adoption behavior, though it in turn may also be dependent on other predictors such as age, exposure, and economic status.

Rogers (and other researchers in the rural sociology tradition) typically measures innovativeness by the point (or points) in a process of community adoption at which an individual adopter has personally accepted some new trait, or set of traits (1962, 1969). This method requires a knowledge of the TIME of adoption which is not always easy to obtain. It is far simpler to employ a list of traits which are in the process of being adopted by community members at the time of the research. Each subject is then given a score corresponding to the number of these traits he has already accepted. This was the technique employed by us. The items used in our index were drawn from those traits on which Indians and Ladinos differed, as reported above, but which were increasingly being accepted by Indians in San Lucas:

1. RELIGION: Change to Reformed Catholicism.
2. COFRADÍA SERVICE: Rejection of further service in the religious hierarchy.
3. DRESS: Change from traditional costume to modern dress.
4. SHOES: Use of shoes rather than sandals or going barefoot.
5. LANGUAGE: Above the sample median on a Spanish-speaking facility rating from zero (no Spanish) to six (Ladino-Spanish).
6. OCCUPATION: Nonagricultural occupation adopted as major economic endeavor.
7. MARRIAGE: Marital union has civil and/or religious sanction.
8. SANITATION FACILITIES: Residence plot contains an outhouse.
9. SWEAT BATH: Residence plot does NOT contain a sweat bath.

Each subject was assigned a total score based on his behavior within each of these nine areas. Three sub-scales are available which tap in more differentiated fashion three areas included within this index: language, dress, and religion.

1. LANGUAGE: The Spanish-speaking facility rating cited above is used in this scale. The ratings were made by two research assistants, one a bilingual Indian and the other a native Spanish-speaking Ladino. Both have had over six years of formal education.
2. DRESS: This scale is slightly different from the dress item in the Innovativeness Scale in that it includes shoes and a "modified" version of modern dress (e.g. long trousers with Indian shirt and/or Indian waist sash). The scale is weighted on a continuum from traditional to modern whereby the adoption of shoes is scored one point, "modified" modern dress two points, and modern dress three points. The range is from zero (traditional dress) to four (modern dress with shoes).
3. RELIGION: This scale also differs from the religion item on the

Innovativeness Scale in that it includes several possible changes in religious behavior: rejection of further *cofradía* service, membership in reformed Catholicism, and a religiously sanctioned marital union. One point is assigned for each of these modifications. The range is from zero (traditional *cofradía* Catholic) to three (a member of Reformed Catholicism who rejects further *cofradía* service and whose marriage has religious sanction).

The correlations among these three measures range from .17 to .48, and with the total Innovativeness Scale from .61 to .70. This further testifies to the internal homogeneity of these indices. Because of its comprehensive coverage, the summary Innovativeness Index has been used as our key measure of this domain.

Measures of various "independent" factors have been grouped into three categories: exposure, age, and economic status.

Exposure

Five indices of exposure to modern ideas and technology were developed. These incorporate the major variables within this domain that have been suggested by previous researchers, plus one which emerged as relevant within this particular research setting. (It was discovered that military service, besides providing a major form of direct exposure to the world beyond the village, also included literacy training. It is thus a double-barreled index.)

1. EDUCATION AND LITERACY: Some formal education completed or literacy claimed.

2. MASS MEDIA USE: The stated frequency of use of newspapers, magazines, and radio. Subjects were then divided into quartiles.

3. MILITARY SERVICE: Years of regular military service in an urban center.

4. TRAVEL:[7] Frequency and extent of travel beyond the local community and particularly to the large urban centers. Subjects were divided into quartiles.

5. POLITICAL AWARENESS:[8] A test of knowledge pertaining to local, national, and international politics. Informants were asked to identify

---

[7] What Rogers refers to as "cosmopoliteness" or "the degree to which an individual is oriented outside his immediate social system" (1969: 147) was operationally almost identical to what we refer to less grandly as "travel." Ideally, however, its definition suggests the possibility of including much more.

[8] Political awareness may be considered an OUTCOME of exposure rather than an index of the amount of exposure to the outside world, though it is frequently so used in the literature.

the local mayor, population size, and geographic subdivisions; past and present national leaders; leaders of selected international powers; and quizzed as to their knowledge of the Vietnam conflict.

An intercorrelation matrix among these five variables is presented in Table 6.

Table 6. Intercorrelations among alternative measures of exposure within a highland Guatemalan community

	1 Education and literacy	2 Military service	3 Travel	4 Mass media	5 Political awareness
1. Education-literacy	X	.36	.32	.39	.49
2. Military service		X	.50	.49	.38
3. Travel			X	.67	.66
4. Mass media				X	.72
5. Political awareness					X

Use of mass media, travel, and political awareness form the core of this syndrome with an average intercorrelation of .68. Military service, education, and literacy are less strongly related to these core elements with an average correlation of .43. These five indices have been combined into a single exposure scale by ranking the forty subjects on each sub-scale, adding the five rank scores received by each subject, and reranking their sums. This combined index has been used as our key measure within this domain.

Age

Subjects were ranked from young to old on the basis of reported age.

Economic Status

Four operationally independent measures of wealth were devised which tap different forms or manifestations of economic status in San Lucas:

1. FARM SIZE: The total amount of land each Indian had available for cultivation. Range is from zero to 128 *cuerdas,* with a *cuerda* being roughly one-fifth acre.

2. RESIDENCE PLOT OWNERSHIP: A binary item; 45 percent of the Indians in our sample claimed ownership.

3. BUDGET: A self-report of the amount of cash each Indian spends in an average month for household expenses. The range was from six to thirty dollars.

4. HOUSEHOLD POSSESSIONS: The approximate total monetary value of all household possessions in a household inventory collected from each Indian family, based on the application of a standard set of values. Range from seven to ninety-five dollars.

A correlation matrix among these four measures is presented in Table 7. Note first that all correlations are positive, suggesting that we are tapping a single conceptual domain. But also note that strongest correlations are between Farm Size and Resident Plot Ownership

Table 7. Intercorrelations among alternative measures of wealth

	1 Farm size	2 Residence plot ownership	3 Budget	4 Household possessions
1. Farm size	–	.53	.14	.14
2. Residence plot ownership		–	.41	.22
3. Budget			–	.57
4. Household possessions				–

For N = 40 a correlation of .26 is significant at the .05 level (one-tailed test).

(.53) and between a subject's monthly Budget and the dollar value of his Household Possessions (.57), whereas the other correlations are substantially lower. This suggested to us that we were actually tapping two fairly distinct forms of wealth: Control over Land (a traditional form of wealth) and Control over Cash (a nontraditional form of wealth). Instead of forming a single Wealth Index, therefore, we constructed two: a Land Index and a Cash Index. These were created by rank-ordering all subjects on each measure, adding the pair of ranks received on the two measures being combined to form the Land Index and the two forming the Cash Index, and then reranking these totals. These two summary indices correlated with each other only .19, which is nonsignificant statistically. As will be seen below, this decision to break wealth up into these two components, traditional and nontraditional, proved to be insightful since they play quite different roles in the modernization process.

A HYPOTHETICAL MODEL OF THE CHANGE PROCESS

Having conceptualized and measured a number of potentially important variables in the change process, the next step is to evaluate their role. Two approaches are possible. The first, and most popular in previous modernization research, employs "multiple regression," a correlational procedure by which all the "independent" variables (the presumed determinants of change) are simultaneously related to the "dependent" variable (the changing behavior we want to explain). The multiple correlation coefficient which results tells us how much of the variation in the dependent variable has been accounted for by the factors (independent variables) we have taken into consideration. The regression equation provides a "prediction formula" by which we can calculate the probable behavior of an individual, given his attributes, and the amount of change in that behavior which we would expect to occur for each unit of change in these attributes. Finally, the "weighting" to be assigned each attribute, which is given by this formula, also tells us the relative contribution of that attribute to our understanding of the behavioral outcome, independent of the contribution of the other attributes. Obviously this is a powerful research tool; Everett Rogers (1962: 287–289; 1969: 301–304) summarizes twenty-seven major studies of modernization in countries at various levels of development which have employed this analytic technique, and he has used it extensively himself.[9]

A contrasting approach — the one we have chosen to pursue in this study — is based on statistical procedures explicated by Hubert Blalock (1961, 1968). This involves systematically generating a tentative causal model of the change process from the pattern of correlations found among our list of theoretically relevant variables. The accuracy of fit between this model and the empirical data can then be tested mathematically, and its characteristics examined logically and in relationship to ethnographic and historical material. As far as we know, this technique has never been applied to data from a field study of modernization. We have chosen to employ it because at this point we are more interested in process than prediction and it fits well the kinds of data we have available.

Any causal reconstruction from correlational data is fraught with

---

[9] There are other statistical techniques such as pattern analysis (configurational analysis) which have quite similar aims.

logical difficulties.[10] It also requires a series of simplifying assumptions about the data themselves which may not be justified (Blalock 1961). So, the task should be approached with caution and the results considered highly tentative until tested with longitudinal data.[11] But at least we can examine the results of this analytic exercise to see if they correspond with theoretical expectations, and perhaps we can eliminate a few alternative models which prove to be empirically inadequate.

Table 8 presents a summary of the Pearson correlations among four key variables selected from our study of changing medical beliefs and behavior in San Lucas: EXPOSURE to modern-Westernized life styles; INNOVATIVENESS, or a predisposition to adopt modern practices based on prior adoption behavior; the adoption of modern MEDICAL PRACTICES; and the abandonment of traditional BELIEFS. We will start with these four because their pattern of relation-

Table 8.   Intercorrelations among measures of key variables in the modernization process in San Lucas Tolimán, Guatemala

	1 Exposure	2 Innova- tiveness	3 Medical practices	4 Beliefs
1. Exposure	–	56	46	—07
2. Innovativeness		–	70	25
3. Medical practices			–	40
4. Beliefs				–

For N = 40 a correlation of .26 is significant at the .05 level (one-tailed test).

ships is easiest to interpret. Notice that the matrix has been arranged so that the level of correlation increases as you move from right to left and from top to bottom, thereby placing the highest correlations adjacent to the central diagonal. This automatically orders the variables in a tentative causal sequence. Figure 1 presents the resulting hypothetical model in somewhat clearer form.

Arrows represent hypothetical causal links. Solid lines represent relationships assumed to be artifacts of these causal links. The figures in

[10]   In another context Graves (1969) has argued against the use of cross-sectional data ordered by means of Guttman Scales as a basis for reconstructing historical sequences. The fact that he is here engaged in a similar form of historical reconstruction simply demonstrates that consistency is not one of his virtues.
[11]   The authors plan to collect such data in a restudy of this community during the summer months of 1971.

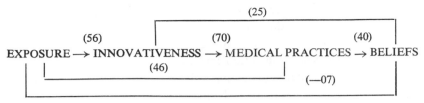

Figure 1. Hypothetical model of the change process in San Lucas Tolimán, Guatemala

parentheses represent obtained correlations between our key measures of each concept in this model.

The basic rule for constructing the simplest type of linear model is that proceeding in any one direction the correlations between adjacent links must always be higher than with more remote links in the causal chain, with the magnitude of the correlations diminishing as one proceeds outward (Blalock 1961: 68). Applying this rule, these four variables order themselves quite nicely: Exposure has its highest correlations with Innovativeness and lowest with Beliefs; Innovativeness and Medical Practices have their highest correlation with each other and lower correlations with Exposure and Beliefs. Thus all links fulfill the general form required for a causal chain.

The DIRECTION of causality operating within a series of variables (indicated in our model by solid arrows) cannot be determined from the pattern of correlations alone, but must be based on some logical property of the variables themselves (Exposure cannot cause Age, etc.) or on historical data. For example, there is no mathematical reason why changes in beliefs cannot lead to changes in medical practices, which promote general innovativeness, which in turn leads a person to seek out increased exposure to the modern world. In fact, such a sequence does not sound totally implausible and may represent an important set of secondary feedback relationships within the change process.[12] But, as the primary sequence, it violates both logic and history.

---

[12] Although Blalock does not deal with this topic in his 1961 book, it can easily be shown mathematically that a linear model is able to include such feedback without any adverse effect on the pattern of relationships among correlation coefficients as long as this feedback follows the same pathways as the original causation, but in a reversed order. If changed beliefs, however, were to have a strong, unmediated recursive effect on exposure, for example, it could foul up the pattern of correlations and thereby obscure the basic model. Blalock's procedures contain no way of handling or even recognizing such eventualities. Fortunately, no such processes appear to be operating in the present instance.

In the present instance we have inferred causal directionality from exposure through the adoption of modern ways, both nonmedical and medical, to changes in beliefs. The reason for this is that two elements in the Exposure Scale, education and military service, clearly predate the adoption of modern medicine, which is a relatively recent introduction into the community. Change in medical practices, furthermore, had proceeded rapidly so that we find roughly three-quarters of the Luceños in our sample using these resources, although as indicated in an earlier section, this does not mean they are not also using traditional resources at the same time. By contrast, all our measures of native epistemology, though demonstrating a wide range of variability in our sample, showed that the majority of these beliefs were traditional in content. Thus changes in beliefs are clearly lagging BEHIND changes in medical practices. In the next section we will further complicate the model by suggesting that the whole process can be touched off by a man's relative age and economic resources, factors which again cannot logically FOLLOW from consequent changes in his beliefs and medical practices.

THE ROLE OF ECONOMIC FACTORS

The role played by economic factors in this process is empirically more complicated. Here we have four operationally independent measures of wealth: Farm Size, Resident Plot Ownership, Budget and Household Possessions. They manifest quite different patterns of relationships with the key variables in our model; the correlations are presented in Table 9. Note first the similarity in the patterns of correlation with the other key variables for the two alternative measures of CONTROL OVER LAND and the two of CONTROL OVER CASH. This further justifies combining each pair into a LAND INDEX and a CASH INDEX, necessary for the statistical manipulations to follow. It also lends validity to any interpretations we may make about the distinct role these two forms of wealth play in the modernization process, because these associations are unlikely to be an artifact of particular measurement techniques.[13]

---

[13] The similarity between the pattern of correlations obtained by means of each pair of operationally distinct measures provides strong support for the validity of the combined indices. Not only have we shown their CONVERGENT validity (by means of their relatively high correlations with each other, averaging .55) and their DISCRIMINANT validity (by means of their relatively low correlations with the other pair, averaging .23), but also now their CONSTRUCT validity by means of their distinct pattern of relationships with a theoretical network of measures of OTHER domains.

Table 9. Correlation between alternative measures of economic status and other key variables

Control over land	Exposure	Innova- tiveness	Medical practices	Beliefs
1. Farm size	.10	—.08	.16	.07
2. Residence plot ownership	.18	.00	.07	.01
3. Land index	.12	—.03	.16	.04
Control over cash				
1. Budget	.36	.24	.18	—.08
2. Household possessions	.53	.35	.25	—.28
3. Cash index	.60	.34	.20	—.22

For N = 40 a correlation of .26 is significant at the .05 level (one-tailed test).

The two distinct patterns of association make good ethnographic sense. Control over Land, of course, is the traditional form of wealth in the agricultural Indian community and appears to be almost unrelated to any aspect of the modernization process. All correlations are small; none approach statistical significance. This is not surprising. A man who devotes himself full time to traditional subsistence agriculture can avoid most contact with the modernizing world around him: he spends his time working his own land, disposes of his surplus through local Indian middlemen or in local markets, and makes his own modest purchases in local markets. In fact, even here he avoids contact, since in the traditional economy his wife performs the bulk of transactions in the marketplace. Women comprise somewhere over 75 percent of all buyers and sellers in most Indian markets.

By contrast, Control over Cash is strongly implicated in the modernization process. This form of wealth requires wage labor, entrepreneurial activity, or the production of surplus goods for sale; therefore, it links the Indian with the regional and, to some extent, the national economy and exposes him in varying degrees to the outside world. This activity, then, is more likely to break down localism and isolation than full-time devotion to traditional subsistence agriculture. The result is that wealth in cash is strongly associated with factors leading to the adoption of modern medical practices.

But note that high cash control is NEGATIVELY associated with a more modern epistemology. The wealthiest Luceños, in terms of monthly expenditures in cash and the value of household possessions, also tend to be the most traditional in their beliefs about the nature of the world. Clearly then, these beliefs can in no sense be considered to serve as a BARRIER to the adoption of modern technology, including Western medicine.

Table 9 shows that the strength of the positive correlation between the Cash Index and other elements in the causal sequence increases as one passes from right to left (this is also true of each of its components). This fits exactly the pattern required for inclusion in the linear change model and appears to be a mathematically logical candidate to place at the left hand end as an initial factor, which activates the whole process.

This we have done, though a qualification is necessary. For most Indians two elements in the Exposure Scale, education and military service, logically precede the acquisition of cash and may, in fact, have contributed to their decisions to follow this particular path to wealth. This again illustrates the fact that relationships from right to left are possible within our model, and add to its complexity and congruence with reality.

TESTING THE MODEL'S FIT WITH THE DATA

To summarize briefly, our model implies that involvement in the CASH ECONOMY appears, at least in San Lucas, to be a prime mover in promoting a more modern way of life. This results in some forms of increased EXPOSURE to people and ideas outside the local community, which in turn fosters a predisposition to INNOVATIVENESS. This then leads to the adoption of more modern MEDICAL PRACTICES, when they become locally available, which in turn begins to break down traditional BELIEFS about the nature of the world. This reconstruction is logically plausible, because the use of modern medical resources brings the Indian into contact with notions of disease causation and curing that are radically different from those accepted in the past, and the latter are inextricably intertwined with the traditional epistemology, which defines the relationship between mortal man and the natural and supernatural world.

One caveat should be introduced at this point, however, to remind the reader of the complexities we are confronting. Clearly, involvement in the cash economy is not the ONLY factor which can lead to exposure to the world outside an Indian's own village, just as exposure is not the only factor leading to Innovativeness. For example, we will show below that AGE also contributes to Innovativeness. Our model does not exhaust all the possible determinants of modernization, even in San Lucas, and there is still much room for the addition of OTHER variables. All we claim at this point is that this is ONE of the paths to modernization operating here. We are convinced it is an extremely important one.

If this causal chain is a valid reconstruction, then we would expect the pattern of relationships among key variables in this model to approximate the following mathematical rules: correlations between nonadjacent links should equal the product of correlations between intervening links, and if we partial out the effect of these intervening links, the nonadjacent correlations should drop to zero. All we are saying here is that the .46 correlation between amount of exposure to modern life and the adoption of modern medical practices is really the result of a predisposition to adopt such practices (Innovativeness) that exposure promotes; the predisposition (Innovativeness) serves as an "intervening variable" between the stimulus (Exposure) and the behavioral response (use of modern Medical Practices). Similarly, changes in native epistemology are considered to result from changes in curing practices, rather than following directly from exposure to a modern way of life or a predisposition to adopt its outward manifestations (Innovativeness). A test of these mathematical predictions is presented in Table 10.

Table 10. Testing the fit between a hypothetical model of the change process in San Lucas Tolimán and the actual correlations obtained

	Predicted	Actual	Difference
Method I			
Innovativeness [I] with Beliefs [B]	.28	.25	.03
Exposure [E] with Practices [P]	.39	.46	.07
Exposure with Beliefs	.16	—.07	.23
Cash [C] with Innovativeness	.34	.34	.00
Cash with Practices	.24	.20	.04
Cash with Beliefs	.09	—.22	.31
Method II			
I with B controlling for P	0	.04	
E with P controlling for I	0	.11	
E with B controlling for I and P	0	.32	
C with I controlling for E	0	.00	
C with P controlling for E and I	0	—.12	
C with B controlling for E, I, and P	0	.21	

Given the crudity of measurement in the social sciences, particularly under natural field conditions, as well as the chance effects introduced by small sample sizes, we should not expect a perfect fit. Unfortunately, there is no accepted statistical procedure for testing the accuracy of fit between such a model as we have presented and the actual correlations obtained (Blalock 1961). But the standard error of correlations of the magnitude we are working with in this case is about .16 (i.e. the standard deviation among successive correlations between two variables, for sample sizes of $N = 40$). If the difference between the expected and the obtained correlation is less than this figure, therefore, the fit can be considered good.

Under these circumstances, the overall fit between predicted and actual correlations in this instance is remarkably good and improves as the number of intervening links in the hypothetical chain decrease. The only real problems are the negative correlations between both Exposure and Cash with Beliefs, each of which results in a fairly substantial deviation from expectations. In fact, these correlations appear to run counter to the postulated modernization process. Why should the Indians with the greatest external exposure hold slightly more traditional beliefs, on the average, than their less-exposed neighbors? And why should those with the highest involvement in the cash economy be even more traditional in their beliefs? This paradox is in need of explanation. If we can identify the factors responsible for this apparent discongruity, their addition to the model as "control variables" might improve its fit with the empirical data.

CONTROL VARIABLES

Our "control variables" are factors which do not form a part of the basic linear model we have formulated, but whose effect on the elements within that model must be compensated for. The possible role of Age may be taken as an example. If older Indians hold more traditional beliefs by virtue of having received more thorough traditional indoctrination, and if older Indians also have had more opportunity to accumulate cash, this could account for the negative correlation between our Cash Index and Modern Beliefs, despite the effects of the modernization process we have just outlined. Consequently, we would like to see if our causal model fits the empirical data better when the complicating role of Age is removed.

Such control over the influence of extraneous variables can be accomplished in either of two ways: mechanically or statistically. In mechanical control we hold some factor constant by examining the relationships between other variables among subjects who are relatively homogeneous with respect to this control variable. For example, we might look at the correlations within our model only among Luceños in their twenties and thirties, and then again among older subjects.

The major disadvantage of this method of control is that it requires a fairly large number of subjects, particularly if it is desirable to control for the influence of two or more factors simultaneously. Statistical control permits the accomplishment of essentially the same thing with smaller samples, by compensating for the influence of these extraneous factors mathematically. All subjects can then be treated AS IF they were the same age. The resulting "partial" correlations between other variables represent the average that probably would have been obtained if we had tested the same model with groups of subjects at different age levels, i.e. if we had used the mechanical method of control.

Table 11 represents the correlations between Age and each of the key variables in our causal model. As suggested in the theoretical section, there are good reasons to anticipate that younger men will be more disposed to adopt the trappings of modern life than those older men, who are more committed to, and rewarded by, the traditional social and prestige hierarchy. Empirically this proved to be true in San Lucas as well, with a -.32 correlation between Age and Innovativeness.

Table 11. Correlations between Age and other key variables in the causal model

	Cash index	Exposure	Innova- tiveness	Medical practices	Beliefs
Age	11	—12	—32	—07	—10

For N = 40 a correlation of .26 is significant at the .05 level (one-tailed test).

But in order to account for the apparent tenacity of traditional beliefs, we are looking for control variables, which have a strong NEGATIVE correlation with modern Beliefs, while at the same time having a strong POSITIVE correlation with some factor near the beginning of our causal chain. As we had anticipated, older subjects do tend to hold less modern Beliefs and have more cash as well. But these relationships are both weak (–.10 and +.11, respectively). As a consequence, when we partial out the effect of Age on all correlations within the model, changes are minor, and a retest of the accuracy of fit with mathematical expectations shows no improvement.[14] Our paradox remains.

[14] As Blalock has noted (1968: 174) a control variable, in order to have any effect on a causal model, must have a reasonably high correlation with at least TWO variables within that model. Age has a statistically significant correlation with only one. Later we will try to explain some of the reasons for this empirical fact as well.

THE ROLE OF ECONOMICS: TWO MODELS OF CASH EXPENDITURES

In an attempt to explain the incongruities in our model, we examined the process by which a man comes to acquire and spend relatively large amounts of cash in the hope that this would provide a basis for understanding his conservatism in beliefs. This proved to be a more fruitful approach. Two complementary models emerged, the first dealing with the subject's economic activity, the second with his ceremonial activity.

In San Lucas a man can acquire cash through three alternate routes: (1) through the production and sale of surplus agricultural goods; (2) through wage labor; or (3) through market activity, i.e. serving as a middleman, buying local surplus, and selling this in nonlocal markets, etc. These routes are not mutually exclusive, of course, and many Indians mix their activities. Nevertheless, an emphasis on one tends to preclude heavy involvement in another. The route chosen by an individual Indian appears to be determined primarily by how much land he has available (owned and sharecropped). If he is land-poor, the sale of his labor or some sort of petty entrepreneurial activity is about his only recourse.

A distinction between wage labor and market activities does not need to be made for purposes of this analysis. First, entrepreneurial involvement is relatively rare, at least in our sample, so that the major nonagricultural activity is wage labor. Second, both nonagricultural wage labor and entrepreneurial activity serve as alternatives to farming and both involve varying degrees of external contact. Consequently, we produced a single Occupation Index composed of the following four steps:

1. Indian who is self-employed on his own land (and/or sharecropped) on a full-time basis (no subsidiary economic activities). (N = 5)
2. Indian who is self-employed on his own land (and/or sharecropped) on a part-time basis but also earns wages as an agricultural worker for someone else. (N = 17)
3. Indian who is self-employed on his own land (and/or sharecropped) on a part-time basis but also earns wages as a nonagricultural worker for someone else. (N = 12)
4. Indian who works full-time as a nonagricultural wage earner for someone else. (N = 6)

The top half of Figure 2 presents the new measure in its relationship with our Land Index and the Cash Index. This part of the model can be interpreted as follows: those Indians without much land are forced to develop alternative economic activities. This interpretation is supported by the strong negative correlation between the Land Index and the Occupational Index (-.59). But both routes produce cash. Since these are largely complementary processes, they tend to cancel each other out when we look at them in relationship to the Cash Index. Consequently, the individual correlations are low (.19 and .22). But a multiple r, in which the contribution of both variables is examined simultaneously, produces a strong positive correlation with the Cash Index (.45).

The role of Age in this process is also interesting. Age has a strong positive correlation with the Land Index (.33) and an even stronger NEGATIVE correlation with the Occupation Scale (-.52). In other words, the younger a man, the less land he controls and, consequently, the less likely he is to engage in agriculture as his major economic endeavor. This makes sense. But whether it is a life-cycle phenomenon or a change occurring in the area as a result of increasing population pressure on already meager land resources (Woods 1968), or a combination of the two, is less clear. However, it is clear that both younger and older people possess a route to monetary wealth (wages on the one hand and cash crops on the other) so that the zero-order correlations between Age and the Cash Index are negligible (.11). This further aids in explaining why Age appears to play so small a part in the modernization process in San Lucas.

We can turn now to a second set of determinants which lead both to increased cash accumulation and the necessity for increased cash outlay: Household Size and Ceremonial Service.

In Guatemalan Indian society the household is the primary social and economic unit. Most commonly this household is composed of a single nuclear family or some simple one-generational extension. Family members pool their energies and resources in all productive and consumptive activities, and likewise share the burden of misfortune. Hence, the larger the family unit, the larger the number of productive individuals, whether engaged in market activities, wage labor, or the creation of agricultural surplus. At the same time, however, a big family results in larger daily expenses for food, clothing, and other household items. Thus Household Size, as measured by the number of persons sharing a common hearth, is quite strongly associated with both a higher monthly budget and a larger inventory of household goods (Cash Index: r = .47).

A brief description of the *cofradía* system (the religious fraternities that are responsible for many ceremonial activities in Guatemala) has already been presented. Within this system there is a hierarchy of services (*cargos*) which represents increasing degrees of responsibility and requires increasing outlays of cash. An index of the level of Ceremonial Service reached by each member of our sample was constructed as follows:

Level One: No Ceremonial Service claimed. (N = 8)

Level Two: Minor service with minimal cash outlay such as supplying fireworks or firewood for a religious celebration. (N = 5)

Level Three: Regular *cofradía* position and/or regular service as a dancer with consequent modest cash outlays for a religious celebration. (N = 11)

Level Four: Major *cofradía* position such as *Mayordomo* in a high-ranking *cofradía* or top spot in any *cofradía*. Considerable cash expenditures involved. (N = 16)

The association of this variable with others is shown in the bottom half of the model presented in Figure 2.

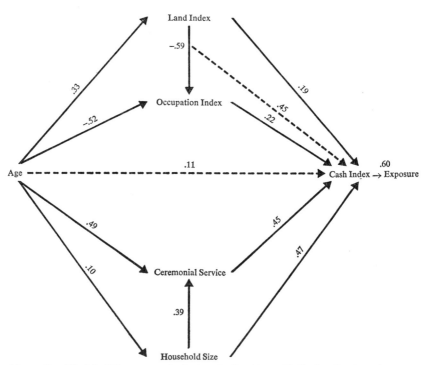

Figure 2.   Model of the economic factors in San Lucas Tolimán, Guatemala

A number of observers have suggested that the civil-religious hierarchy in Middle American Indian communities serves as a leveling mechanism whereby those who have accumulated wealth in the community are "pressured" into serving civil and religious positions, which require ever-increasing cash outlays. Some have argued that this serves to redistribute surplus wealth and maintain a nonstratified, classless society (Tax 1953; Nash 1958b; Carrasco 1961). At the same time, however, there is reason to suspect that the status and prestige attained through service in the hierarchy may be translatable into additional wealth so that some form of socioeconomic stratification, passed through family lines, can develop. Cancian (1965) has outlined an example of this in the Mayan highlands of southeastern Mexico. That our data suggest this for San Lucas is shown by the .45 correlation between level of Ceremonial Service attained and wealth as measured by the Cash Index. Thus, the direction of causality between Ceremonial Service and wealth is probably not unidirectional but includes a strong feedback effect in both directions. Participation in the *cofradía* increases wealth, and vice versa. In any case, service in the upper levels of the civil-religious hierarchy requires large cash expenditures and those men in the community without economic resources of one sort or another will not qualify to serve at this level.

In addition to economic resources, our empirical data suggest two further important factors in the level of Ceremonial Service achieved: Age and Household Size. Since this is a time-ordered sequence of activities, the older a man is, the greater the probability that he has achieved a relatively high level of service (r = .49). The level of achievement also appears to be a function of the size of a man's household. Since the family is the primary economic unit in Guatemala, it is actually the family that climbs the ceremonial ladder; the larger the family, the more resources that are available when the time comes for expenditures. Although the adult male head of household occupies the *cofradía* position, his sons (and sometimes brothers and more distant relatives) aid him with cash and labor outlays, while his wife and daughters have important duties in the preparation of ceremonial dinners and in catering to respected guests at festivals. And, as they all share in the labor, they share the status and prestige acquired through high levels of community service. In this kind of system, every FAMILY knows its position in the community *vis-à-vis* every other (Nash 1958b). That family size is an important facilitator of high levels of Ceremonial Service in San Lucas is shown empirically by the .39 correlation between our sample index of Household Size and level of

Ceremonial Service achieved by the household head.

Age and Household Size are relatively unrelated (.10), perhaps because their actual relationship is curvilinear. In any event, they account for fairly independent portions of the variance in Ceremonial Service, so that their multiple r is .60.

Except for the Land Index, these various economic factors form a syndrome of influences which are positively associated with relatively large amounts of Cash, while at the same time being negatively associated with modern Beliefs, via the influence of the *cofradía* system (Table 12). These, then, can serve as a group of control variables which account in large part for the statistical paradox that we found in our earlier test of the causal model.

Table 12. Correlations between control variables and other key variables in the model

	Cash Index	Exposure	Innovativeness	Medical practices	Beliefs
1. Land Index	19	12	—03	16	04
2. Occupation Index	22	35	20	05	—20
3. Ceremonial Service	45	18	—10	—18	—23
4. Household Size	47	14	09	00	—24

For N = 40 a correlation of .26 is significant at the .05 level (one-tailed test).

SUMMARY

A glance back at Figures 1 and 2 may serve to summarize and clarify what has been a rather complex exposition at points. Briefly, in San Lucas, as in many other parts of Indian Guatemala, traditional beliefs about the nature of the world show a remarkable persistence (Siegel 1941; Tax 1941; Tumin 1952; Adams 1957; Nash 1958a; Reina 1960; Hinshaw 1966; Tax and Hinshaw 1970). In San Lucas, however, these beliefs are beginning to fade in response to the adoption of modern medical practices which are incompatible with them at many points. These changes in medical behavior, in turn, are strongly related to a predisposition toward innovativeness, which has been fostered by increased exposure to the outside world. Such exposure is promoted in part by involvement in the cash economy, which leads to increased contact with people and ideas outside the local community.

This economic activity can come about in either of two ways. First is the more traditional route involving the use of significant amounts of land to produce agricultural surpluses above subsistence needs. Generally speaking, this is the choice of the older men. The second route is through full- or part-time wage labor, market activities, or some combination of them. This is the typical choice of the younger man. Consequently, it is not age but relative economic success, whether in traditional, modified traditional, or nontraditional activities, which sets a person on the path to modernization.[15]

But economic success is strongly linked to traditional beliefs via the *cofradía* system. The wealthier a man becomes, the further he is expected to advance in the religious hierarchy; the greater his participation in this system, the more he is exposed to traditional beliefs. In San Lucas, as in other Indian communities in the western highlands of Guatemala, it is in large part the *cofradías* which serve as the mainstay of the traditional way of life and the ideas which underlie it. The *cofradías* integrate the celebration of the various holy and secular festivities that comprise the annual cycle of events: the *cofradías*, as opposed to official Catholicism (and Protestantism), perpetuate the syncretism of pagan and Christian deities and practices which began after the Spanish Conquest: high-ranking members of the *cofradía* structure *(principales)* perform traditional rites such as engagements, marriages, and the investiture of sacred office. And it is in the *cofradías* where pagan deities are worshipped and where shamans conduct many of their age-old divination and curing ceremonies. In short, the *cofradías* are the essential backbone of traditional Indian culture.

Consequently, the relatively affluent Indian is subjected to competing and, in many cases, incompatible influences. On the one hand, through the cash economy he is increasingly exposed to modern ideas and practices; on the other his ceremonial responsibilities are reinforcing a traditional epistemology. Undoubtedly these forces are sometimes experienced as conflicting, and we suspect this is one im-

---

[15] We suspect that personality variables such as achievement motivation and feelings of personal control might be found to be further important determinants of economic success. Because this represents an early link in the modernization chain, however, these psychological variables would be found to have little direct effect on adoption behavior. This corresponds to Rogers' findings (1969: 305) which would help explain what otherwise might appear to be a disappointing empirical fact.

Figure 3. Hypothetical model of the change process in San Lucas Tolimán, Guatemala controlling for the influence of extraneous factors

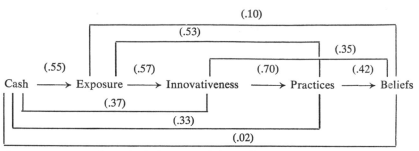

Arrows represent hypothetical causal links. Solid lines represent relationships assumed to be artifacts of these causal links. The figures in parentheses represent third order partial correlations between key measures, controlling for Occupation, Ceremonial Service, and Household Size.

Table 13. Testing the fit

	Predicted	Obtained	Difference
Innovativeness with Beliefs	.29	.35	.06
Exposure with Practices	.40	.53	.13
Exposure with Beliefs	.17	.10	.07
Cash with Innovativeness	.31	.37	.06
Cash with Practices	.22	.33	.11
Cash with Beliefs	.09	.02	.07

portant reason why the *cofradía* system is being abandoned by many.[16] In any event, in the meantime it helps to explain why the wealthier men in this community also tend to retain traditional beliefs despite their increasing acceptance of modern medical practices.

Only one statistical task remains. Now that we have discovered several sources of the paradoxical negative relationships between wealth in cash and traditional beliefs, we need to control for these effects to see if the resulting pattern of correlations within our hypothetical model better fits mathematical expectations. Three of the four control variables discussed in the last few pages were employed: Occupation, Ceremonial Service, and Household Size. These are the three with the strongest positive associations with our Cash Index and negative association with Belief. Figure 3 presents our basic linear model with these three muddling variables controlled. The third-order partial correlations have then been subjected to the accuracy of fit (Table 13) with mathematical expectations as we did with the orig-

[16] Luceños are aware of these conflicts. They realize that many of their traditional beliefs and behaviors as expressed in the *cofradía* are looked down upon as

inal zero-order correlations.[17] Note that now all correlations are fairly close to expectations; the greatest deviation is .13, still well within the .16 range suggested by us as representing a good fit. Note particularly that the correlations between Exposure and Cash with Beliefs are now both low but positive, as the model predicts, and within .07 of mathematical expectations. We conclude that our efforts to account for the one area of poor fit in our original model have proved successful and that the model as now presented is probably a pretty good representation of what is actually going on in the community.

CONCLUSIONS

A large number of theoretically important variables have been incorporated in this model of the change process in San Lucas, and the result has been a rather complex analysis. But these variables in no sense exhaust all the possible determinants of the changes which are taking place. For example, other than our indirect measure of Innovativeness, we have not incorporated any psychological variables, although other theoretists have considered some, such as Empathy (Lerner 1958), Need-Achievement (McClelland and Winter 1969), or feelings of personal control (Erasmus 1961), important. That our model has a high degree of internal mathematical consistency, furthermore, should also not be seen as an argument for its exhaustiveness. The very fact that the correlations between adjacent variables are far from unity and are attenuated as one proceeds outwards argues for the operation of unconsidered and unmeasured influences. There is still plenty of opportunity for other researchers to demonstrate the simultaneous relevance of other variables.

But within the compass of the factors which have been considered, some conclusions seem warranted:

1. Neither exposure to the outside world, nor the predisposition to entertain new ideas (Innovativeness) which it promotes, appears to

---

backward by Ladinos and progressive Indians. In addition, they cite the costly expenditures in time and money, internal arguments, lack of interest in the old ways, and the heavy ceremonial drinking required of them as reasons for discontinuing *cofradía* service. Cognitive dissonance theory (Festinger 1957) suggests that this disjunction between belief and behavior will give rise to pressure for their resolution in some manner. This will bear watching as modern medicine increases in popularity locally.

[17] For computational simplicity only the first method for testing accuracy of fit was employed; the second method would have required calculating sixth-order partials.

DIRECTLY undermine traditional beliefs. Rather, these beliefs appear to be highly resistant to change until they are found incompatible with changes in BEHAVIOR. This is in line with all we know about the relationship between beliefs and behavior as seen in many psychological studies of "attitude change" (Kiesler, et al. 1969).

2.   The traditional epistemology in Guatemala, as in many parts of the world, has at its core beliefs about the causes of health and illness which support and serve as the rationale for traditional medical practices. The introduction of modern medicine, which is based on quite different beliefs about disease causation, is apparently undermining these traditional beliefs even in spheres which are not obviously health-related.[18] The fact that modern medical services have not been available in most Guatemalan villages until fairly recently may help account in part for the "conservatism" in the traditional Guatemalan world view which has been widely commented on by anthropologists. Since there appears to be relatively little resistance to the use of modern medicine by Guatemalan Indians, however, one can predict that further changes in beliefs may follow now more quickly.

3.   The strong relationship between traditional beliefs and *cofradía* service is not surprising. What is more interesting is the link between traditional beliefs and other factors, such as wage labor and household size, that are correlated with *cofradía* service by virtue of their contribution to the accumulation of cash. (Unexplained is why the Land Index is not also negatively correlated with modern beliefs.) This then produces the paradox that the same thing which fosters modernization — involvement in the cash economy — also leads to the reinforcement of traditional beliefs via expectations of religious service. This is probably another factor contributing to the slowness of change in belief systems in Guatemala. But this also creates psychological conflicts for Guatemalan Indians, conflicts which are felt most keenly by rich men in San Lucas. (We have case material to illustrate its consequences.) Young men making choices about their future, however, also experience this conflict in anticipation, and many decide never to enter *cofradía* service and thereby avoid these pressures. Although this is a situation peculiar to Guatemala, we suspect that it is not unique, and it would be interesting to look for among modernizing peoples in other parts of the world.

---

[18]   Efforts at syncretism would be a fascinating focus for observing these cognitive conflicts working themselves out, and it will also be interesting to observe how long these efforts persist.

4.   The distinction we drew between traditional and modern forms of wealth has not usually been made in the modernization literature. We suspect this may be responsible for some of the empirical confusion concerning the relationship between wealth and modernization. For example, Maher (1960) found his conservative subjects to have the highest wealth in traditional symbols; wives, pigs, and shell ornaments. But his progressive subjects were actually the richest in Australian shillings. Similarly, many researchers have found wealthy natives to be among the first to adopt modern farm practices (Rogers 1969: 296ff.). Clearly, "wealth" in itself is not the critical factor. What is important to consider in each case is the ROLE that different forms of wealth may play in promoting or inhibiting the modernization process.

5.   Age is another factor that has played an ambiguous empirical role in the past. There are good theoretical reasons to expect the young to be more receptive to new ideas, and in fact we found a significant relationship between youth and innovativeness in San Lucas. But there was almost none between youth and modern medical beliefs and practices. Our examination of the relationship between age and alternative economic pathways explains both the reason for our overall low correlations and the important role that age actually plays in the modernization process in San Lucas despite these low correlations with the outcome.[19]

6.   The preceding point illustrates one important theoretical and empirical advantage of a causal-processual model, such as we have developed, over more commonly employed multiple regression techniques. When "explanation" is based on regression formulas, the researcher is led to conclude that those factors with low beta weights, i.e. little independent correlation with the outcome (criterion measure) after all other factors in the formula are controlled, have little explanatory importance. But as the mathematics of the causal model we developed here should indicate, variables which are remote in a causal chain not only have relatively low zero-order correlations with outcome variables, but these correlations are even further reduced, often to zero when intervening variables are controlled. Consequently, they would make essentially NO independent contribution to a multiple re-

---

[19]   In the Philippines Madigan (1962: 148–151) found a curvilinear relationship between age and the adoption of modern farming methods, with middle-aged men being the most receptive. As a result his overall LINEAR correlations were also low. A causal model such as we developed might help explain WHY this curvilinear relationship was found, rather than leaving it as a curious empirical fact.

gression formula, even though they are found to play an important role in some causal sequence. A researcher must be careful not to discard theoretically important variables from his analysis simply because their correlation with his criterion measures are found to be low. Sometimes another type of analysis will prove more fruitful.[20]

7. Finally, this analysis has attempted to blend traditional ethnographic description with more formal quantitative procedures and model building in a way which we hope has proved fruitful for both enterprises. The use of clearly defined operational definitions of our concepts and the mathematical manipulation of our data is an important path to the discovery of subtle relationships that might not be apparent to an ethnographic observer. In this case, for example, Woods, who knew the community well, learned things about the process of modernization in San Lucas that he had not suspected or understood at the point when the data were collected. At the same time, however, it was his intimate familiarity with the research community that enabled him to help Graves construct meaningful indices of key concepts to be investigated, to interpret and make sense of the relationships that emerged, and to direct them to the solution of an apparent empirical paradox. The point seems obvious and would not be worth laboring if it were not for the fact that both anthropologists and their more quantitatively oriented colleagues in other social sciences are apt to ignore the substantial contribution that each can make to the other.

REFERENCES

ADAMS, RICHARD N.

1951   Personnel in culture change: a test of a hypothesis. *Social Forces* 30:185–189.

1952   *Un análisis de las creencias y práticas médicas en un Pueblo Indígena de Guatemala*. Publicaciones Especiales del Instituto Indigenista Nacional 17. Guatemala.

1957   *Cultural surveys of Panama-Guatemala-El Salvador-Honduras*. Pan American Sanitary Bureau Scientific Publications 33. Washington D.C.

1960   "Social change in Latin America today" in *Social change in Latin America today*. Edited by R. Adams. New York: Vintage.

[20]   Actually, regression analysis and causal models are often usefully viewed as complementary statistical strategies. In another paper Graves hopes to explicate this point, illustrating their mutual contribution to the same analysis.

BARNETT, HOMER G.
1941 Personal conflicts and culture change. *Social Forces* 20:160–171.
1953 *Innovation: the basis of cultural change.* New York: McGraw-Hill.
BLALOCK, HUBERT M., JR.
1961 *Causal inferences in nonexperimental research.* Chapel Hill: University of North Carolina Press.
1968 "Theory building and causal inferences," in *Methodology in social research.* Edited by Hubert M. Blalock, Jr., and Ann B. Blalock. New York: McGraw-Hill.
BLALOCK, HUBERT M., JR., ANN B. BLALOCK
1968 *Methodology in social research.* New York: McGraw-Hill.
BROOM, LEONARD, *et al.*
1954 Acculturation: an exploratory formulation. *American Anthropologist* 56:873–1000.
BRUNER, EDWARD M.
1956 Cultural transmission and culture change. *Southwestern Journal of Anthropology* 12:191–199.
CANCIAN, FRANK
1965 *Economics and prestige in a Maya community.* Stanford: Stanford University Press.
CARRASCO, PEDRO
1961 The civil-religious hierarchy in Mesoamerican communities: pre-Spanish background and colonial development. *American Anthropologist* 63:483–497.
ERASMUS, CHARLES J.
1952 Changing folk beliefs and the relativity of empirical knowledge. *Southwestern Journal of Anthropology* 8:411–428.
1961 *Man takes control: cultural development and American aid.* New York: Bobbs-Merrill.
FESTINGER, LEON
1957 *Theory of cognitive dissonance.* New York: Harper and Row.
FIRTH, RAYMOND
1951 *Elements of social organization.* Boston: Beacon Press.
1959 "Acculturation in relation to concepts of health and disease," in *Medicine and anthropology.* Edited by Iago Goldstein. New York: International University Press.
FOSTER, GEORGE M.
1962 *Traditional cultures and the impact of technological change.* New York: Harper and Row.
GILLIN, JOHN
1951 *The culture of security in San Carlos.* Middle American Research Institute Publication 16. New Orleans: Tulane University Press.
GLUCKMAN, MAX
1940 Analysis of a social situation in modern Zululand. *Bantu Studies* 2(14):91–146.
GONZÁLEZ, NANCIE L.
1964 Beliefs and practices concerning medicine and nutrition among lower-class urban Guatemalans. *American Journal of Public Health* 54:1726–1734.

GRAVES, THEODORE D., NANCY B. GRAVES, MICHAEL J. KOBRIN
  1969   Historical inferences from Guttman Scales: the return of age-area magic? *Current Anthropology* 10:317–338.
HAGEN, EVERETT E.
  1962   *On the theory of social change*. New York: Dorsey Press.
HINSHAW, ROBERT
  1966   "Structure and stability of belief in Panajachel." Unpublished doctoral dissertation, University of Chicago.
KEESING, FELIX M.
  1952   *Culture change*. Stanford: Stanford University Press.
KIESLER, CHARLES A., BARRY E. COLLINS, NORMAN MILLER
  1969   *Attitude change: a critical analysis of theoretical approaches*. New York: John Wiley.
KUSHNER, GILBERT, *et al.*
  1962   *What accounts for sociocultural change?* Institute for Research in Social Science. Chapel Hill: University of North Carolina.
LERNER, DANIEL
  1958   *The passing of traditional society*. Glencoe: The Free Press.
LINTON, RALPH
  1936   *The study of man*. New York: Appleton-Century-Crofts.
  1952   "Cultural and personality factors affecting economic growth," in *The progress of underdeveloped areas*. Edited by F. F. Hoselitz. Chicago: University of Chicago Press.
MADIGAN, FRANCIS C.
  1962   *The farmer said no*. Community Development Research Council. Dilman, Luzon City: University of the Philippines.
MADSEN, CLAUDIA
  1965   *Mexican folk medicine*. Middle American Research Institute. New Orleans: Tulane University.
MAHER, ROBERT F.
  1960   Social structure and cultural change in Papua. *American Anthropologist* 62:593–602.
MANDELBAUM, DAVID G.
  1941   Culture change among the Nilgiri tribes. *American Anthropologist* 43:19–26.
MC CLELLAND, DAVID C., DAVID G. WINTER
  1969   *Motivating economic achievement*. New York: The Free Press.
MC CONNELL, WILLIAM A.
  1965   "Characteristics of innovators and early adopters." Unpublished papers, University of Colorado.
MOORE, WILBERT E.
  1963   *Social change*. Englewood Cliffs: Prentice-Hall.
NASH, MANNING
  1958a   *Machine age Maya*. Chicago: University of Chicago Press.
  1958b   Political relations in Guatemala. *Social and Economic Studies* 7: 65–75.
  1969   "Guatemalan Highlands," in *Handbook of Middle American Indians*, volume seven. Edited by E. Z. Vogt. Austin: University of Texas Press.

OGBURN, WILLIAM F.
1922   *Social change.* New York: Viking Press.
PAUL, BENJAMIN D.
1955   *Health, culture, and community.* New York: The Russell Sage Foundation.
1969   "San Pedro la Laguna," in *Los pueblos del lago Atitlán.* Edited by Sol Tax. Guatemala: Seminario de Integración Social.
PAUL, LOIS, BENJAMIN D. PAUL
1963   Changing marriage patterns in a highland Guatemalan community. *Southwestern Journal of Anthropology* 19:131–148.
REDFIELD, ROBERT
1941   *Folk culture of Yucatan.* Chicago: University of Chicago Press.
REINA, RUBEN E.
1960   *Chinautla, a Guatemalan Indian community.* Middle American Research Institute Publication 24. New Orleans: Tulane University.
ROGERS, EVERETT M.
1962   *Diffusion of innovations.* Glencoe: The Free Press.
1969   *Modernization among peasants.* New York: Holt, Rinehart and Winston.
ROJAS-LIMA, FLAVIO
1969   "Consideraciones generales," in *Los pueblos del lago Atitlán.* Edited by Sol Tax. Guatemala: Seminario de Integración Social.
RUBEL, ARTHUR J.
1960   Concepts of disease in Mexican American culture. *American Anthropologist* 62:795–814.
SCHWARTZ, LOLA ROMANUCCI
1969   The hierarchy of resort in curative practices: the Admiralty Islands, Melanesia. *Journal of Health and Social Behavior* 10:201–209.
SIEGEL, MORRIS
1941   Resistance to culture change in western Guatemala. *Sociology and Social Research* 25:414–430.
SIMMONS, OZZIE G.
1955   Popular and modern medicine in Mestizo communities of coastal Peru and Chile. *Journal of American Folklore* 68:57–71.
TAX, SOL
1937   The municipios of the midwestern highlands of Guatemala. *American Anthropologist* 39:423–444.
1941   World view and social relations in Guatemala. *American Anthropologist* 43:27–42.
1946   *The towns of Lake Atitlán.* University of Chicago Microfilm Collection of Manuscripts on Middle American Cultural Anthropology 13.
1953   *Penny capitalism: a Guatemalan Indian economy.* Institute of Social Anthropology Publication 16. Washington, D.C.: Smithsonian Institution.
1969   *Los pueblos del lago Atitlán.* Guatemala: Seminario de Integración Social.

TAX, SOL, ROBERT HINSHAW
1970   "Panajachel a generation later," in *The social anthropology of Latin America*. Edited by W. Goldschmidt and H. Hoijer. Los Angeles: University of California Press.
TUMIN, MELVIN
1952   *Caste in a peasant society*. Princeton: Princeton University Press.
VOGT, EVON
1960   On the concepts of structure and process in cultural anthropology. *American Anthropologist* 62:18–33.
WAGLEY, CHARLES
1950   *The social and religious life of a Guatemalan village*. Memoirs of the American Anthropological Association Publication 71.
WALLACE, ANTHONY F. C.
1962   *Culture and personality*. New York: Random House.
WEBER, MAX
1953   *The Protestant ethic and the spirit of capitalism*. New York: Charles Scribner and Sons.
WHITE, LESLIE
1949   *The science of culture*. New York: Grove Press.
WOLFF, ROBERT J.
1965   Modern medicine and traditional culture. *Human Organization* 24:339–345.
WOODS, CLYDE M.
1968   "Medicine and culture change in San Lucas Tolimán: a highland Guatemalan community." Unpublished doctoral dissertation, Stanford University.
1969   "San Lucas Tolimán," in *Los pueblos del lago Atitlán*. Edited by Sol Tax. Guatemala: Seminario de Integración Social.
1970   Medical innovation in highland Guatemala: the case of San Lucas Tolimán," in *Stranger in our midst*. Edited by Peter Furst. Los Angeles: University of California Press.

Endemic Goiter, Salt, and Local Customs in Central America: Prevention of a Preventable Disease

HAROLD B. HALEY

An example of the cultural aspects of control of a preventable disease is the use and nonuse in Guatemala and Central America of iodized salt as a control measure to prevent endemic goiter.

The word goiter means an enlargement of the thyroid gland. There are many kinds of goiter, but here we are primarily concerned with endemic goiter, which is defined as "the presence of localized or generalized thyroid enlargement in over 10 percent of the population" (Selenkow and Ingbar 1970). The World Health Organization estimated in 1960 that approximately 200 million people in the world were goitrous (Selenkow and Ingbar 1970). In 1969 Kevany estimated that thirteen million people in Latin America were goitrous (Kevany 1969). In 1953 four of the six countries in Central America had defined areas in which more than 50 percent of the population had endemic goiter (Food and Agriculture Organization 1954). Since use of iodized salt in the United States became widespread, the incidence of endemic goiter has been estimated at 2–4 percent of the population (DeGroot 1971). Some areas where endemic goiter flourishes are the Andes Mountains, central New Guinea, parts of Switzerland, the Baltic plains, Zaïre, and parts of Central America.

The most important cause of goiter is a deficiency of iodine in the salt and water, but there are also other causes. Chemical substances called "goitrogens" induce enlargement of the thyroid gland. Part, if not all, of the action of goitrogens is to inhibit iodine absorption or utilization and therefore may be remedied by high iodine intake. Such substances have been found in the water in Colombia, in the milk of cows eating certain grasses in Tasmania and Finland, as thiocyanates in legumes in central Africa, and in turnips, soybean flour, and other legumes in some areas. A less well defined cause of endemic goiter is variation in individual susceptibility, either genetically induced (Covarrubias, et al. 1969; Degrossi, et al. 1969) or because of conditioning by previous diet. Although these other causes are present, iodine deficiency in soil and water, and therefore in individual iodine intake, is the primary cause of endemic goiter. Local deficiency could be compensated for if populations ingested many foodstuffs from areas in which soil and water were iodine-rich. However, communities with high incidence of goiter "have little communication with urban areas, transportation facilities are very limited, and migration levels are low. Little exchange of products occurs and practically all of the foodstuffs that compose the basic diet are produced locally" (Kevany 1969).

Control measures have been based primarily on adding iodine to the diet, most commonly in salt and occasionally in bread. This has been effective in the United States and many other countries. In some limited areas, where iodination of salt has not been practical, the injection of iodinated oils is being used as a control measure.

For most people with endemic goiters, the disease is not a serious health problem. Nevertheless, there are a number of reasons for control. A large neck mass is abnormal, unusual, unsightly, and worrisome. It causes compression of the trachea, which makes breathing difficult, and in some cases affects speech because of pressure on the laryngeal nerves. Along with this, a high incidence of cretinism, mental retardation, and deaf mutism accompanies endemic goiter.

Adding iodine to the salt supply of a country has many cultural aspects, ranging from technology to education to government to evaluation of the results. In some countries or regions, control measures have been successful; in others, they have failed — usually because of inadequate implementation, which was most often due to political, social, or economic factors. Experiences in Central America, particularly in Guatemala, for the last twenty years outline some of the cultural aspects of control of this disease.

GOITER CONTROL IN CENTRAL AMERICA

Prior to the early 1950's, goiter was a widespread disease in much of Central America. "In Guatemala, surveys carried out in 1952 indicated an average prevalence of endemic goiter of 38.5 percent" (Béhar

1968). In Guatemala and adjacent countries, it was common to see people with huge neck masses walking down the streets in apparent good health. A large percentage of the children of school age had goiters. Dr. Howard Mahorner published a paper showing a dog with a large goiter from the Quetzaltenango area of Guatemala.

When the Institute of Nutrition for Central America and Panama (INCAP) opened in 1949, one of the first problems they tackled was iodine deficiency goiter. INCAP's first idea was to add iodine to the salt used in Guatemala in the same iodized form used in the United States. However, because the salt usually consumed in Guatemala is nonrefined sea salt, the iodine leached out and no effect was found. After research, it was recommended that stable potassium iodate be added to the salt (Arroyave, et al. 1956).

Commercial salt in Guatemala comes from at least three sources: the Pacific Ocean, rivers, and brine wells. The largest amount is called "salinas" salt. A salina consists of a large concrete slab, similar to a parking lot, near the Pacific Ocean. Between this concrete slab and the ocean is a large dike with culverts. During the dry season from November to March, the culverts are opened at high tide and sea water rushes into the salina. The culverts are then closed and the water evaporates, leaving a salt brine on the concrete floor. The culverts are then reopened and the area reflooded. When several inches of salt have accumulated on the concrete slab, the salt is shoveled into carts and carried into long sheds for processing. During the wet season, the clear white salt is carried through machines that distribute potassium iodate evenly throughout the salt. Because potassium iodate is insoluble, it stays in the salt after it has been mixed. The salt is then loaded into large sacks and shipped by rail to various parts of Guatemala. The law states that all salt sold in Guatemala must be iodated sea salt from the salinas. This is enforced by government inspection and sampling. With the use of potassium iodate in the salt, the results have been spectacular. Goiter is now a relatively uncommon disease in Guatemala. A survey conducted in 1965 showed an average prevalence of 5.2 percent. There appears to have been no significant increase in thyrotoxicosis, thyroid cancer, or other untoward effects (Béhar 1968).

There are two other sources of commercial salt in Guatemala that account for small pockets of goiter still being observed. One of these sources is river salt. In Sacupulas, a village in the Guatemalan highlands, river salt is obtained from salt beds in nearby Río Chixoy. Culturally, this is an ancient source of salt. Archaeological evidence has shown that the ancient Maya, in the Petén area of Guatemala, traded for Río Chixoy salt more than 1,200 years ago (Thompson 1964). In 1972 one could purchase gray river salt from this source for $.09 per pound in local markets such as Aguacatán in Huehuetenango.

Another commercial source is brine salt. In 1967 one could purchase brine salt in the Cuchumatanes Mountains. In the village of San Mateo Ixtatán, there is a brine well. Each day, Indian women would go to the well, climb down a ladder, and be met by a man who would check off their names. They would then be allowed to fill two large pottery jars with brine water from the well. In their homes they placed one jar over the fire to evaporate the water, adding more brine well water until the jar was filled with salt. The pottery was then broken off and a large block of pure white salt remained. This was brought to nearby markets, such as the one in Santa Eulalia, and sold. Side by side in the markets one could see the legal, standard, packaged, iodated, commercial salt and the lower-priced brine salt. (An anthropological vignette is seeing the brine salt being broken into chunks for a purchaser by a small child using an ancient Mayan celt, or hand axe.) There may also be areas where very small producers of noniodinated sea salt sell their product.

The presence of three different types of noniodated salt, arising from local sources and affecting only a very small part of the population, is tolerated. Occasional cases of goiter are seen in these areas.

In an adjoining country close to the Guatemalan border, school children were examined in 1964. Little evidence of goiter was found: bootleg Guatemalan iodinated salt sold in the local markets in this country had apparently decreased the local incidence of goiter. A reverse trade route was seen where noniodinated salt from yet a third country was smuggled into Guatemala and sold at a lower price in a few local markets, with goiter resulting.

Iodinization is now national policy in all Central American countries. In some countries all salt is iodated; in others only salt directed for human consumption is iodated. This provides another possibility for variation. In 1969 it was considered that this policy was fully implemented in only two of the six countries (Kevany 1969).

Currently El Salvador is using iodated salt. In Honduras, local commercial salt is salinas salt. I have the impression that early in 1973 some noniodated salt was being used. In some Honduranian homes one may see United States iodized salt being used as table salt while the cheaper salinas salt is used for cooking. In Honduras some goiter is seen, particularly in older women. There is an impression that more people with goiter may be seen in villages where more noniodated salt is used.

CULTURAL ASPECTS OF CONTROL OF PREVENTABLE DISEASE

Principles

Control of a preventable disease on an area-wide or population basis is expensive, difficult, and requires mobilization of tremendous community resources. To accomplish this, a number of conditions must be met:

1. The disease must be widespread. A small number of cases are better controlled on an individual and local basis.

2. The disease must be serious. If the disease does not entail significant loss of life or good health, use of major resources of the community on such a condition might divert resources away from more important conditions.

3. The disease must be preventable to a significant degree, if not entirely. There are many approaches to prevention. Infectious diseases are a good example of a disease complex that may be controlled or prevented by many different approaches, depending on the specific natural history of the disease and its specific agent.

a. Some infectious diseases are controlled by controlling the insect vectors that transmit the disease to humans, e.g. mosquito control to prevent malaria or yellow fever.

b. Other infectious diseases are best prevented by control of transmission routes. Pasteurization of milk and vaccination of cows prevent bovine tuberculosis in man.

c. Still other infectious diseases are best prevented by vaccination of subject populations to prevent such diseases as measles, smallpox, tetanus, etc.

d. A fourth approach in control of infectious diseases and sequelae includes better diagnostic measures in order to specify particular treatment. For example, certain areas of the United States have a high incidence of streptococcal diseases with a corresponding high incidence of rheumatic fever sequelae. The differential diagnosis of viral sore throats and tonsilitis from streptococcal disease is impossible on clinical grounds. The correct diagnosis is important because viral sore throats do not respond to antibiotics, while streptococcal do.

In order to prevent the rheumatic fever sequelae, streptococcal infections must be vigorously treated with antibiotics. Therefore, control requires establishment and access to good bacteriological facilities for making specific diagnoses, education of physicians to their use, and subsequent guidance of therapy to prevent rheumatic fever.

Some control measures have been controversial, i.e. the addition of fluorides to water supplies to control dental caries in the United States.

Addition of iodine to salt, as described in this paper, is the most widespread use of adding a nutritionally important substance to the diet of entire populations in order to eliminate a deficiency disease. Current proposals to add retinol to sugar in Guatemala represent a way of handling another deficiency disease whose levels in the total population would be altered by addition of this precursor of Vitamin A to the sugar supply.

Specific items must be considered in implementing a control program:

1.   Is appropriate technology available to accomplish the program?

2.   Has the control program been analyzed in terms of finances and benefit? After a decade of effort expended on widespread use of chest X rays as a mass screening device to detect tuberculosis and other pulmonary disease, cost-benefit analysis has now shown that individual case finding is too expensive for the economic resources of the community.

3.   The universality of application and completeness of coverage of the object of control is important. What educational, legal, economic, or other measures are necessary to accomplish this control?

4.   The relationship of the control measures and the disease process to the total culture is important in determining whether or not a program will be successful. The total economy of the culture is involved. In a health situation other health parameters become important. Nutrition is an important example because, if malnutrition is widespread, the population is more susceptible to other diseases. Malnutrition will also affect the immunological responses of the subject if immunological procedures are being used. The total civil engineering and sanitation facilities are important to any control program for infectious diseases.

5.   Control programs will require participation of both public and private sectors of the culture. For the private sector to be motivated positively it must be included in planning. This appears to have been one factor in the success of control programs in Guatemala (Béhar 1968).

Methodology

Control measures will not be feasible unless applicable technology is available. A technique that has worked in one area may be inadequate in another. In that case, further technological development becomes necessary. Distribution facilities for the technique employed are of great significance and will involve commercial marketing, governmental units, etc.

Techniques should be monitored and enforced. Is the technique being used as planned? How does one enforce this?

Results

Any program must have a specific evaluation system. Measurable end points must be defined in advance. Regular, consistent measurement of accomplishment of goals in terms of end points must be made. Can a planned program accomplish its mission? This is the key question.

Have conceptual or technological advances in other areas found a better way to accomplish the same goal? For example, cholera vaccine has not been uniformly effective. Researchers have found treatment more effective. Now, the question is: Which is the most effective way of controlling cholera — vaccination or treatment? Similar questions are being asked about typhoid.

Cost-benefit analysis continues to be important. Were the original estimates unrealistic?

What complications, either foreseen or unforeseen, have occurred as a result of the control program? The cases of poliomyelitis resulting from live virus contamination of early poliomyelitis vaccine are one example. What exceptions and variations have occurred?

Specific Cultural Considerations

It is critical that the control measures work within and become a part of the culture of the subject population. With widespread malnutrition, for example, protein supplementation of the diet must be accomplished within the culture itself. A local or foreign government distribution of materials may be of value in specific therapeutic circumstances, but it will not be acceptable on a widespread population base. The protein supplement must be included in normal commercial and living patterns and must develop acceptability in that area. Then consumer cost becomes a major factor in accomplishment of the goals in a given program. Adding iodine to a universally used food like salt puts it into usual commercial channels. The education of the public and the governments involved may very well be the most important factor in success of a control program.

A special problem is the loss of the initial drive and enthusiasm for the new project. In the Papanicolaou smear programs this has been evident from both patients and doctors. For the patient, returning to her doctor's office every year for the pap smear is a nuisance. For the physician, the incidence of finding a positive case is low, and because he has done hundreds and not found a treatable new case, the initial drive to continue doing them is not strong. It is important that access to the control measure be easy and almost automatic.

Another problem is that conflict can occur between private individual desire and the public good.

We are left with the problem of individual cases that, for medical reasons, should not consume the relatively high amount of iodine contained by iodized salt. These cases, if they really exist, are very few and should be dealt with by allowing the individuals involved to use noniodized salt, which they could obtain under medical prescription (Béhar 1968).

DISCUSSION OF ENDEMIC GOITER CONTROL

At the time when control measures were initially implemented, endemic goiter was widespread, in terms of both geography and population. As previously stated, the seriousness of goiter problem rests in (1) the cosmetic and health effects of a large mass in the neck and (2) the related conditions of cretinism, myxedema, mental retardation, and deaf mutism resulting from thyroid enlargement. The moderate seriousness of endemic goiter is balanced by its wide prevalence and its relative ease of control. There are many factors involved in the etiology of endemic goiter. Iodine deficiency is not the only one, but it is the most important and the most easily corrected. Cost is significant, but in terms of population benefit it would seem bearable. The universality of coverage would be 100 percent, if other sources of salt did not exist. Brine wells, river beds, and smuggling all provide salt from outside the system. Nevertheless, only a small percentage of the population is affected by the extraneous salt sources.

When this program was established, technological problems were encountered. The previously developed technique of adding iodide did not solve the problem. Additional technological development was required and was accomplished. By introduction of the controlling substance into the normal commercial products, distribution within the culture became standard and easy. A specific enforcement program was established by the government. Commercially sold salt is analyzed and its iodate levels determined. The availability of other types of salt has been observed in some markets.

Is the problem solved? Basically, it is solved. Compared to years ago, people with evident goiters are rarely seen in general public today. Specific analyses of population segments have been completed and much lower prevalence has been reported.

In dealing with induced changes in thyroid function, questions are raised as to possible complications. Are there increases in the incidence of thyrotoxicosis (hyperthyroidism) or cancer of the thyroid? So far, there has been no increase in cancer of the thyroid. In Guatemala there may have been some increase in thyrotoxicosis, but not enough to be a significant factor. The literature of endemic goiter control in other parts of the world has shown that thyrotoxicosis can be increased temporarily under this type of a program. Exceptions and variations due to other salt sources have been described. Some goiter still is found, probably attributable to unrecognized dietary goitrogens.

REFERENCES

ARROYAVE, G., O. PINEDA, N. S. SCRIMSHAW
 1956 The stability of potassium iodate in crude table salt. *Bulletin of the World Health Organization* 14:183–185.
BÉHAR, M.
 1968 Progress and delays in combating goiter in Latin America. *Federation Proceedings* 27:939–944.
COVARRUBIAS, E., J. BARZELATTO, R. GUILOFF
 1969 "Genetic questions related to the goiter endemia of Pedregoso (Chile)," in *Endemic goiter*. Edited by J. B. Stanbury. Washington, D.C.: Pan American Health Organization.
DE GROOT, L. J.
 1971 "Diseases of the thyroid," in *Cecil-Loeb textbook of medicine* (thirteenth edition). Philadelphia: W. B. Saunders.
DEGROSSI, O. J., *et al.*
 1969 "Characteristics of endemic goiter in a Mapuche Indian tribe in Chiquillihuin, El Malleo, Province of Neuquén, Argentine Republic," in *Endemic goiter*. Edited by J. B. Stanbury. Washington, D.C.: Pan American Health Organization.
FOOD AND AGRICULTURE ORGANIZATION
 1954 *Report on the Third Conference on Nutrition Problems in Latin America, Caracas, Venezuela, 1953*. Food and Agriculture Organization Nutrition Meetings Report Series 8. Rome.

KEVANY, J. P.
    1969   "Prevention of endemic goiter in Latin America," in *Endemic goiter*. Edited by J. B. Stanbury. Washington, D.C.: Pan American Health Organization.
SELENKOW, H. A., S. H. INGBAR
    1970   "Diseases of the thyroid," in *Harrison's principles of internal medicine* (sixth edition). New York: McGraw-Hill.
THOMPSON, J. E.
    1964   Trade relations between the Maya Highlands and Lowlands. *Estudios de Culturas Mayas* 4:13–49.

Effect of Rural-Urban Migration on Beliefs and Attitudes Toward Disease and Medicine in Southern Peru

A. QUINTANILLA

The Indians living in the high plateau of southern Peru belong to two different linguistic groups: Kechua-speaking and Aymara-speaking. From the point of view of conceptualization and practices related to disease and medicine there are no major differences between them, and in the subsequent discussion no attempt is made to distinguish between the two populations.

One of our working hypotheses is that disease and medicine in the Kechua-Aymara world are understood by the Indian within relatively coherent conceptual frames of reference. Even though the Indian interpretation of the causes and nature of disease falls, to a great extent, in the realm of magic thinking, it has a certain coherence and logic. The categories of disease among the Kechuas and Aymaras of Puno have been well described by several authors, particularly Frisancho (1972). I do not intend to repeat those descriptions here except as necessary to illustrate certain postulates. A few broad generalizations can be offered.

1.   In the Indian culture diseases are defined in accordance with a certain primitive nosology. In this nosological classification, some diseases are categorized as a cluster of symptoms and signs with more or less defined causes, treatment, and prognosis. Another group of diseases are identified not by a set of symptoms but rather by a common etiology, usually magic. This will be discussed further.

2.   Indians are not entirely opposed to Western medicine. In fact, it is accepted that Western medicine may have some usefulness along with traditional medicine. Modern medicine has made inroads into what once was the exclusive domain of the local healer or witch doctor *(laikka* or *jampicuc)*.

The integration between traditional conceptualization and treatment of disease and Western medicine has evolved slowly, over many years, and in this way without noticeable disruption of the traditional beliefs. 3.   Their system is coherent inasmuch as their concept of diseases integrates well within the context of their whole cosmic interpretation. The explanation of the causes of disease makes sense within their conceptual world, and treatment is the logical application of remedies designed to neutralize or counteract the forces believed to be the causes of disease.

THE IDEA OF DISEASE IN THE RURAL KECHUA-AYMARA WORLD

In order to study the impact of migration I will review briefly some concepts of disease and medicine held by the Indian in the rural community as opposed to the Indian transplanted to the city. I refer to the Indians who are minimally exposed to the Westernizing influence of the coastal city as the rural Kechua-Aymara world. Spread over a vast area, grouped in small hamlets or in isolated communities, with no knowledge or only minimal knowledge of the Spanish language, they present to a marked degree the theoretical characteristics of the *Gemeinschaft* [community]. Rural, communal, patriarchal, preliterary, homogeneous, ruled by custom and tradition, isolated, their economy is one of subsistence, static and self-sufficient.

As pointed out by Martínez (1961), this Indian has developed a more or less clear distinction between diseases which are amenable to the therapeutic tools of the physician and those which are not. These categories correspond more or less to diseases believed to be caused by natural agents and those of preternatural or magic causation, for which the physician has neither powers nor insight.

Examples of some of the diseases listed by Martínez as due to natural agents and treatable by physicians are the following:

Costado: Disease believed to be due to exposure to cold or a chilling wind; it is characterized by chest pain, cough, and sometimes hemoptysis. (It probably includes most forms of pneumonia, pleuritis, epidemic pleurodynia, occasional cases of herpes zoster, intercostal neuritis and other diseases characterized by chest pain.)

Puraka usu: Abdominal pain believed to be the result of by dietary indiscretions. (It may include any of the myriad of diseases where the presenting symptom is abdominal pain.)

Caju usu: Disease characterized by persistent cough and thoracic pain; it affects mainly children and is believed to be caused by cold. (It probably includes most cases of whooping cough, as well as banal bronchitis.)

Nayra usu: Encompasses diseases of the eyes characterized by reddening, soreness, pain, and lacrimation which in rare cases may lead to blindness; it is believed to be due to wind, heat, or smoke. (It includes most cases of conjunctivitis, keratitis, uveitis, and probably many other diseases of the eyes.)

Of more interest is the group of diseases which are not considered amenable to Western medicine. The following are important examples in this category: (a) A group of closely related disease entities or variants of the same entity, variously known as *jallpa jappiskka* (Kechua), *orakke mankantihua* (Aymara), *urahuena kkatua, katkja* (also Aymara); (b) *Animu karkkuska* (Kechua), *ajayu sarakkata* (Aymara), *susto* (Spanish).

Phenomenologically I call them disease entities because that is what they are within the context of the Indian conceptual universe. If we put ourselves in the position of the Indian, with his cognitive elements and mechanisms of causation rooted in magic thoughts and beliefs to which he strongly adheres, we cannot help but see them as disease entities. This is important, because a disease entity is a defined type of health disorder which calls for specific diagnostic and therapeutic measures.

Jallpa kappiskka (Kechua), *orakke mankantihua* (Aymara): In a myth common to many primitive peoples, the earth, the mountains, the springs, and rivers have a spirit which under certain circumstances may take possession of a person and cause him to become sick. *Jallpa kappiskka* applies particularly to possession by the spirit of the place where one lives. The clinical manifestations are loss of appetite, general malaise, muscular aches, nausea, vomiting, and headache. Since these are universal symptoms, it is obvious that *jallpa kappiskka* can correspond to almost any of the diseases as we know them. The singularity of *jallpa kappiskka* as a nosographic entity is given, for the Kechua-Aymara, by the specific causation as indicated by Frisancho (1972). In reality, probably the majority of cases of *jallpa kappiskka* are infectious diseases and most of them viral, particularly in children. Those cases of *jallpa kappiskka* manifested chiefly by gastrointestinal disturbances may correspond to simple acute gastroenteritis, whose viral etiology has been recently established. Many cases are functional disorders such as irritable colon. Others correspond to shigellosis, salmonellosis, and staphylococcal food poisoning. Occasionally, more serious or even fatal surgical intra-abdominal conditions may be responsible for the disease.

Animu karkkuska (Kechua), *ajayu sarakkata* (Aymara), *susto* (Spanish): The disease is believed to result from detachment of the spirit or abandonment of the patient by his soul, which wanders aimlessly in the area where a frightening episode took place. The person who lost his soul develops symptoms which are remarkably reproducible and allow the diagnosis to be made easily, often without the benefit of coca adivination by the *laikka*.

It is noteworthy that this syndrome has been described in virtually all Latin American countries and even in the United States (in Texas), among Spanish-speaking people of Mexican descent (Rubel 1964: 268). There is a remarkable coincidence in the description of the disease by different authors. The patient has a restless sleep, nocturnal fears, lack of appetite, loss of weight, loss of interest in attire and personal hygiene, depression, and introversion (Sal y Rosas n.d.; Martínez 1961; Frisancho 1972; Rubel 1964; Vellard 1957). The treatment, with minor local variations, consists basically in the identification of the place where the soul was lost and the performance of a ritualistic ceremony in which the *jampicuc* or *laikka* entices the soul to follow him from the place where it is wandering to where the patient lies so that the two are reunited; all this is accompanied by the proper incantations and magic ritual to assure the success of the treatment.

EFFICACY OF THE NATIVE HEALER

The *laikka's* approach to disease reassures the Indian and allays his anxiety because it is the logical answer to his concept of disease. The crucial difference between the Indian's concept of disease and ours is not so much in the kind of factual knowledge but in the mental categories in which we believe.

In our quest for explanations, modern medicine has painstakingly established the physical causes of an ever-growing number of diseases. The primitive mind, on the other hand, has solved its quest for the cause-effect relationship by attributing causality to forces which we call magic but which for the primitive mind are in a way more real and credible than our medical answers. Belief in the explanations offered by Western medicine requires a high degree of faith in explanations which are utterly meaningless except for the initiated. Today, germs and microbes are commonplace concepts for the occidental layman, but there was a time when it was not so and to believe in them required an act of faith far greater than to believe in the spirit of the earth doing harm to a child. Today there is a host of diseases for which modern medicine is beginning to describe the causative mechanisms in terms of molecular diseases, auto-immunity, failure of self-recognition, immune complexes, membrane phenomena, messenger RNA (ribonucleic acid), and what not. In these areas even the average medical practitioner does not understand what the specialist is talking about, let alone the layman. Yet, the medical practitioners and the layman believe the conclusions of the researcher because modern medicine has such a distinguished record of accomplishments that it is easy to believe.

For the Indians who live in isolated huts in the high plateaus of southern Peru, this act of faith is neither easy nor warranted. They have undoubtedly observed that in certain cases the Western doctor has a greater rate of success than the local healer (*laikka, jampicuc,* or *yatiri*), but this observation has not shaken their faith in the healer, because they have also observed that in certain diseases the modern physician was utterly incompetent while the *laikka* was often successful. In consequence, the popular wisdom has concluded that some diseases are amenable to treatment by physicians while others are not, as previously described.

Acceptance of the physician in a limited role has not been disruptive because it resulted from the slow realization of his powers over certain types of maladies. Modern medicine was never forcibly imposed upon the Indians — the option was open to the sick Indian and his family. The Indians opted to seek the physician's help only when they had reason to believe that he would be more successful than the healer, while they called the *laikka* for those diseases caused by spirits, mountains, the earth, or malefic actions of witchcraft or *brujería* (Spanish). For these disease entities the Western physician is considered, and correctly so, hopelessly ill equipped to handle.

When modern medicine was made available in the rural communities of Puno, the Indian was not deprived at any time of the local healer, who was available as he had always been, and with him the comfort and security offered by a man who can understand the obscure forces at work and can command healing powers. Whether or not the healer's treatment is effective depends on as many variables as our own therapeutics. Failure to achieve a cure does not necessarily diminish the prestige of the healer, just as unavoidable failures do not destroy the prestige of our clinicians.

Many of the disease entities which are not considered within the realm of occidental medicine are psychiatric disturbances, particularly certain forms of neurosis. It seems likely that most cases of *susto* and *animu karkkuska* are neurosis of anxiety with organic manifestations con-

ditioned by the firm belief prevalent in the group that the episode of fright
WILL produce such symptoms. *Susto* in infants is more difficult to
interpret, and probably encompasses a variety of conditions. To the best
of my knowledge, patients with *susto* do not have organic disease, and
their manifestations are only the functional disturbance associated with
neurosis of anxiety (López Ibor 1950; Álvarez 1958). It is noteworthy
that the concept of detachment or loss of the soul is akin to the sensa-
tion of *déspersonalization* (French) or loss of "self" (Dugas and Montier 1910). It is well known that neurotic manifestations may assume
peculiar and reproducible characteristics conditioned by the culture of
the group. The symptoms can be learned and the pattern transmitted by
imitation. The clinical picture, reproducible and similar in patient after
patient, can be explained because there are institutionalized expectations
of behavior of the person with *susto,* analogous to the institutionalized
expectations of the sick role as described by Parsons (1952: 436).

Examples of similar syndromes peculiar to certain groups are the
ufufunyane of the Zulu-speaking peoples and the *ukuphosela* of the
Xhosa (Loudon n.d.: 137); the possession syndromes described among
the Teita by Margetts; and the frustration syndrome of the island of Ti-
kopia (Firth 1959: 328). There are even epidemics of *susto*, as there are
of *ufufunyane*, and as there were epidemics of dancing mania in medieval Europe (Rawnsley 1962: 49).

Given the psychiatric nature of the disease, it is not surprising that
the *laikka* should be more successful than the Western physician in treating this disease entity. The physician is likely to be lost in a sea of obscure symptoms, will want to have a variety of laboratory tests, and will
finally be unable to establish a precise diagnosis, much less effect successful treatment. In contrast, the *laikka* will be speaking the same conceptual language as the patient; he will establish rapport with him at a
deep emotional level and, through powerful suggestion, will usually succeed in ridding him of his imaginary symptoms.

EFFECT OF MIGRATION TO THE WESTERNIZED CITIES
OF THE COAST

Indians have been migrating to the coastal cities for many years. When
the impoverished lands of the *altiplano* (high plateau) cannot support
more than one family, the growing children are forced to abandon the
native village and seek a better living in the Westernized cities. The profound psychological and sociological impact of migration and the slow

process of adaptation termed by some Peruvian sociologists as the process of "cholification" (i.e. the Indian becoming a *cholo,* or acculturated) have been described many times. I will not delve into these changes except as concerns their effect upon health and medicine.

Rotondo has pointed out that one of the salient traits in the Indian migrating to the city is an excessive, almost pathologic fear of becoming sick. We have confirmed this observation. In a survey among a group of natives of Puno villages who had migrated to Arequipa within the previous five years, the following question was asked: "What are you most afraid of?" The number one fear was of falling sick. Not even the loss of job was feared so much. This cannot be explained solely by the financial implications of sickness. In Peru, any impecunious person is eligible for medical attention in the hospitals supported by the Ministry of Health. The same fear of sickness is frequently observed among Indian girls working as domestics in the city. In most cases the fear is unwarranted, because in the event of disease, the family will take the necessary steps to assure her medical attention. In general, primitive people are more aware of how precarious the state of health is, and the everpresent possibility of disease causes a great deal of anxiety; however, in the case of the migrant Indians, there is more to it than that.

One clue to the nature of this fear is provided by our observation that the diseases or symptoms of disease which were most feared were not necessarily those of serious physical nature. Often there was more concern over minor skin blemishes, questionable reddening of the eyes, questionable paleness, etc. Many of these "symptoms," often imperceptible to myself, caused the individuals great anguish. A girl insisted on going back to her native village to seek a cure for darkening of her skin which I could never detect. A young man left his job and returned to his village because of some vague aches and insomnia. Another girl was extremely worried about a "spot" in her eye which I could never see. Cases like these were seen time and again.

On the other hand, I have often seen Indians in the city who have arrived at the hospital *in extremis,* who had continued to work until they physically could not stand on their feet because they had not paid much attention to the progressive worsening of their condition.

The explanation for this anomalous perception of the severity of one's disease seems to be related to the Indian's categorization of diseases as amenable or not amenable to Western medicine. If they fear that their disease may be one of those which is not due to natural agents, and therefore not understood by physicians, they become extremely worried and feel abandoned among people who lack insight in the problem.

Migration to the cities in itself seems to increase the incidence of the psychiatric maladies described above, perhaps in relation to the cultural clash.

It is noteworthy that the *ufufunyane* syndrome of the Zulus occurs with higher incidence among those who live and work on farms run by Europeans (Loudon n.d.: 137). Another example of the same pattern is the case of laughing disease, which occurs in epidemics among tribes of Lake Victoria. This is a form of hysteria which is much more prevalent among girls receiving education in Christian schools (Lambo 1954: 162), probably in relation to the change in cultural setting.

Another factor of the cultural clash which compounds the Indians' fear of disease is their inability to play the sick role in the urban setting, a role which would have been expected and approved in their native community. They rapidly learn that their symptoms are considered imaginary and that reassurance and support will not be provided by the outside world, so they will have to brood over their troubles alone with themselves.

The urban lack of resources to cope with their traditional diseases may be extremely disruptive and incapacitating, to the point that sometimes they cannot think about anything else, and yet will be reluctant to communicate their fears.

REFERENCES

ÁLVAREZ, W.
    1958   *Practical leads to puzzling diagnoses.* Philadelphia: Lippincott.
DUGAS, LUDOVIC, FRANÇOIS MONTIER
    1910   La déspersonalization et la perception intérieure. *Journal de Psychologie* 7.
FIRTH, R.
    1959   *Social change in Tikopia.* London: Allen and Unwin.
FRISANCHO, D.
    1972   *Creencias y supersticiones relacionadas con las enfermedades del altiplano puneño.* Puno, Peru: Los Andes.
LAMBO
    1954   *Transcultural psychiatry.* Boston: Little, Brown.
LÓPEZ IBOR, JUAN JOSE
    1950   *La angustia vital.* Madrid: Paz Montalvo.
LOUDON, J. B.
    n.d.   *Social aspects of ideas about treatment in transcultural psychiatry*
MARTÍNEZ, H.
    1961   Enfermedad y medicina en Pillapi, Bolivia. *Revista del Museo Nacional* 30:178. Lima.

PARSONS, T.
1952   *The social system.* London: Tavistock.
RAWNSLEY, K.
1962   *Sociology and medicine.* Sociological Review Monographs 5.
ROTONDO, H.
1960   *La personalidad básica del mestizo peruano.* Lima.
RUBEL, A. J.
1964   The epidemiology of a folk illness: *susto* in Hispanic America. *Ethnology* 3:268.
SAL Y ROSAS, FREDERICO
n.d.   El susto. *Revista de Sanidad de Policía.* Lima.
VELLARD, J.
1957   La conception de l'âme et de la maladie chez les Indiens américains. *Traveaux: Institut Français d'Études Andines* 6:5–33.

A Transubstantiated Health Clinic in Nepal: A Model for the Future

WILLIAM STABLEIN

The following paper is the partial results of my fieldwork in Kathmandu, Nepal from 1969 to 1972. During the process of observing, and participating in, the Buddhist rituals of the Karmarāj Mahāvihāra monastery, I assisted the now deceased Dr. Bethyl Fleming in the designing of a health clinic that ostensibly was to administer health to the monks and priests of the monastery and to their relatives.

Other than to report my ethnography, the purpose of this article is to attempt a model approach to designing health delivery systems for Tibetan-speaking peoples in the Himalayas.[1] The approach with little structural variation could possibly be applied to high-altitude peoples in general. I will consider the material in four stages: (1) the need for medical care and the health resources as they existed in 1972; (2) what the dominant cultural factors are in Tibetan communities that need to be considered in such a project (here I will sketch the methodology used in my research with a note on ethnic diplomacy); (3) the actual delivery, in the discussion of which I will point out the significance of ritual and how it was related to the clinic; and (4) the efficacy of the clinic and our own soft approach.

---

[1] That is, the *bhoṭīyas*, as they are called in Nepali, Hindi, and Sanskrit. This term refers to those Nepalis whose ethnic origins are within the boundaries of Tibetan culture. For the most part they live in the high-altitude regions of Nepal. They include the regions of Mustang, Dolpo, Nub.ri and extend as far south as Dorpatim and Pokhara. Tibetan refugees are also included in *bhoṭīyas*.

NEED AND HEALTH RESOURCES

In 1969 most of the thirty-nine monks and priests at the Karmarāj Mahāvihāra, which is located at the top of a famous pilgrimage complex in Kathmandu valley called Svayambhunath, were stricken with either chronic intestinal problems, tuberculosis, or, quite often, depression. Most of the monks and priests were from Nang Chen, a province in eastern Tibet where the life-style for the lay community revolved around the cycles of the *ḥbrog.pa* [nomadic pastoralists] (Ekvall 1968) and where disease, according to my interviews, seldom manifested itself in chronic physiological conditions. Indeed, in the region of Nang Chen there were no mosquitoes and very few flies. The monks and priests may have tended to overrate the perfection of life in their own country but their exaggerations were symbolic of their health conditions in Kathmandu valley. The shock of having moved from the high altitudes of Tibet to the monsoon region of Kathmandu valley was an undertaking of traumatic dimensions. It is fortunate that they had at least a few Nepalese patrons and an occasional convert.

The resources for medical care in Kathmandu are what might be expected (Colson 1971: 229–231). There are governmental health services, primarily Bir Hospital in downtown Kathmandu, and its adjoining tuberculosis clinic headed by Dr. Malla.[2] Although this is a fine hospital, expected cross-cultural conflicts, which are too sensitive and extensive to mention here, caused the Nang Chen Tibetans to take advantage of its services infrequently. It was not until 1972, mainly because of the personal intervention of Dr. Malla, that the monks and priests began to go to his chest clinic. This is a very efficient clinic, and because of its free services, we were able to begin treatment on five monks who had serious cases of tuberculosis. Two of them, who were referred to the Mission Tuberculosis Sanitorium in Bhaktapur, received very fine treatment under the guidance of Dr. Roche and his staff. This was not free, however, and the monks hesitated to be a burden on their own clinic,[3] from which the funds ultimately would be withdrawn. The other major service was Shanta Bhavan Mission Hospital, which was only free to those whom the social services department approved. Until our clinic had worked out a special system

---

[2]   When there was no one left to administer the clinic, Dr. Malla graciously assumed the responsibilities.

[3]   Actually the hospital was free for those patients who had no possible funds. As our clinic had some funds but not a large reservoir, Dr. Roche was kind enough to commit the hospital to paying half the expenses. It was an enormous help and no doubt greatly prolonged the life of a few good men.

of health delivery in coordination with Shanta Bhavan, the monks had great difficulty in receiving treatment. Again it was a cross-cultural problem and not the fault of the hospital. Bir and the mission hospitals were used widely by the purely Nepalese-speaking peoples.

When we talk about resources for medical therapy, the Western systems as a rule stand in sharp contrast to the indigenous ones, although a study done in Kerala and the Punjab has suggested that there are numerous indigenous medical practitioners who used Western medicine, including penicillin injections (Neumann 1971: 140–141). Among the Tibetan refugees in Nepal no such practitioner exists, and few Tibetan indigenous doctors are known for their special skills in the strictly Ayurvedic sense. Tibetan medicine, as well as traditional Nepalese curing systems, is very fluid. There are the herbal vendors, the Ayurvedic shops, at least one Muslim doctor, and the community of hierophants who perform ritual curing rites. The average Tibetan has little access to any of these sources except for the ritual curing. Throughout history ritual curing has had the power to accommodate other systems. Hence the Tibetan hierophant will more often than not have a knowledge of herbs and medicines; this is not, however, readily apparent to the outsider, who only sees him performing ceremonies and does not notice the special attention given to the substances in the ceremonial circle (Stablein 1976). And it is in this sense that the monks and priests of our clinic were their own resources. It was inconceivable that, because the hierophant and his assistants had a knowledge of medicine, the people whose country they were living in could have a better system, system here meaning ritual *(cho.ga)*.

Curing ceremonies were performed everyday and on rare occasions ceremonies to make pills *(ril.bu)* were performed; these were called the "very hidden practices concerning the ambrosic sacred substances."[4] Because the goal of these ceremonies was to transform ordinary matter into a curing ambrosia, its power of accommodation can readily be understood. There are curing ceremonies which destroy effigies: the effigies can be personifications of the disease or even a representation of an individual who was believed to have inflicted the donor of the ceremony with some disease.[5] There are other ceremonies that use a large image constructed in the likeness of the donor to attract the

---

[4] dam.rdzas.bdud.rtsiḥi.sgrub.thabs.gsang.chen.

[5] The black magic aspect is legitimized by aiming the incantations, instruments, and counter-medicines not at the individual *per se* but at the hatred, lust, greed, and so on that is possessing the individual. Hence, there is really no black magic in Buddhism.

disease. At a peak moment in the ceremony the image, i.e. a scapegoat, is burned; hence, the diseases are thought to be nullified. These ceremonies are usually performed for seven days or more. There are smaller ceremonies, which do not make use of the effigies, but are structurally the same as the above and are performed sometimes every day. There are even smaller ones, such as the one in which the hierophant places his foot on the devotee and simultaneously utters the appropriate curing *mantra*. The ceremonial resources for medical therapy are varied and extensive. In high-altitude regions they are the dominant methods of curing. Even in Kathmandu, where there are other resources, the ceremonial circle remains the most popular.

Ceremonial medicine, in comparison to other forms of therapy, is mainly based on the belief system and, although it is socially restrictive, it has a proclivity for accommodating other forms of ceremonies and in general all symbolic constructs which lend themselves to the curing process. The problem among the monks and priests in the Karmarāj Mahāvihāra was not to convince them that there were two hospitals available to them in Kathmandu but rather to lead them through the symbolic constructs of another culture. I was often asked by Tibetans in their first visit to Shanta Bhavan: "Where was the ceremony?" "Where are the divinities?" and "Was this the method of curing that Christian people adhered to?" Quite often the cultural conflict inherent in visiting the hospital produced more negative than positive effects. Hence, the need for a small clinic system is not only based on the need for health delivery in general but also on the cultural factors that lend to an efficient administering of medicine.

THE DOMINANT CULTURAL FACTORS FOR A CLINIC SYSTEM

The first problem in designing a clinic system is to find a place to construct the clinics. It raises a very important issue of proxemics. In Tibetan-speaking areas of northern Nepal the villages are more often than not set apart and below the monastic complexes. The exception is in Kathmandu valley where the Karmarāj Mahāvihāra as well as the temple complex at Bodhnath are in the midst of Newar-Tibetan communities. If the clinic is in close proximity to the monastic complex, it takes on the aura of sacredness. The monks and priests, because they are the community leaders, would of course prefer this close proximity. If the clinic is lower in elevation and with the villagers, they have less control over what is obviously a very powerful force in their community. Our own clinic, called the "Karma Clinic," was actually inside the monastery on the same top floor on which the pontiff of the entire sect stayed when he visited Kathmandu. Hence, the Karma Clinic had a transubstantiated aura.

On the less positive side a clinic placed within the confines of a monastery acquires sectarian dimensions and may sponsor ill feelings among various ethnic groups in and around the same area. It is quite common in Nepal to have four or five potentially contending groups within one area. As this was the case with the Karma Clinic, we were fortunate indeed to have Dr. Fleming, a superb diplomat as well as doctor, in charge of the clinic. Credit in this regard also goes to the head of the monastery, Sabcu Rimpoche, for inviting those emergency cases in the neighborhood to attend the clinic. Unfortunately, the donations to the clinic could barely cover the expenses of medical supplies for those associated with the monastery.

Diplomacy (Badeau 1970: 303–312) is significant in another aspect, such as why we were so willing to help design a health clinic. Because I was a scholar from the West interested in Tibetan medical systems, my own ulterior motive was clear (although I never found in Tibetan communities the same degree of negative value judgments attached to the phrase "ulterior motive" as Americans, particularly, I think, attach to it). The teachings and assistance I received from the Nang Chen Tibetans in their own cultural context were on the same level as blessings given to someone who asked for them; therefore, it was as if they were helping one sentient being to climb the ladder to salvation. In return, as any donor would do, I made my offering, which was my assistance in the creation of the Karma Clinic. It was simply one type of offering, and here we come to the core of my ethnographic methodology.

METHODOLOGY FOR ETHNOGRAPHIC INQUIRY

The most dominant cultural event in the Nepalese and Tibetan communities is ritual (*pūjā*, Tibetan *cho.ga*). Every act of any biological, astrological, or cultural consequence is immediately preceded, and most often followed, by ritual.[6] It is ritual which programs the community

---

[6] Basically, ritual is a set of relatively flexible behavioral rules that regulates and controls, in particular, the aggressive tendencies of individuals and groups. There are transubstantiated rituals where the material culture in some aspect takes on a sacred or mystical quality, and there are rituals where the material culture is an end itself. We might call the latter **Skinner rituals.**

in its approach to life's problems. In the ritual approach the universe and man are neatly classified into a hierarchical, structural, cultural system. The flaws, problems, and toxic elements that enter this system are nullified, neutralized, or, more properly, transubstantiated through the techniques of ritual. And furthermore, if there is an unconscious stratum in culture, as Lévi-Strauss contends, then its symbolism in its material aspect lies in the ceremonial circle. Yet, at the same time, the devotee carries the ceremonial circle within him wherever he goes. In a sense it is one of many adjustment mechanisms that maintains his biopsychological clock which regulates his approach to the world.

In my participation in and observation of curing rituals, which took place just one level below the clinic, I made the assumption that there was no common ground in my cultural outlook and the Tibetan one; but in order to experience and understand as much as possible, I opened myself to being reprogrammed. Assuming the validity of the biocomputer theory of man, I ostensibly accepted the power of ritual to recondition my biocomputer to share the Tibetan ritual experience. Using this approach, I came to realize that note-taking was a hindrance in obtaining the sharing-experience level of existence. I found that repetition, tapes, textual aids, and memory sufficed until such a time when I could sit down alone and write.

My theoretical framework for analyzing my friends' attitudes toward the Karma Clinic was partly based on their known attitudes and approaches to the other health resources mentioned above and their own life-style, which centered around ritual, i.e. the ceremonial circle. The clinic offered an excellent medium by which to compare and contrast the two attitudes, Western and Tibetan, toward health and disease.

As I became more adept at sharing experiences, I realized that the clinic functions were regarded as a ritual-like affair and conducted by good thought *(sems.yag.po)*. The doctor, unlike many other Westerners, was calm, slow in movement, very orderly, and compassionate. It was often said that she, although in reality a Christian, could be a Buddhist, i.e. a *nang.pa* [inner one] as well. In other words, they shared with the doctor enough *sems.* [thought], which had outward manifestations, to think of her and the clinic as an intricate part of their own ritual. The medicine cabinet with its mysterious and powerful pills that was placed beneath a picture of the doctor was a transubstantiated spot. That the clinic was a ceremonial circle in its own right where there mingled two systems of ritual was crucial, not only for the success of the clinic but also for a large part of my ethnography.

THE HEALTH DELIVERY AND THE
CEREMONIAL CIRCLE

The close proximity of the clinic with its apparatus of healing went a long way toward inspiring confidence in the monks. The fact that the Western scholar friend, myself, was living only a quarter of a mile away and was seeing them everyday at the monastery, eventually sharing many of their experiences, also was an aid in gaining their confidence. That is, they believed in the clinic's efficacy and in the doctor's power, having faith that all they had to do was call for help and they would receive it. When the doctor came once a week, as in their ritual proceedings, she would come not as an ordinary secular doctor but as a *sman.lha* [medicine divinity], which is what she was called.

Usually a ceremony was being conducted at the same time the doctor arrived and some of the monks would leave their own ceremonial circle on the bottom floor to be examined. One of the monks would bring water to the clinic for cleansing. From the monks' point of view this was akin to their own ritual purification *(bsang.sbyang)* which took place at the beginning of every major ceremonial phase. The doctor's presence was like the presence of a deity, which corresponded to the Tibetan priest who had the quality of *nga.rgyal.bzung.ba* [his inner face ritually blends into that of the deity himself] — a necessary prerequisite for any healer. The stethoscope, gauze, scissors, and any type of utensil were referred to as *bsrung.ba*, which ritually designated that part of the ceremony that invests the participants with the protective qualities of the divinities (who have their own instruments of war to fight disease). The patients would line up according to their social ranks: the head priest first, then his assistant, the teacher, and so on down to the youngest and least trained. After the doctor made her diagnosis, she would distribute the medicine which was likened unto *dam.tshig.gi.rdzas* [the distribution of transubstantiated food] during and after a cere-mony. More often than not the monks would take the medicine into their own ceremonial circle just one flight down the stairs where they would utter the *sṅags* [sacred utterances] and blow the transubstantiated powers on the Western pills. That is, in this case the medicine func-tioned as both Western medicine and Tibetan religious medicine. When the clinic period was over, the doctor and myself would be invited to a luncheon with the head priest; this was in conformity with the structure of ritual proceeding in general. Near the end of every ritual *(tshogs.gi.-ḥkhor)* the participants shared in the transubstantiated food designating the body, speech, and mind of the highest divinities. When the doctor left the monastery, it was not unlike the last stage of ritual *(gshegs.su.-gsol.ba)*, which politely sends the divinities away, ostensibly completing the ritual process.

THE EFFICACY OF THE KARMA CLINIC
AND SUMMARY

When the Karma Clinic began administering in 1969, the thirty-nine monks and priests were almost all sick, i.e. all except four when interviewed had complaints concerning either the eyes, ears, nose, stomach, or lungs. The complaints were always followed by "I was never sick in Tibet." In further interviews I decided that this meant that in Tibet there was not the same degree of aggravation, stress, and deprivation which they felt in Kathmandu Valley. After two months, the chronic complaints had dwindled to just a few cases. These cases were all sent to the Shanta Bhavan Lab during the first two weeks and had been diagnosed as having tuberculosis and liver ailments. After the second month, the general health of the monastery had improved almost 100 percent. The problem then turned to preventative medicine, which involved matters of hygiene. To help, an American Buddhist contributed enough money to rebuild and repaint the monastery. Part of this money went to reconstructing the latrine; this proved to be effective in lowering the number of occurrences of intestinal infections.

The positive results of our work were very much due to the doctor's recognition of the useful aspects inherent in the subcultural system in which she had placed herself. Although it was not apparent at first, it became clear that the clinic had become an intricate part of another medical-cultural system. The clinic was neither in competition nor estranged from its environment, and it became the focus of respect along with the monks' and priests' own ritual objects and divinities. It also became clear that the head priest himself functioned as a shaman-like healer with his own ceremonial circle and was given professional respect from the doctor as well as myself. In 1971 when the head priest had a severe case of high blood pressure, he terminated the doctor's medicine and went into retreat for three weeks where he was able to reduce it to almost normal. The doctor and I, even though there were somewhat obvious rational reasons for his improvement, thought it was quite extraordinary. The monks however took the powers of the head priest for granted. Yet, the head priest as well as the monks thought the Western medicine quite powerful, but were critical that it did not provide a lasting cure; they were also somewhat skeptical of the effects it would have on one's afterlife. The latter problem was solved by accommodating the Western approach in their own ritual complex and the former, we came to understand, was purely a reaction to the stories they heard about the miraculous cures by Western medicine. Naturally, they were let down.

The most significant conclusion to be drawn from my research is that an effective clinic system in Nepal, especially among high-altitude peoples, should seek out ways to accommodate itself to the indigenous system of medicine. The point is that it will not be strictly an Ayurvedic system but rather a ceremonial process, which may or may not have accommodated certain Ayurvedic features. It is a soft approach that rests on the assumption that a gradual, untraumatic social change will take place only in the indigenous system's absorption and accommodation of the foreign elements. Once a new system is transubstantiated into the indigenous ritual, it can "comfortably" administer health and make the kinds of changes which are tolerable to the environment.

REFERENCES

BADEAU, JOHN S.
    1970   Diplomacy and medicine. *Bulletin of the New York Academy of Medicine* 46:303–312.
COLSON, ANTHONY C.
    1971   The differential use of medical resources in developing countries. *Journal of Health and Social Behavior* 12:229–281.
EKVALL, ROBERT
    1968   "Fields on the hoof nexus of Tibetan nomadic pastoralism," in *Case studies in cultural anthropology*. New York: Holt, Rinehart and Winston.
NEUMANN, ALFRED K.
    1971   Role of the indigenous medicine practitioner in two areas of India: report of a study. *Social Science and Medicine* 5:141–142.
STABLEIN, WILLIAM
    1976   "A descriptive analysis of the content of Nepalese Buddhist Pūjās as a medical-cultural system with reference to Tibetan parallels," in *The realm of the extrahuman: ideas and actions*. Edited by Agehananda Bharati. World Anthropology. The Hague: Mouton.

Traditional African Medicine

KAMUTI KITEME

For four hundred years, European peoples have misrepresented, insulted, and abused African traditional medicine. They have called it "black magic," "witchcraft," and "tribal fanaticism." They have referred to African traditional doctors and psychiatrists as "witch doctors," "witches," "wizards," "men possessed by the devil," and "medicine men." This was partly due to ignorance and partly due to the white people's chronic cultural superciliousness which notoriously leads them to treat other peoples' cultures as inferior.

The fundamentally universal concept of medicine is prevention and cure of diseases and illnesses. Thus, the focus of all medicine among human beings has been (and still is) to devise cures for mental and physiological diseases which would otherwise cause the oldest and the most dreaded of all man's enemies — death. African medicine serves precisely this purpose. No distortions and name-calling will ever negate the fact that Africans managed to survive without the white man's "aspirin," "laxatives," and "pills" for hundreds of generations — and the majority of us still do.

African traditional doctors are experts of the mind. They are psychiatrists and psychotherapists. They have immense wisdom, sagaciousness, expertise, and knowledge regarding the African psyche, mentality, society, tradition, and social problems. They counsel on marital and personal problems, psychosomatic and organic diseases, bringing up children, and responsibilities of men and women in society. Kings, elders, leaders, men, women, and children see doctors for advice, treatment, and cure.

African traditional doctors use the "placebo effect" extensively. In addition to administering the medicine orally, they instruct patients to wear small or large "curative" objects whose "healing effects" are directly controlled by the doctor himself. There are literally hundreds of these "curative" objects prescribed by the African doctors for all kinds of problems and diseases — headaches, lovemaking, search for wealth, malaria, stomachaches, blindness, wounds, good omen, good relations with other people, lunacy, and other mental and nervous disorders.

Actually, the procedure is composed of complex psychological mechanisms related to the POWER OF THE WORD from a doctor's mouth. The doctor's "word" is more powerful than the "medicine" itself. And so he can, at any time, change the healing power of any given object to treat totally different diseases successfully. Parenthetically, it is because we believe man has power over objects and idols that African traditional societies never practiced idol worship. The idol's function, meaning, and purpose (unlike the single meaning of the Christian Cross) can always be changed by man's POWER OF THE WORD to meet different needs at different times.

Moreover, the traditional medical man is a priest as well as a country doctor. He interprets the metaphysical wonders that God provides; he analyzes the relationships between the Deity and His people; he advises the people on how to pray to the Creator during the times of misery, and how to thank Him for our happiness. The doctor-priest speaks to God on our behalf — for only he can understand the mysteries surrounding God.

In short, the traditional doctors seek to create harmony between the body and the mind and with the world around us. They are custodians of our culture and tradition. And they are responsible for the sane and orderly existence of our communal societies.

In addition to psychoanalysis, African doctors recognize "organic infection" and they seek the means to cure it. It is the professional duty of the traditional doctor to know different types of plants and minerals and the prospective medicines they produce. It is quite usual for a medical student to study and to analyze the medicinal value of over 200 different pharmacological herbs before he can qualify as a full doctor. He often grinds the bark, roots, leaves, or flowers of ten or twenty herbs and mixes them together to get the required dose of medicine. Sometimes the bark or leaves from one herb are strong enough to constitute a powerful prescription.

It is significant that the use of herbs for medicines is still found among African descendants in the West Indies, Brazil, and the southern

United States. In Haiti, for instance, the Creole word is *Docteu feuilles* [literally, "leaves doctor"]. My visit to a Haitian "leaves doctor" revealed very similar medical practices to those described in this paper. It should also be pointed out that other indigenous peoples around the world have used (and still are using) herbs for medical purposes.

The training of African doctors is a life-long enterprise. Usually, a child inherits the profession from his/her parent through apprenticeship, starting as early as the age of two years. The process is complex, and as a rule it is all kept secret. Only the apprentices are gradually introduced to the mysteries of a doctor's life and knowledge. The doctor's tools and bag are all sacred and "dangerous." Only a "trained hand" has permission to handle them.

The complicated teaching is divided into different age grades, examinations, and graduations. It starts by simple observation of the doctor at work. As the apprentice grows up, he/she is given responsibilities such as diagnosing illnesses, "putting his hands in the doctor's bag" without ill effects, searching for herbs in the forest, and sometimes doing the actual doctoring.

Clearly, then, NOT ALL doctors have the same qualifications. The older the doctor is, the more graduations he has gone through and the more knowledge he has. One way to be upgraded from one level to another is to disappear in the forest alone and to meditate about medicine for several days. During this time, the apprentice does original research on medicinal herbs. He thinks about the most clinical way of approaching and dealing with patients; he "talks to birds" and other animals so as to discover their world and life; he fasts in order to identify with the hungry and the poor; and he "talks" to the forefathers who begot him and who accumulated medical knowledge for himself, his family, and his society.

When he returns home, he can only share his experience and discoveries either with graduates of the same grade level or with the older and more experienced doctors. No younger doctors (let alone the ordinary people) may know anything about it.

More advanced graduations are known to include sacrificing one's blood to God, complete self-denial, excrutiating self-torture, daring and dangerous acts of bravery such as challenging a lion with bare hands, and yoga-like exercises to orchestrate one's soul, body, spirit, and mind with the environment. The most valuable and coveted knowledge, examination of the inner self in relation to others and an analysis of natural medicine, means a temporary hermit's life and requires the strength gathered by a prolonged and mysterious solitude.

The African traditional doctors are given a code of ethics and morality. For example, only a bad doctor (whom we incidentally refer to as a witch doctor or wizard or witch) uses his/her medicine to kill. The doctor's knowledge must be used exclusively for saving lives. A doctor who accumulates much wealth might be suspected of preying upon people's illnesses. Thus, he may only charge a moderate fee and determine it according to the patient's ability to pay.

European-trained doctors today confirm that the traditional medical experts have a profound knowledge of the human body and anatomy. This is demonstrated by a usually careful diagnosis beginning with the history of the disease, followed by a thorough examination of the body — a kind of physical checkup. He palpates the different parts and looks for tender spots. He feels the beating of the heart, the position of the inner organs, checks the eyes and ears, and smells the mouth for bad breath. Sometimes all this takes days unless, of course, it is an emergency situation. By this time the doctor is so well acquainted with the patient's body and mind that he can quite accurately identify what part of the body is ailing.

Once the disease is unmistakably identified, the doctor explains the problem to the patient. Prescription is given only if the particular herbs or minerals are easily obtainable in the area. Otherwise the doctor gives already prepared medicine. There are no nonprescription "health aids" such as "pain killers," "diet pills," and "vitamin additives," such as people easily find at every American drug counter.

During the recuperation period, members of the family, friends, relatives, and everybody in the community come to see the patient, to bring gifts, and to wish him/her well. Practically every minute the sick are surrounded by people who constantly give them moral support, courage, and hope for recovery and survival. Incidentally, whether we are sick or in good health, the communal nature of our traditional societies is somewhat synonymous to group therapy, collective sharing, mutual assistance, and individual responsibility for the welfare of the whole group.

It is quite clear that the African country doctor-priest has much more to offer for our people's health than what we "educated" people have given him credit for. He deserves our respect for his knowledge. We should do research regarding his use of herbs, minerals, and his expertise in psychotherapy among our people. We should work together to complement each other in our common efforts to improve the health of the masses. Africans have a tremendous potential for making valuable contributions to the world in medicine and psychology. We will never disseminate this medical knowledge until we learn from our indigenous medical men and decipher the exact nature of the mysterious African medicine for the rest of mankind.

SECTION FOUR

Theoretical Aspects of
Medical Anthropology

Introduction

JOHN HENRY PFIFFERLING

I will present very briefly the major theoretical issues that were raised. We can divide the discussion and the papers in the Pre-Congress Conference into several areas. One of these would be a concern with a methodological problem: how do you record illness description or illness material? Where does an illness episode begin and end? What are the significant sectors to be observed in this episode? And what do these descriptions mean from a cross-regional or a cross-cultural perspective? Some agreement was reached concerning whether illness data should be retrospective or prospective, the consensus favoring prospective data—which has rarely been done in most medical anthropological fieldwork. We should never forget the biases that exist when you are using recall data, particularly in ethnomedical data description.

The second area would concern whose view of illness is significant — the patient, the patient's family, or any concentric circle of friends, kin, etc., any network group, the curer's perspective, etc. At what level of local specificity should one stop in eliciting illness description? Whose view of reality should be considered in describing illness: the patient's medical belief system? the curer's? or the observer's synthesis? This again brings into discussion the problem of emic and etic differences (insiders' and outsiders' differences) and all the middle grounds in between, which we will probably have to live with.

The third area is: what knowledge base should the medical anthropologist have in describing illness cross-culturally? Or in one culture? In this context Western medical (classificatory or analytical) categories can be contrasted to folk-elicited (inductive) classifications. The question is: are these perspectives mutually exclusive, and does a bias from enculturation in a Western categorical scheme unduly affect the observer's ability to record non-Western medical data? Particularly, when you think even of many anthropologists — some being physicians and anthropologists, some being just anthropologists with a folk knowledge — what do Western medical categories mean in their data collection?

The fourth area is: what is the nature of the category "medical"? And, what components constitute relevant medical behavior from other sectors of behavior (ideological, cosmological, religious, economic, etc.)? What kind of boundary mechanism exists for "medicine" — both in the Western and non-Western medical world?

A final area of concern is: how can illness entities be compared for their "morbidity" from one culture to another using a Western analytic framework? In attempting to prepare material for eventual inclusion in "invariant" illness categories, several problems should be mentioned. These concern the nature of the application of epidemiological rates and techniques to populaces. A serious problem is the comparability of anthropological samples and epidemiological samples (which are rarely contiguous) with the nature of biological illness and social illness. And, of course, can this division really be made? These are all open questions we are working on and may eventually find some kind of beginning answers to.

Editor's Note: In this section on the theoretical aspects of medical anthropology we are including the papers of John Pfifferling, "Medical anthropology: mirror for medicine"; Simon Messing, Ph.D., "Emics and etics of health problems in Ethiopia"; the co-authored paper of K. L. Bhowmik, Ph.D. (University of Kalyani), and J. Basu Roy Chowdhury, Ph.D. (Institute of Social Studies, Calcutta), "Sociocultural barriers to technological change: an anthropological approach"; and the brief communication to the Congress by Or. Luis A. Vargas (Universidad Nacional Autónoma de México). On this fourth session of the Pre-Congress Conference, Dr. Haley commented: "We deliberately put it last because we think it is important to take a further look at some theoretical aspects of medical anthropology. John Pfifferling gives the outline.

Medical Anthropology: Mirror for Medicine

JOHN HENRY PFIFFERLING

Fabrega, in a recent extensive analysis of medical anthropology, feels that there are several areas of incipient theoretical importance that need to be extensively covered (1972). These areas are the nature of illness invariants, the clarification of the interaction between culture and biology, and the nature of the illness episode cross-culturally.

In order to construct any model of health care that should have significance beyond the local community we must have adequate illness episode data. Fabrega feels that we have few adequately described illness episodes in the ethnographic record (1972: 179). A common framework of orientation in the collection of the case histories should include the following:

Any illness episode makes possible a careful description of the factors leading to the recognition of an altered behavioral or biological state, to the illness behavior itself and the manner of onset, progression, and resolution of the illness episode, to an assessment of the contribution of different apparent etiological factors, and to a careful analysis of the meaning given the behavior by the members of the group. A careful inspection of the rather extensive reports of illness problems in various cultures will disclose that these rather basic ethnographic elements of illness episodes are usually overlooked. The greater the number of case analyses of this type, the more we will be able to learn about factors influencing behavioral reactions. A follow-up of individuals who have had these reactions, a survey of the frequency and distribution of occurrences, and specification of the social context and of how the behavior differs from other behavioral reactions that may or not be viewed similarly by members of the group would allow a better understanding of the meaning of these reactions (1972: 179).

In the collection of these data the investigator is constrained by an anthropological paradox. When we describe illness episodes we are almost invariably describing completed situations and, in fact, using categories that we find fit the situation. Fabrega feels that retrospective illness analyses are insufficient in properly relating culture and cognition. He then calls for more case histories of the illness-episode type. However, other semantic problems must also be considered. Should etiology be defined from our perspective in Western disease classification or from the local community's perspective? From a native standpoint, what degree of consensus or professional expertise shall serve as a baseline for accepting the etiologic agent or agents? Within every concentric sphere of social relations, definitions of what are considered "seen" as part of the illness episode may serve as a starting point. Depending on which viewpoint one takes (either emic, etic, or some middle ground), different considerations loom as matters of greatest import. Time-bound episodes are well known to be culturally specific and this may also influence our view of them. The semantic clarity of terms like onset, progression, and resolution is extremely vague when one crosses cultural and linguistic borders, and this fact further complicates the description of illness. These terms may be of much practical significance in prevention and intervention and should be utilized in plans for the delivery of care.

To the medical laity, notions such as discharge of medical outcome are reified far beyond what is generally understood by physicians themselves. There is currently no acceptable criterion for medical outcome (resolution), in our culture; why should one expect this for other cultures? If, after investigation, one does find community (or subcommunity) consensus concerning illness resolution, what significance does this have for medicine or anthropology?

Fabrega recommends that ethnomedical data should be analyzed in terms of or with reference to external systems of meaning (Western medicine), and that these systems bear directly on the domain under investigation (1972: 183). A basic question: is do they have to be compared, and is our Western classification system any less arbitrary or nomothetic than the local system? It is strange that there should be little or no investigation by anthropologists of the Western classificatory system. When one compares terminology (from a putative system) used in different decades of the twentieth century, a remarkable amount of faddism is noted. This is also associated with treatment, both in types and general-illness consideration. Our classification system variously uses body parts, organ systems, modes of transmission, disease agent(s), psychological phases, and a host of other arbitrary labeling signs (MacMahon and Pugh 1970: 51). If we seriously consider comparing noncomparable categories, we raise some epistemological ghosts.

If one disregards the thorny problem of classification and concentrates on trying to link the behavior of certain personnel and patients with biological parameters of illness, we may be able to bridge the gap between biology and culture. In this area Fabrega suggests that a typology of illness based on adequately described illness episodes might allow anthropologists to develop models of medical care (1972: 187–188). Fabrega then offers nine tentative dimensions of behavior that should be recorded. They include detailed description of the social ecology of the illness (incorporating behavioral and chronological components of the illness) and local etiologic ideas. If fieldworkers incorporate Fabrega's dimensions of illness behavior consistently, we may have a data base upon which to construct theoretical models of medical care. However, as no standard nomenclature exists in medical anthropology, as opposed to psychiatry or international health, we have only to hope that every fieldworker will follow Fabrega's dictates (see American Psychiatric Association 1968; Freedman, et al. 1972: 201–216).

One partial answer to the preceding problem is the adoption of consistent quantitative measures in the description of illness episodes. Until a refinement of the illness category is available, one can still record numbers of cases, since those cases are considered locally important. If individual describers of illness in other cultural contexts apply equivalent or Western arbitrary categories, this research can be used in seeking to establish illness invariants. Such a system is epidemiologic and makes cross-cultural studies of illness possible.

The epidemiologist attempts to describe geographic pathology: the determinants and distribution of disease entities. The terminology of an entity can be variously very specific or very general. Thus, the epidemiology of drug abuse can be written before we discover the causative agent(s) of drug abuse. In the same mode, an epidemiology of lower-back pain can be described without a specific diagnosis of sciatica, etc. Epidemiologic studies can serve as clues to the severity or nonseverity of a particular entity.

Our approach to the investigation of illness is based upon two variables. One of these is that adequately described data are necessary for generating and testing hypotheses about unknown causal factors in the distribution of disease. These data must be collected prospectively. The investigator must observe and describe what occurs in the context of the defined illness-treatment episode. Care must be taken to record group (situational) factors. For example, what is the social position of the individual at the time of his illness history and prior to it, and what is his illness history? This body of data would add up to a careful case history. An attempt can be made to categorize these factors by having adequate demographic and social data available at the time of observation of this illness episode. One must be prepared to relate this episode to others in the culture. In this way a time factor is added to the case-specific statement. The accumulation of case-specific material enables the investigator to construct case-general statements for the population. By working as an anthropologist, one can record locally defined illness episodes, relate them to locally defined treatment modalities, and produce a culture-specific picture of local illness.

The second conceptual variable that must be recorded is the time-place-person trilogy of traditional epidemiological investigation. Characteristics describing the TIME at which the persons were afflicted should be enumerated. Do cases occur in relation to season, time of month, day, or in relation to some other temporal concept that is culturally different from a Western physician's expectation? An example would be the relationship between the illness and the local cosmological, calendrical, or religious system. Characteristics describing the PLACE in which the afflicted persons were found should be enumerated. Do cases occur more often in rural rather than in urban environments, in higher-altitude or lower-altitude settings, in areas of greater population density or less?

Characteristics describing the PERSON OR PERSONS afflicted must be enumerated. For example, at what stage of the life cycle are they? What are their age, sex, occupation, education, socioeconomic class, marital status, position in relation to birth order, and a host of other demographic aspects that could impinge on their susceptibility to illness or some class of association?

These two variables, situational description (Fabrega's "social ecology") and regard to the epidemiological trilogy (time, place, person) should, in our formulation, be sufficient criteria for constructing an epidemiology of an unknown illness. The methodology should be applicable to smaller- and larger-scale societies and should enable fieldworkers to compare locally defined illness rates.

If one has a complete demographic census, construction of population-at-risk categories can easily be computed. Where local terminology extends to contiguous regions, estimates of illness can be sampled on larger populations than the small anthropological community. Even in small populations, intervention by directed action (public health) or by natural experiments should enable some assessment of changed prevalence rates. Without some follow-up observation of the population, the sampling problem inherent in anthropological studies can hardly be corrected. Within a specified period of time incidence rates can be computed in this way for folk illnesses. These rates can be used in the construction of a morbidity profile for the community. Such a profile would indicate the distribution of certain conditions of locally defined behavior (and their treatment) among a population.

We suggest that by adopting this formulation, workers in Western medicine (particularly in the areas of multifactorial etiology) may be released from the burden of applying terminology to a problem that is not yet ripe for such specificity. Only when tests of sufficient rigor are available to discriminate a specific diagnosis should we use a particular term. We will thus be able to rethink some of our hallowed categories, report on the mode of discrimination, and through this feedback system evaluate our treatment for a general (as yet undiagnosed) ailment. The pressure of early terminological diagnosis can thus be lifted somewhat from a conscientious physician. As Weed suggests, a list of the patient's problems "should not contain diagnostic guesses; it should simply state the problems at a level of refinement consistent with the physician's understanding, running the gamut from the precise diagnosis to the isolated, unexplained finding" (1971: 25).

The ramifications of this approach extend to many disciplines. If the anthropologist can enable clinical and social medicine to understand the whole patient (individual and population), much needless resentment can be relieved. If we can accurately describe health and illness behavior from the patient's perspective, we can begin to formulate health therapies that do not conflict with local values (Paul 1955; Simmons 1953: 67; Hochstrasser and Tapp 1970: 247). If we can establish a methodological baseline that is consistently applied, we can collect data that are useful in formulating generalizations (possibly invariants) about sickness and health cross-culturally (Kiev 1968: 153; Mechanic 1969; Hanson 1970: 1446).

The Western physician, by adopting an epidemiologic perspective, including an awareness of cultural factors, may be able to approach patients with multiple problems in a less constrained way. And as cultural blinders are lifted, social and psychiatric problems should be considered integral rather than alien in handling total health care.

The combined perspectives of anthropology and epidemiology

should lead us to a rethinking of classification, etiology, and the role of social factors in illness. By perceiving all illness from a biosocial orientation, the multicausal framework is seen as a needed theoretical model. The role of social science in medicine is thus both practical and theoretical (Cassel 1964: 1484).

REFERENCES

AMERICAN PSYCHIATRIC ASSOCIATION
  1968   *Diagnostic and statistical manual of mental disorders* (second edition). Washington, D.C.: American Psychiatric Association, Committee on Nomenclature and Statistics.
CASSEL, JOHN
  1964   Social science theory as a source of hypotheses in epidemiological research. *American Journal of Public Health* 54(9):1482–1488.
FABREGA, HORACIO, JR.
  1972   "Medical anthropology," in *Biennial review of anthropology 1971*. Edited by Bernard J. Siegel, 167–229. Stanford, Calif.: Stanford University Press.
FREEDMAN, ALFRED M., HAROLD KAPLAN, BENJAMIN SADOCK
  1972   *Modern synopsis of comprehensive textbook of psychiatry*. Baltimore: Williams and Wilkins.
HANSON, F. ALLAN
  1970   The Rapan theory of conception. *American Anthropologist* 72: 1444–1447.
HOCHSTRASSER, DONALD L., JESSE W. TAPP, JR.
  1970   "Social medicine and public health," in *Anthropology and the behavioral and health sciences*. Edited by Otto von Mering and Leonard Kasdan, 242–271. Pittsburgh: University of Pittsburgh Press.
KIEV, ARI
  1968   *Curanderismo, Mexican-American folk psychiatry*. New York: Free Press.
MAC MAHON, BRIAN, THOMAS PUGH
  1970   *Epidemiology: principles and methods*. Boston: Little, Brown.
MECHANIC, DAVID
  1969   "Illness and cure," in *Poverty and health: a sociological analysis*. Edited by John Kosa, Aaron Antonovsky, and Irving Kenneth Zola, 191–214. Cambridge: Harvard University Press.
PAUL, BENJAMIN DAVID, *editor*
  1955   *Heath, culture and community*. New York: Russell Sage Foundation.
SIMMONS, OZZIE G.
  1953   Popular and modern medicine in mestizo communities of coastal Peru and Chile. *Journal of American Folklore* 66:57–71.
WEED, LAWRENCE L.
  1971   *Medical records, medical education, and patient care*. Cleveland: Case Western Reserve Press.

Emics and Etics of Health Problems in Ethiopia

> Of children, the worst is the bastard;
> of foods, the toughest is beans;
> of clothing, the poorest is a thin shawl;
> of housing, the poorest is a lean-to;
>
> [but] from the enemy, the bastard son will defend you;
> · toward better days, the bean will let you survive;
> in [warm] daytime, the shawl will clothe you;
> till a better is built, the lean-to will shelter you.
>
> AMHARIC PROVERB

The concepts "emic" and "etic" can serve not only as heuristic tools of analysis in linguistics, but as paradigms for ethnological research in the field of health.

In the following examples the etic paradigm is represented by the attempt to measure the effectiveness of rural health centers (in addition to a series of medical tests) in terms of raising general aspirations. Several questions bearing on education and on desired changes were asked during the baseline research prior to the functioning of the new health centers (Messing 1965) and again about four years later in the restudy (Spruyt, et al. 1967). The same questions were also asked in four control communities that were not to receive a health center. All questions were asked of heads of households whose locations had been drawn at random from a map prepared by the sanitary engineer of the research team. The questions were interspersed among those on demography and attitudes and practices relating to health and economics. Thus the etic paradigm was modelled on the requirements of precision of the standard sociological questionnaire.

The emic paradigm was modelled on the ethnological method of "participant observation" and collected as community reports (Messing 1972). This approach was to serve as a check on the accuracy, validity, and relevance of the etic measurements. The methods of observation were sensitive to volunteered expressions and actions of the respondents, their families, and neighbors. In this way their dominant phenomenology of "subsistence anxiety" was discovered (Messing i.p.). Emic research follows more inductive, less structured methods, thus achieving more holistic realizations, which are essential to any successful program of development.

THE ETIC PARADIGM: RESPONSES TO THE QUESTIONNAIRE

While the large majority of the respondents were illiterate, most responded in the affirmative to the question: "Do you want your son to have education?" Since this aspiration was already so high at baseline, it was unlikely that an effective health center would raise it significantly higher, and the question therefore had little usefulness for measuring health-center effectiveness in the broader range of aspirations.

An additional question on education had been designed to test whether the notion of "education" involved some realistic planning on the part of the head of household, or only a pious hope. The question asked was "What level of education do you hope your sons should achieve?" The results are shown in Table 1.

In general, most heads of households had only vague aspirations, rather than expectations or concrete plans for the education of their sons (for their daughters it was not even a vague aspiration as yet). In four communities, the response "as much education as possible" was the vague response most frequently encountered. "No education desired" and irrelevant responses coded as "offset" were numerous in MayChew and Korem, which suggests that educational opportunities there were regarded as hazy and unrealistic (since the previous question, "Do you want your son to have an education?" had been answered in the affirmative). The Somali populations of Aware and DegehBur were special situations due to political-nationalistic disturbances (which also rendered a restudy there impossible). Expressed aspirations for a son's education there were higher than in the other communities, but the high response expressing the desire to send their sons to college on the part of illiterate fathers was hardly a realistic response. More likely it

Table 1. Responses on education, baseline survey 1962/1963 (in percent)

	MayChew (x*)	Korem (y*)	Hosaina (x)	Durami (y)	Metu (x)	Hurumu (y)	DegehBur (x)	Aware (y)
Needed at home		2	6	8		4		
Should have 4 years of education	2	4	4	4		6	10	19
Should have 8 years of education	4	10	4	6	2	2	30	9
Should have 12 years of education	10	6	6	6	6		8	19
Should go to college	8	16	10	6	4	12	24	21
Should have as much education as possible	16	10	20	22	62	34	6	7
Should have education according to ability or willingness	14	4	10	16	4	6	2	
Should have education as long as the government wants to educate him	6	4	2	4	6	6		
No education desired	32	30	20	16	8	22	14	23
Don't know	8	14	18	12	8	8	6	2

*   x = health-center town.
    y = control town.

was an expression of Somali humor with strangers and love of fantasy. (It should be noted that three to four years of education are generally regarded as minimal to provide permanent literacy.)

In the resurvey of 1965/1966, no basic changes were noted (see Table 2). The school in MayChew had just been greatly expanded and this had aroused considerable envy in the control town of Korem.

Another attempt to measure general aspirations asked a more direct question: "What would be the most important improvement for this community?" The results are shown in Table 3. The only responses not listed in this table were the irrelevant ones coded as "offset." These were negligible in number except in the Somali population of Aware and DegehBur, where political responses were expressed in a general way.

The high proportion of "don't know" responses in all the other communities reflects the feeling among rural and small-town people in Ethiopia that common people should not concern themselves with the expression of aspirations. These feelings were reflected in side comments during interviews (see below).

Table 2.   Comparison of baseline survey 1962/1963 and resurvey 1965/1966 (after Spruyt, et al. 1967: 45)

	MayChew (xª)	Korem (yª)	Hosaina (x)	Durami (y)	Metu (x)	Hurumu (y)
Baseline	4.00	3.30	4.10	4.40	4.60	4.20
Resurvey	4.56	4.81	4.42	4.43	4.13	3.75
Change	+0.56	+1.51	+0.32	+0.03	—0.47	—0.45
Differenceb		—0.95		0		0

ª   x = health-center town.
   y = control town.
b   Between the changes, when comparing health center and control communities; sign denotes position of health-center community.

Table 3.   Responses on community improvement, baseline survey 1962/1963 (in percent)

	MayChew (x*)	Korem (y*)	Hosaina (x)	Durami (y)	Metu (x)	Hurumu (y)	DegehBur (x)	Aware (y)
Hospital or health center	12	6	6	4	12	30	32	35
Doctor or qualified dresser	4	6	4	6				
Clean water	12	12	38	12	34	6	10	
Clean town	14	14		12	14	16		21
Better road		2	2	2		2		
Telephone or electricity						2		
School							16	7
Economic growth	4	2	4	20	10	4	14	12
No answer				2				
Other	4	2	6	12	12	4	6	5
Don't know	50	54	40	30	18	34	16	5

*   x = health-center town.
   y = control town.

The desire for medical and school facilities in DegehBur and Aware apparently reflects sophistication among Somalis who frequently cross the border into what had recently been British or Italian Somaliland, now the Somali Democratic Republic. The high response in the control community of Hurumu was probably due to the local desire to have medical facilities like those in Metu, in the same province. Desire for water was high in places that frequently suffered shortages of water and did not necessarily emphasize the desire for clean or pure water.

In the resurvey of 1965/1966, no basic changes were noted except for a more depressed outlook in the control community of Korem, which had in the meantime suffered a famine (see Table 4).

Table 4. Comparison of baseline survey 1962/1963 and resurvey 1965/1966 (after Spruyt, et al. 1967: 45)

	MayChew (x^a)	Korem (y^a)	Hosaina (x)	Durami (y)	Metu (x)	Hurumu (y)
Baseline	1.74	1.98	2.64	2.48	3.34	2.62
Resurvey	2.12	1.57	2.20	2.69	2.44	1.59
Change	+0.38	—0.41	—0.44	+0.21	—0.90	—1.03
Difference[b]		+0.79		—0.65		0

a x = health-center town.
   y = control town.
b Between the changes, when comparing health center and control communities; sign denotes position of health-center community.

In the etic design of the questionnaire, increases in aspirations were expected as a consequence of health-center programs. It had been felt that effective health education, improvements in environmental sanitation, etc. would promote a desire for higher standards in other areas. But the programs were hampered by many difficulties (Messing 1970).

THE EMIC PARADIGM: PARTICIPANT OBSERVATION
AND HOLISTIC ANALYSIS IN ETHNOLOGY

From the brief foregoing comments it is clear that even a simple presentation of figures would be unintelligible or misleading without at least a minimum of local or regional holistic and ethnological explanations.

The emic paradigm proposes to move deeper into the phenomenology of the respondents. The opportunity to do so was at hand in the field when respondents volunteered their feelings that related to their total (holistic) situation in ways not foreseen by the designers of the questionnaire. For this reason the "participant observation" method of ethnology may provide more accurate and valid data than the more precise but possibly less relevant methods of sophisticated random sampling with carefully prepared (*a priori*) pigeonholes.

Observation of attitudes relating to education shows that in rural and small-town Ethiopia children constitute a sizeable portion of the labor supply from the age of five years onward. This includes farming (such as guarding the crop from birds) and escorting cattle. Even if schools are available, peasants often employ their sons up to the age of eleven years before enrolling them in the first grade (Messing 1957, 1968). Therefore the expressed desire for education is often hypothetical, at most an approach to "ideal culture" rather than to "real culture," expectation, or planning. This is very shaky ground on which to construct measurements for the effectiveness of health centers.

Responses in answer to the "improvements desired" question elicited even more pessimistic comments, usually accompanying the "don't know" response:

— "I am poor, who would inform me?"

— "I am not a judge, nor do I hold office."

— "We are like cows that eat grass, that's all we know."

Frequent comments mentioned the government, for example:

— "The government knows."

— "Whatever the government wants to do is good."

Observation shows that minimal food consumption by the sharecropper peasant, his thatched hut and ragged clothing, and the frequent desertion of wives due to poverty, is related to attitudes of pessimism. When a local or regional famine, epidemic, or locust invasion loads the survival problems beyond the bearable point, the mental condition is one of subsistence anxiety (Messing i.p.). In the small towns that exist as market centers for the rural hinterland, the largest single occupational group is often made up of divorced peasant women who survive there as home brewers of beer and pay for their rent and clothing through prostitution if still young and fairly attractive. Subsistence anxiety leads to such discounting of health (Messing i.p.) that etic measurements of health-center effectiveness become invalid (in a statistical as well as a medical sense).

CONCLUSION

The etic assumptions underlying Western measurements of health-center effectiveness were found to be naive and invalid. The etic phenomenologic paradigm viewed the health center as a castle from which staff would ride out to slay the dragons of nonscientific practices, without regard to the holistic problems of survival of the rural majority population.

The emic paradigm begins at the other end of the human spectrum, applying participant observation and collecting inductive data. What it lacks in precision and quantification, it more than gains in accuracy and quality of ethnological information. Future assumptions underlying changes that would affect the majority of a population should begin with the study of survival patterns and "subsistence anxiety," not with sophisticated census definitions borrowed from highly industrial and literate societies.

REFERENCES

MESSING, SIMON D.
1957　"The highland-plateau Amhara of Ethiopia." Unpublished doctoral dissertation, University of Pennsylvania.
1965　Application of health questionnaire to pre-urban communities in a developing country. *Human Organization* 244:365–372.
1968　Some human factors, problems and possibilities in developing Ethiopia. *Human Factors* 10:559–564.
1970　Social problems related to the development of health in Ethiopia. *Social Science and Medicine* 3:331–337.
1972　*The target of health in Ethiopia.* New York: MSS Information Corporation.
i.p.　Discounting health, the issue of subsistence and care in an undeveloped country. *Social Science and Medicine.*
SPRUYT, D. J., *et al.*
1967　Ethiopia's health center program — its impact on community health. *Ethiopian Medical Journal* 5:1–87.

Sociocultural Barriers to Technological Change: An Anthropological Approach

K. L. BHOWMIK and J. BASU ROY CHOWDHURY

The development of anthropology as a study of MAN AND HIS WORKS has traversed a long route over centuries that has given the present-day anthropologists many useful and effective tools and methods to unveil the truth of man and his affairs. These methods and tools of anthropological tradition have not been utilized only by the bearers of this discipline; the fellow-workers of the natural and social sciences have also employed these methods and tools for collecting data and interpreting facts of their respective interests. Hence, we propose that the employment of an anthropological approach in delineating the roles of sociocultural barriers which stand in the way of a smooth technological change will be of much use.

Anthropological studies of the day may broadly be classed under two different approaches: microscopic and macroscopic. In a microscopic approach, the scholar works with a very specific problem at a very well defined place. In deciding upon the size of the group that he studies, the scholar thinks of the group in which he may personally establish all necessary contacts with members of the group so that nothing stands in the way of collecting and understanding the explicit and implicit meanings of the situations, interactions, and values. Thus he gives more emphasis to the smallness of group, area, and problem. He goes to the bottom of the problem and unearths the reality of it. In a macroscopic survey the problem is not very closed in nature nor is the area of investigation small in size. The scholar goes horizontally over a wider region of human habitation and interactions and approaches respondents from various walks of life so that nothing stands in the way of the scholar. Consequently, he is able to collect and understand all consequences of the situations and to develop a color film around the problem by employing various shades for all notations of variability of the problem.

The methodological aspects of the research projects conducted by the Institute of Social Studies have been discussed in a number of workshops organized by the Institute. These discussions have revealed that the employment of a macroscopic approach preceded by a microscopic approach and followed again by a microscopic approach is much more meaningful in studying some problems of sociocultural bearing. The object of this paper is to see how this combined approach helps in detecting the sociocultural barriers which stand in the way of introducing a technological change to a community of rural West Bengal. The study was conducted on the acceptance of allopathic medicine by the Muslims in a rural region of lower Bengal.

In the first place, a study following the microscopic approach was carried on in the village Ramakantabati which is inhabited by fifty-three Muslim families and four Hindu families. Those Hindu families living in the village Ramakantabati belong to the lowest rung of the Hindu hierarchy and exert little or no influence in the sociocultural orientation of the Muslims of this village. This village is situated at a distance of two furlongs away from the Dakshin Barasat market where allopathic medicines can be had at dispensaries of five private medical practitioners, one charitable dispensary, and three medical shops. Besides these, there are some grocers' shops where some popular allopathic medicines to relieve headache, scabies, indigestion, acidity, etc are available. The village Ramakantabati is located very close to the metalled road which passes through the Dakshin Barasat market. Thus the Muslims of the village of Ramakantabati do not have any difficulty in obtaining quickly a supply and service of allopathic medicine in adequate quantity. In reality, it is seen that there are forty-six families which do not like to depend on allopathic medicine. Of these families, there are forty families which have never used allopathic medicine. Of the families which have ever used allopathic medicine, there is no family which has not tried any other medicine or magico-religious trick before knocking on the door of a practitioner of allopathic medicine. It shows that the Muslims of the village of Ramakantabati are noted for their general aversion to allopathic medicine. As to the cause of their aversion they speak of the bitter taste of allopathic medicine, the physical pain involved in getting injections, and the fear of operation. Some of them have expressed a doubt as to the composition of allopathic medicine. They say that the manufacture of allopathic medicine is devoid of any and all religious prescriptions. Thus some of them strongly believe that the acceptance of allopathic medicine may lead them to become unfaithful to their own religion.

Next we study the problem with a macroscopic approach. A structured questionnaire was developed on the basis of the knowledge acquired from the study of village Ramakantabati and it was administered to all the Muslim families residing in all the villages of Dakshin Barasat region. The analysis of the data reveals that the attitude of the Muslims of this region towards the acceptance of allopathic medicine is not as negative as one finds with the Muslims of Ramakantabati. In the region under study there are six villages including Ramakantabati where Muslims are found. These villages altogether have 520 families. Two hundred forty-seven families do not like to depend on allopathic medicine. Of these families, there are 215 families which have never used allopathic medicine in their respective families. Of the families which have ever used allopathic medicine, there are 126 families where the family heads have first gone to a practitioner of allopathic medicine before trying any other medicine or magico-religious tricks. This picture developed from the macroscopic survey does not corroborate the picture that we get from Ramakantabati through a microscopic survey.

A detailed analysis of the situations reveals that there is a differential attitude reported by the Muslims of different villages towards the acceptance of allopathic medicine. The highest acceptance is reported in the village of Baneswarpur (82.05 percent) followed by the villages of Abdul Karimpur (76.47 percent), Mastikari (62.32 percent), Padmerat (60.57 percent), Nurullapur (35.56 percent), and Ramakantabati (24.53 percent). This has necessitated the undertaking of a microscopic survey in order to unearth the causes which have developed this differential attitude. On inquiry, it has been found that the only Muslim practitioner of allopathic medicine has his residence and chamber in Dakshin Barasat. He belongs to Dhali social group which has a lower social standing in their community. The Muslims belonging to higher social groups do not like to take medicine from this man of lower social standing, and at the same time most of them do not like the idea of calling a Hindu physician to their house. This Muslim physician belongs to a faction of Padmerat village which maintains more connections through extravillage factional alliances with Mastikari, Baneswarpur, and Abdul Karimpur. This is believed to have brought more and more patients from these villages to Mr. Dhali. The Muslims of Ramakantabati are very conservative and depend more on *hakimi* [Muslim medicine] than on allopathic medicine. These people have more marital alliances with the Muslims of Nurullapur. As a result of such close interactions, the lower amount of acceptance of allopathic medicine by the people in Ramakantabati has greatly influenced the acceptance of allopathic medicine by the Muslims of Nurullapur.

It is evident from the above discussion that the Muslims of the Dakshin Barawat region have different attitudes towards the acceptance of allopathic medicine. Some of them are very traditionally oriented and do not like to accept innovations in their sociocultural dynamics of the life process. The acceptance, as well as nonacceptance, of innovations in the Muslim community is being regulated by factional alliances, lineage affiliations, and personal relations with agents of change. To conduct this type of study effectively requires the undertaking of a macroscopic survey preceded by a microscopic survey and again followed by a microscopic survey.

Reflections

LUIS ALBERTO VARGAS

In its relatively short history, medical anthropology has been approached from at least three different fields: that of the medical practitioner, of the cultural anthropologist, and of the physical anthropologist. This has given medical anthropology such a broad field that it has now become difficult to decide on its limits and goals. Fabrega (1972) has stated a definition in which "neither concepts, methods, nor aims are critical, but rather the content of the work that is performed. A medical anthropology inquiry will be defined as one that (a) elucidates the factors, mechanisms, and processes that play a role on or influence the way in which individuals and groups are affected by and respond to illness and disease, and (b) examines these problems with an emphasis on patterns of behavior." Newman's paper on "Ecology and medical anthropology" (1964) should serve as a good example of the physical anthropologist's approach to the field. Alland's paper on "Medical anthropology and the study of biological and cultural adaptation" (1966) is an excellent example of the ways in which the anthropological study of medical problems can contribute "as a major link between physical and cultural anthropology, particularly in the areas of biological and cultural evolution." Finally, Beltrán's book (1955) on health programs in the intercultural situation can be considered a classic on the uses that the medical profession can make of medical anthropology.

Much of the work done in medical anthropology seems to be undertaken with the idea of testing and developing anthropological theory, but also many papers deal with applications of anthropological knowledge in medical settings, particularly in the field of public health.

In order to clarify the scope of medical anthropology, the scope of medicine must be understood. We feel that medicine can be viewed and practiced with two complementary approaches, aside from basic research: as applied to groups of people and as a person-to-person relationship. In both cases two kinds of problems develop: one is the different approach and conception of health, disease, and medical treatment of the recipients and purveyors of medical care, and the other is the need of the medical practitioner to focus the patient or patients within the "normal" frame of the human species and of his group in the biological, psychological, and sociocultural perspectives. Since human variability in these three spheres is so great as to make every person unique, medical anthropology can be viewed as a means by which the medical profession can have a better understanding of both the individual patient and the group with which it works. It can be easily understood that with this point of view apparently unconnected fields of research claiming to belong to medical anthropology make sense, such as constitutional medicine, forensic physical anthropology, ethnomedicine, ethnopsychiatry, folk medicine, etc.

For instance, most of the so-called "normal standards" of growth, arterial blood pressure, nutritional requirements, etc. are based on studies made in Europe or the USA and they are applied indiscriminately to other human groups. Of course these are useful indicators, but human variability must be taken into consideration. Growth curves of Mexican and North American children are similar, but not identical, even in well-nourished groups, and a particular child can be labeled as undernourished using the curves of a group different from his own. Physical anthropologists have many contributions to make in this field.

The cultural aspects of medical practice have been far more studied by anthropologists — at least in Mexico — and the literature on different conceptions of health, disease, and medical care is continually growing. This is one of the most important means by which doctors trained in the Western tradition can have an efficient holistic practice with individuals and communities. Unfortunately this information has been rarely used by public health services and individual practitioners — again, at least in Mexico — and most of the time they are viewed as the "primitive and exotic customs of Indians."

It seems that apart from its theoretical interest, medical anthropology can be seen as an important aspect of applied anthropology that must be incorporated into the medical curricula from the earlier years, before medical students become an immutable part of the medical establishment with deep-rooted ideas on how, why, when, and whom they must heal.

REFERENCES

AGUIRRE BELTRÁN, GONZALO
 1955 *Programas de salud en la situación intercultural.* Mexico City: Instituto Indigenista Interamericano.
ALLAND, ALEXANDER
 1966 Medical anthropology and the study of biological and cultural adaptation. *American Anthropologist* 68:40–51.
FABREGA, HORACIO, JR.
 1972 "Medical anthropology," in *Biennial review of anthropology, 1971.* Edited by Bernard J. Siegel, 167–229. Stanford, Calif.: Stanford University Press.
NEWMAN, MARSHALL T.
 1964 Ecology and medical anthropology. *American Journal of Physical Anthropology,* n.s. 22:351–354.

Vox Populorum:
Congress Commentaries

Vox Populorum:
Congress Commentaries

DR. HALEY: At this point, I would hope that either somebody will have an irresistable urge to open the discussion or, if not, we can present this summary of comments. There are several issues or questions that seemed of greatest importance to us as we thought about it:

1. As a further definition of what is medical anthropology, if one looks at social psychologists, medical sociologists, and cultural anthropologists, where does the uniqueness of each lie? We have some thoughts on it, but I think it is fair enough to say that we did not answer that question definitively.

2. Following the lines that Mr. Pfifferling just talked about, what are the feelings about methodology?

3. The research that is done by anthropologists; are there additional things that should be done to help the subjects of the studies of the anthropologist to improve the quality of their living?

4. This leads to a very important question through all of anthropology, but certainly in medical anthropology — what is the role of the anthropologist? Researcher, or action implementor?

5. Are there particular defined areas of research that can be seen now that the state of the knowledge is such that says, "This is where we should be going"?

6. Are there recommendations that this session should bring to the Congress as a whole? Or to any other appropriate body? I have no need to restrict the discussion to those subjects, but I don't think we can cover them all. Our time is too limited. But these are the things that have come to our minds as seeming to be of considerable interest.

There is something I might like Dr. Kochar to say something about. In talking about anthropology as a discipline, Dr. Kochar has worked on a coding classification system in medical anthropology that would seem to be one of the ways of establishing identifiable areas, if not boundaries, and I wonder if he would like to say something to us to open the discussion with his thoughts on medical anthropology as a field, and particularly, what contributions could be made in classification and organizations.

DR. KOCHAR: I would have preferred to wait until comments from the audience were forthcoming because of the fact that what you have referred to as my attempt to list our areas of research is nothing new. It is very well known. It has been listed in very many ways in bibliographies and summaries and reviews. This work was done primarily as a personal effort to line up my reading and thinking in the field of medical anthropology. But since you have called me, I'll very briefly mention the broad basis for this outline. In the field of medical anthropology we can identify very broad dimensions which have been mentioned in a number of reviews, since the very, very illuminating review of Dr. Polgar in an article in 1963 which appeared in *Current Anthropology*. At that time he used a number of titles and subtitles in the paper. Later views have used different types of classification for reviews of the field of medical anthropology. Particularly with reference to Dr. Polgar's paper, comments were made by some people that the titles were too diverse. Well, medical anthropology is diverse in its nature; the impression that there are too many different areas with which anthropologists are coping is a natural conclusion.

What I attempt is to describe a basis on which these different areas could be labeled. I identify four major dimensions of medical anthropology. One would be disease sectors in which one could have sub-classification of genetic, ecological, social, and others. Another dimension would be disease management. Within this we can have two broad categories of modern and traditional systems. Within each we can probably have subclassifications. The third dimension is that of illness and health state. This "illness and health" can be seen from two points of view: the state of illness and the illness behavior that results. And the fourth dimension which has NOT been much emphasized in the literature is that of social milieu; the social milieu in which all these different things are happening. I find it useful to distinguish two common types of milieu — the milieu of the traditional societies, societies in which the health, public health, and medical problems are of a much different nature than the milieu of the modern society or the urban societies where the problems of public health are of a slightly different nature. And within these areas the interrelationship between these different dimensions can constitute a basis of classification. It's very crude and I am very apologetic that I have been called to explore it here with the audience because I haven't really given very serious thought to this theme. Thank you.

DR. SONUKA (from Nigeria, temporarily at Harvard): It seems to me from the summaries of the papers that were given at the conference on medical anthropology of the Congress that you people had that there is still an overemphasis on culture in medical anthropology. And this carries the implication — a very elitist one — that problems of health — let me explain it to you: that it is the culture of the masses specifically that constitutes the more crucial obstacles to improvement in public health. For example, there is the notion of the urban, traditional model. We seem to lose sight of the fact that since the rise of capitalism, primitive or traditional societies have been destroyed. That kind of categorization can no longer be used critically. Medicine has become a commodity in all of these new states in which medical anthropologists do research or go in to search for cultural obstacles. The fact is that at least in the pre-capitalist era the font of medical knowledge available to these communities was available to everyone, whereas in the present situation, even given the rise of the fund of medical knowledge, the availability of medical knowledge is determined by the ability of the individual to pay for it. These kinds of factors did not appear to emerge from the activities of the medical anthropology session in its pre-Congress papers. I think this is a serious limitation if we just continue to focus on culture. It has other kinds of consequences concerning the image that we hold about the proletarian peasant majorities of our epoch. At least I feel this is true in terms of the country from which I come — Nigeria.

Medicine has been heavily implicated in the whole capitalist process, so that problems which the masses face with regard to health can more accurately be decoded and resolved by commenting on the capitalistic and socialistic structure and waging a war against that kind of social system. Thank you.

DR. QUINTANILLA (from Peru, and now Chicago): The preceding speaker has established a distinction which is basically an economic distinction between the approach of Western medicine and the approach of traditional medicine. I don't know the case of Nigeria. But Professors Leeson and Frankenberg established that in Lusaka, Zambia traditional medicine is more expensive than Western medicine. The same situation applies in Peru. Traditional medicine is much much more expensive. As a matter of fact, to pay a healer, a *laica* or *huampicu*, as they are called in the Peruvian mountains, they are obliged to pay with a cow, several pigs — which are extremely high, expensive commodities. What happens, I think, is that rather than being a difference in economic terms, the difference is in sociological terms.

The person who goes to the traditional healer expects — and obtains — a great deal more than the one who goes to the Western physician. The one who goes to the Western physician may attain phsyical health, but does not get the social reinforcement and understanding of his own deep beliefs. He does not obtain the whole set of psychological and sociological reinforcements which the local healer gives. And he is willing to pay for that. For him it doesn't matter if he pays a cow or several sheep. While the other fellow, just to cure, let's say pneumonia with penicillin, may ask for a certain amount of currency which is not justified according to the categories of the patient. I think that is a closer approximation of the situation from the economic viewpoint.

DR. RÖMER (from Yugoslavia, speaking in German):   We have been working with aborigines in Australia and we have been able to determine that the aborigines in Australia resort to the use of clay to cure many diseases, and especially those relating to pregnant women. We have noticed that large numbers of pharmaceutics were found in the clay that these women used. At least it was felt that that was the case, but then we realized that this was not quite accurate and that we should ask ourselves, therefore, what are the reasons why this custom of eating clay still exists. Here we have really hit the nail on the head with regard to colloids and aluminum substances which are neutralizers in cases of hyperacidity — as happens frequently among pregnant women.

Professor Stumpf and Dr. Hallman have undertaken studies after an epidemic of cholera in my country, and Professor Stumpf was in favor of the ingestion of clay as a medication against cholera. I think it is interesting to state that a factory of pharmaceuticals in Hungary recently has decided to manufacture two preparations based on clay. In that case, also, we have noticed that the ethnology might be studied. These could be extremely interesting surveys. Now, as to problems relating to diet, which are not strictly medical problems, we have here (for tasting) clay from Australia, and those of you wish to see clay from Australia have to come close to us and examine it or taste it, if you wish.

DR. HALEY: Dana Raphael has comments on the last two reactions from the audience. Dana has been interested in geophagy and in the ethics of cultural examination.

DR. RAPHAEL: I hope everybody can understand: this is a kind of poor man's Gelusil that Dr. Römer is talking about. I think this is a very technical paper and must really be discussed. I am very grateful that we are doing both; medical anthropology is both medical and anthropology. But I think Dr. Sonuka's statement, a political statement, is one of the most important statements that we have to deal with. It took anthropology about a hundred years to get into the question of ethics and politics and the political aspects of the ethics of human beings. I think medical anthropology is about ten years old — Dr. Polgar's paper dates from about 1963 — so it only took us ten years. So, you see, we are improving. The political statement that we have to have ethics in dealing with all of these questions is a very important one. We've already called for — in the medical anthropology meeting — consideration of the whole issue. The whole political, ethical issue. And I would like to invite you, as well as other people, to discuss it.

MISS SHEILA COSMINSKY: I'd like to add something to that. While I agree with Dr. Sonuka that the emphasis has been on traditional culture as an obstacle, I think there is an increasing realization of, and there are an increasing number of studies on, the agents of change, on the ideology and organization of Western medicine as obstacles to change. This, then, does not put the blame on the developing people — as has been the bias in the past. And I know in my own paper, I discussed some of the problems in WHO or modern medical programs in terms of barriers to change. I just want to say that there is, I think, an increasing realization and perhaps, hopefully, a sophistication in terms of expanding that area of research.

MR. JOHN MARSHALL (Human Reproduction Unit, WHO, Geneva, Switzerland): I hesitate to interrupt the discussion about the political and ethical implications of medical anthropology, but I may not have another chance. In the discussion about the indigenous pharmacological properties, that was mentioned before, I suggest that this would be a good point at which to mention that the WHO is interested in research on indigenous contraceptive and abortifacient agents. We would like to hear from you if you have information about indigenous methods of fertility regulation, because we are interested in understanding the acceptability of new methods (we are trying to design technology for people that they will accept and think we can learn from what they have been using). Moreover, there will probably soon be a lab that will screen biomedically and through primate studies the effectiveness and toxicity of indigenous fertility regulating methods. And, if we can be provided with about ten (the equivalent of ten) human doses of indigenous fertility regulating methods, we might be able to see what is in them and if and why they work. Thank you.

DR. REINA TORRES DE ARRUSO (from Panama, speaking in Spanish): I'm an ethnologist and I also work with social anthropology. Recently at the University of Panama we have been working jointly with the medical school and the Department of Anthropology in the humanities. We are working, I say, in a program which seeks to find the causes for the high incidence of hypertension and stroke, especially among Negro groups working in Panama. This has been done jointly with the University of Texas. So, recently I have become very interested in medical anthropology. Of course, I had some background in this field, I had studied the situation regarding deliveries among Indian women and also had studied groups of the Chavanismo women in Panama. Therefore, these are the experiences I have had up to now in the field of medical anthropology.

I should like to make a general comment on the topic to say that we cannot overemphasize a cultural approach to problems of medical anthropology. We have to think in terms of applied medical anthropology because we will always have to bear in mind the approach of the individual with regard to belonging to a cultural group. In dealing with a given disease, for instance, certain groups, I think, are fatalistic with regard to certain diseases. On the other hand, there are attitudes or approaches in other cultures where diseases are not considered to be diseases but rather a part of life — part and parcel of life. Now the approach of a given individual *vis-à-vis* a certain disease has to always be taken into account. It should be the object of detailed study, so that we can have truly applied medical anthropology. And to be able to do something with regard to the medical activity is the function of medical anthropology.

DR. HALEY: We have about ten minutes left, so I think it is important that each speaker limit himself to about a minute. I think Dr. Katz has had his hand up for a while. Dr. Katz.

DR. KATZ: Yes, I would like to speak about some of our experiences in the Alaskan Arctic, in particular, working with the Eskimo populations. In the past, the delivery of health services in the Arctic area has been provided by the U.S. Public Health Service. In certain areas of Alaska, particularly around the Bering Straits, there are many villages that did not receive the kind of medical attention that they felt was useful for their purposes. In other words, the health services that they were given did not fit their definition of health.

Specifically, they asked us to come in and help with their formation of a native health corporation, the Norton Sound Health Corporation. It was founded in Nome, Alaska, to serve sixteen villages. This was initially funded by the U.S. Office of Economic Opportunity in this country; it is now funded by the Department of Health, Education, and Welfare.

The point is that it actually survived and has been extremely viable. What it has done is to try to define health according to the people's definition, that is, according to the Eskimo's definition of what they desire. It has put their priorities in the top position and tried to organize the delivery of health services around their particular priorities. We have attempted to train health aides particularly. This has been so successful that there are now thirty-five villages in Alaska that are having health aides trained specifically by the Health Corporation.

Essentially, we have designed services from an anthropological point of view. I believe that these in and of themselves have been extremely sensitive to a number of the issues raised by several of the previous speakers, in trying to design both the biological and social aspects of medical care. If anybody would like to discuss this further with me some time, I would be happy to talk about it. I do not want to take any more of your time to do that. Thank you.

DR. POLGAR: Thank you very much. Several speakers were kind enough to refer to a rather inadequate review article that I wrote in *Current Anthropology* some ten years ago. I think it is very important to recognize that medical anthropology dates much further back than the appearance of that article and I think that a great deal of the emphasis in that article may be classified as a post-World War II ef-florescence of certain kinds of medical anthropology which, as Julius

Roth has called it, had a pretty strong "management bias." And I think that part of the earlier medical anthropology, of which I think we are now seeing a great deal of revival, had a much closer link to attempts to provide health care in various ways to segments of the population in Europe, in Latin America, in other countries which did not quite as strongly emphasize the barriers on the client's side. This earlier medical anthropology was also much more involved in trying to reform the medical care system from the inside.

I think that amongst our ancestors we should certainly recognize Dr. Virchow in the nineteenth century (I believe) and many other medical reformers who were physicians and anthropologists as well. And so I hope that you will not merely take these remarks as an unnecessary diversion in personal modesty, but a reminder that we can and we should look to the more long-term history of medical anthropology which did not, in fact, suffer as strongly from this cultural bias to which Dr. Sonuka made very appropriate reference.

DR. HALEY: I have tried to make one real quick comment in regard to this elitist comment. I am impressed with the fact that in the so-called elitist culture in the United States, without regard to a system one way or the other, we have some major problems in health care delivery that I think are tremendously culturally oriented, and that is in the whole field of public health and preventive medicine. For example, we have fewer children getting polio vaccinations than we did ten years ago, more women getting pap-smears, etc.; these are cultural things that are not part of political ideology and have, I think, an appropriate place in medical anthropology. Second statement: I believe that our conference on Friday (31 August 1973) was oriented to culture *per se*, without definition as to whether it was "elitist" or not, but rather what are the cultural relationships between how all people receive their care, and whether we can improve it from the cultural or medical standpoint.

MRS. RAIKS: I'm from England. I would like to refer back to a paper that was mentioned after Nugi's paper. And that was a reference that was made to the study that was done by Leeson and Frankenberg in Zambia. And the person (Dr. Quintanilla) who quoted the study said that because of the importance of traditional medicine, people preferred to go to a traditional healer than to use Western medicine. This sounds as though people are preferring to go to the cultural healer over Western medicine. I think that is a figure taken very much out of context. Western medicine very often doesn't work in developing countries and is ineffective because there is so little of it. Money spent on health care in Zambia, and also in Tanzania, is about a dollar per head of the population per annum, compared to something like $150.00 per head per annum in England, and something like $480.00 per head per annum in the States. So, Western medicine is not effective for the population in places like Zambia and other developing countries.

JULIA OPTI (School of Public Health, University of North Carolina): I'd like to make an observation about medical anthropology in general. It seems to me there are two major aspects to medical anthropology: one is the theoretical and the other is the applied. And we have been dealing only with the theoretical aspects here. This is the aspect that the medical staff at the hospitals, etc. feel very comfortable with. As long as we sit at the typewriter and we write down what should be done and what are the problems involved, this is fine. But as soon as the anthropologist says, "I'd like to take an active part in patient care or in health delivery to the patient," the hospital staff gets very upset and says that there is just no room for anthropologists in hospitals or in medicine today. I think that we should try to deal with this aspect of medical anthropology as well.

DR. PFIFFERLING: I think we are dealing with this aspect. I've just been hired by the Veterans Administration to be, if you wish, a clinical anthropologist, being a part of the team involved in delivery of health care to the patients and taking cognizance of the cultural kinds of factors. There is a whole conference in New Orleans (November 1973) of people who are hired as clinical anthropologists who are part of the therapeutic delivery team. Many physicians are aware of this hiatus and are hiring or getting consultation and this for many years from anthropologists. So, it is not that we are with ourselves just recently. I think, medicine is certainly aware of this.

DR. HALEY: I think it also has a relation to the developing roles like hospital epidemiologists. These things are, as you say, "a drop in the bucket," but at least there is a bucket catching a few of the drops. Let us hope that we will continue to progress in this direction. The gentleman back here.

DR. VIRGIL VOGEL (from the U.S.A.): I'm interested in this question of the cultural bias of the observer of primitive medicine. I think there is some substance to the charge of this cultural bias. I think this is shown in the long delay that took place before primitive medical drugs — drugs that were used by primitive people — were finally accepted in white medicine. It wasn't until 1970 that anybody bothered to even list them. There were two hundred botanical drugs that were used by North American Indians that were accepted in the American pharmacopoeia or the national formulary. But the interesting story is the long delay before they won acceptance. Coca, for instance, was not accepted scientifically until 1885.

Primitive medicine is too often regarded as merely a "quaint" branch of folklore. Yet, it was from primitive medicine or folk medicine that we learned of digitalis, oral contraceptive pills, innoculation, the dietary basis of scurvy, cinchona, and discovered medical uses for South American curare. It is our civilization that has been hurt by this cultural bias, by this unwillingness to admit that primitive peoples might have something to offer scientific medicine. Even in writing *American Indian medicine*, which I published in 1970, I found a great deal of resistance to the proposition that I presented there: that Western medicine has actually learned something from primitive medicine.

DR. HALEY: One very brief comment. We've got less than two minutes left.

DR. LUIS VARGAS (from Mexico):   We now have a small group of those interested in medical anthropology in Mexico. And so far, our definition of medical anthropology has been a functional one. We have always thought that medicine should see patients as people. That is to say, as an integrity of physical, social, and psychological aspects. Thus, medical anthropology has to focus on man in his wholeness, in his totality. And, so far, our definition has worked, since we have taken into account the physical and anthropological views of man in his variability in our country. We hope to have started a small revolution having medical practitioners understand that man is very complex and he has to be considered as a biological, cultural, and social individual in order to understand him and offer him good medical care.

DR. HALEY: Four quick points to close:
1. Dr. Vargas: a year from now the Americanista meeting is in Mexico City — invite us to meet with you!

DR. VARGAS: Yes, we are having this meeting, the International Congress of Americanistas, in which both Dr. Cijas and I are very interested in having a group in medical anthropology. We are working on this, and we hope that you will keep this in mind for next year and join us in September 1974.

DR. HALEY: I have submitted a title that I hope will fit in with your plans — a paper entitled, "Amuletos."

DR. VARGAS: Of course.

DR. HALEY:
2. There have been a number of references (by Dr. Polgar, Dr. Raphael, and others) as to the state of development of medical anthropology. Dr. Lucille Newman, in the Department of International Health of the University of California at San Francisco, now has established a doctoral program in medical anthropology. This is a first. This is something that you should know about. There are people in the room who are getting their degrees in cultural anthropology who would like to have had an opportunity to go on in medical anthropology. I only hope that as we develop more structures, we will still keep movement and not be encased in cement in the foundations of those structures.
3. In the big green folders that you were given are about twenty abstracts for the session on Medical Anthropology. Obviously, we have been talking about reports on many more papers. Some of this [difference] reflects conference chairmen of other sessions referring papers to us. In some cases, such as my good friend on the left, the editor, his was one of the last abstracts in, and it was too late to get into the program — so if this happened to you, you are at least in good company.
4. I think many of us feel that we could use another hour or two. There are many whom we have talked to and we would have liked to have heard more of — Dr. Stablein, Miss Urdaneta, for example; there are others whom I don't know, who I'm sure would have added to the knowledge of all of us. Thank you for coming. It has been a pleasure to work with you.

Post Scriptum

It has been indeed a most pleasant and academically rewarding year of work in the field of medical anthropology. Since this volume could not have been possible without the energetic and dynamic cooperation of Harold Haley, M.D., I think it most appropriate that he be given the last word on the subject of medical anthropology in this volume.

FRANCIS X. GROLLIG, S.J., PH.D.

While reviewing these and other Anthropology Congress papers and discussions, I concluded that when comparing Western medicine and traditional healing, we will find more emphasis in traditional healing on two media. One is the use of ritual; the other is the responsibility and involvement of the community as a whole (and/or the family as part of the community) in the care of the patient.

The use of ritual for the sake of ritual by the *curandero* plays an important part in the therapeutic process. In Western medicine, ritual is less important. Placebos are used in both and recognized as such by all practitioners. Some observers of American medicine try to attribute some of our practice to ritual. The gown, mask, and gloves of the surgeon are considered ritualistic mystique by some sociological writers who apparently haven't heard of bacteria and the prevention of infection. I don't see the need in Western culture for increased use of ritual.

On the other hand I believe Western medicine can learn from traditional healers in their supportive incorporation of the family and community in the care of individual patients. Isolation, breaks in contact with society, and loss of a future are common aspects of serious illness in Western cultures. This also relates to the role of the elderly in our society. We can learn from other healing systems whose practices in these areas appear wiser than ours.

HAROLD B. HALEY, M.D.

Biographical Notes

RAYMOND C. BAUMHART, S.J. (1923–   ) has been President of Loyola University of Chicago since July, 1970. He had previously served Loyola as Dean of the School of Business Administration (1964–1966), Acting Vice-President for the Medical Center (1968–1969), and Executive Vice-President of the University (1968–1970). A member of the Society of Jesus since 1946 and a Catholic priest since 1957, he studied at Northwestern University (B.S., 1945), Loyola (B.A., 1950; Ph.L. *cum laude*, 1952; S.T.L., 1958), and Harvard University (M.B.A., 1953; D.B.A., 1963). He served as a trustee of St. Louis University (1967–1970) and Boston College (1969–1973), and was on the Advisory Council of the Center for the Study of Applied Ethics at the University of Virginia (1969–1973). At present he is on the Board of Directors of the Jewel Companies, Inc. (since 1973) and on the Council of Better Business Bureaus (since 1971). He has written extensively on business ethics, writing the book, *An honest profit: what businessmen say about ethics in business* (Holt, Rinehart, 1968), and co-authoring *Cases in business ethics* (Appleton-Century, 1968).

JANET BELCOVE (1954–   ) was born in Chicago. She has spent two summers excavating the Koster Site under the direction of Northwestern University (1970, 1971), has done field research with Southern Methodist University in Taos, New Mexico (1972), and has spent a year studying at the University of Durham, England (1973–1974). She is presently a senior at the University of Illinois. She is primarily interested in philosophical anthropology and intends to pursue this interest in graduate school.

K. L. Bhowmik (1938–) is Director of the Institute of Social Studies, Calcutta, and Editor of *Society and Culture*. He is also a Reader in Bidhan Chandra Krishi Viswa Vidyalaya. He received his M.Sc. in Anthropology from the University of Calcutta and a Ph.D. from the same university with a dissertation on the structure of the society of the Dule Bauries, a particularly interesting caste in West Bengal. His publications include three books, *Tribal India, Fertility of Zemi women in Nagaland*, and *Fertility of Muslim women in lower Bengal* (written with Dr. Chowdhury), as well as about a hundred papers. Member of the Executive Committee of the Indian Anthropological Association and a member of the Indian Science Congress Association, his present research interest is in the field of demography, particularly in the area of fertility.

Alifeyo Chilivumbo is at Chancellor College, Limbe, Malawi.

A. B. Chowdhury.   No biographical data available.

J. Basu Roy Chowdhury (1937–) is Director of the Rural Reconstruction Division of the Institute of Social Studies in Calcutta and Associate Editor of *Society and Culture*. He received his M.A. from the University of Calcutta in Political Science. He has co-authored one book, *Fertility of Muslim women in lower Bengal*, and written about fifty papers. He is also Chief Executive *cum* Secretary of the Kalikata Bustee Pragati Sangstha, a group of organizations serving the people of Calcutta. His present research interest is focused on leadership and the diffusion of innovations. He is Secretary of the Academy of Folklore in Calcutta and a member of the Board of Editors of *Lokasanskriti* and *Folklife*.

Francis Clune, Jr. (1930–) studied anthropology at the University of California at Berkeley, receiving his B.A. in 1957. He continued his studies at U.C.L.A. with the Ph.D. awarded in 1963. He is now an Associate Professor at S.U.N.Y. College at Brockport. His interests are in medical anthropology, technology, and the archaeology of the Pacific.

Sheila Cosminsky (1941–) is Assistant Professor of Anthropology at Rutgers University, Camden. She received her B.A. from Brooklyn College (1962), her M.A. from Washington State University (1964), and her Ph.D. from Brandeis University (1974). Her special interests include cultural influences on illness and medical care, interethnic relations, nutritional anthropology, and sociocultural change, with emphasis on these problems in Central America and Africa. Recent publications include: "Utilization of a health clinic in a Guatemalan community" (in *Proceedings of International Congress of Americanists*, 1972) and "The evil eye in a Guatemalan Mayan community" (in *The evil eye*, edited by C. Maloney, in press).

C. G. DEAN. No biographical data available.

HARVEY E. DOORENBOS. No biographical data available.

JOSEPH A. GAGLIANO (1930–) was born in Milwaukee, Wisconsin. He studied at Marquette University, where he received his B.S. in 1954 and his M.A. in 1957. In 1961, he received his Ph.D. in Latin American History at Georgetown University. He is Professor of History at Loyola University of Chicago, where he has taught Latin American History since 1962. His special interests include Andean history and Latin American social history.

MIGUEL F. GRACIA (1923–) was born in Havana. He received his Bachelor's of Science and Letters in 1941 and graduated as a Doctor in Medicine from the Havana University Medical School in 1955. He completed a rotating internship in General Medicine and Surgery at St. Vincent Hospital (Worcester, Mass.) in 1956. From 1956 to 1959, he was Resident Physician in Psychiatry at Westborough State Hospital (Westborough, Mass.), at which time he presented a series of staff lectures on the history of psychiatry, hospital administration, and group psychotherapy. He did psychiatric out-patient work for several years at different hospitals in Massachusetts and was Clinical Director of Montana State Hospital in Warm Springs, Montana (1964–1974). In 1964, he completed a summer course at the School of Alcohol Studies at the University of Utah. He has been a member of the Montana Governor's Committee for the Aged (1963–1964) and Psychiatric Consultant of the Third Judicial District of Montana (1962–1972). He has written several papers, some of which have been published, on geriatrics, alcoholism, deafness and mutism, and on north American Indians. He is at present Director of a forensic psychiatric service.

THEODORE D. GRAVES (1932–), formerly Professor of Anthropology at the University of California, Los Angeles, is currently Captain James Cook Fellow of the Royal Society of New Zealand. Professor Graves received his Ph.D. in Anthropology from the University of Pennsylvania and, before going to U.C.L.A. in 1969, engaged in interdisciplinary research for ten years at the Institute of Behavioral Science, University of Colorado. He is best known for his psychological studies of American Indian drinking behavior and the adjustment of urban migrants. In addition to work among various U.S. miniority groups, he has also conducted research on the social psychology of modernization in Latin America, East Africa, and, currently, the South Pacific.

FRANCIS XAVIER GROLLIG, S.J. (1922–   ) is Professor and Chairman of the Department of Anthropology at Loyola University of Chicago. His broad academic background includes A.B. (Classics) and A.M. (History) from Loyola University; Ph.L. (Philosophy) and S.T.B. (Theology) from West Baden College; and Ph.D. (Anthropology) from Indiana University in 1959. He became a Jesuit in 1940 and was ordained a priest in 1953. His extended sessions for ethnological fieldwork include (for one year) Guatemala in 1958 as a grantee under the Buenos Aires Convention and (for six months) Peru in 1961 under a Fulbright Research grant. Besides other numerous papers and publications, he has presented papers at the session of the International Congress of Americanists in Vienna (1960), Mexico (1962 and 1974), Madrid (1964), Buenos Aires (1966), Lima (1970) and Rome (1972); and at the International Congress of Anthropological and Ethnological Sciences in Chicago (1973). He is the co-editor with Dr. Sol Tax of *Serial publications in anthropology*, 1973.

VINIGI L. GROTTANELLI (1912–   ) graduated in Economics (1933) and Law (1935) from the University of Turin. Curator and then Director of the Museo Nazionale Preistorico-Etnografico in Rome from 1944 to 1967 and Lecturer of Ethnology in the University of Rome since 1957, he is now Professor of this discipline in the same university and Director of its Institute of Ethnology. He was a Visiting Professor at the University of Pittsburgh in 1964. He has been a Member of the Executive Council, International African Council, London from 1946 to 1967, and a Vice-President of IUAES from 1964 to 1973. An author of numerous publications based on his own field research (in Ethiopia, 1937–1939; in Somalia, 1951–1952; and in Ghana, 1954–1973) and on general anthropology (as an editor and co-author of *Ethnologica*, three volumes, Milan, 1966–1967), his main interests include African ethnology and cultural dynamics.

HAROLD BERNARD HALEY (1923–) received his M.D. degree from St. Louis University in 1946 and did his surgical residency and research fellowship at Harvard. From 1955 to 1969, he was in the Department of Surgery at Loyola University in Chicago and from 1969 to 1972 was at the Medical College of Ohio. Since 1972, he has been Associate Dean and Professor of Surgery of the University of Virginia. Since 1964, he has had extensive interests in Latin America and has studied nutrition and anthropology — primarily in Central America, but he has also done some work in Peru and Bolivia. His research interests include studies of attitude formation in physicians, evaluation in medical education, and medical anthropology in underdeveloped countries.

KAMUTI KITEME is an Associate Professor, Black Studies, Department, City College of the City University of New York. Formerly, Dr. Kiteme edited *Afro-Vision*, the newsletter of the Pan African Students' Organization in the Americas. His articles on the Black experience have also appeared in sixteen Black newspapers in the U.S.A., the West Indies, and Africa. More recently, Dr. Kiteme has published articles in *Ebony*, *Essence*, and the *Negro History Bulletin*, and has written a book, *The effects of European education upon African culture* (1974). His father is a traditional African doctor.

VIJAY KOCHAR. No biographical data available.

FRANKLIN O. LOVELAND (1941–) was born in Cincinnati, Ohio. He received his A.B. in Economics from Dartmouth College in 1964, his M.A. in Social Relations from Lehigh University in 1967, and is presently completing his doctorate in Social Anthropology at Duke University. He has been an Instructor in Anthropology at Gettysburg College since 1971. He is primarily concerned with the study of cosmology in the lower Central American culture area from the perspective of symbolic anthropology. His field research studies include a study of symbolic communication among the Shouters of Trinidad (1966–1967) and a study of the cosmology of the Rama Indians, a tropical forest people of Eastern Nicaragua (1969–1970).

SIMON D. MESSING (1922–) is Professor of Anthropology at Southern Connecticut State College, New Haven. As a member of the Public Health Demonstration and Evaluation Project, he did research in rural Ethiopia for six years. Born in Germany, he received the Ph.D. from the University of Pennsylvania (1957). Publications include work on marketing in Ethiopia, culture and mental health, editorship of a monograph on "Rural health in Africa," and a paperback *The target of health in Ethiopia* (MSS Information Corp., New York, 1972).

T. NAWALINSKI.   No biographical data available.

KIVUTO NDETI is in the Department of Sociology, University of Nairobi, Kenya.

MARY LASSANCE PARTHUN (1936–   ) was born in Dubuque, Iowa. She studied at Clarke College, where she received her B.A. in Sociology, and at the University of Ottawa, where she received the M.S.W. degree. She has since worked extensively in various areas of professional social work and has studied and lectured in the field of anthropology at Trent University, Peterborough. At the time of this writing she was Consultant in Social Work at a provincial training school in Ontario.

JOHN HENRY PFIFFERLING (1943–   ) was born in Lancashire, England. He studied at the City University of New York (B.A., 1965; M.A., 1967) and at Pennsylvania State University. He is currently Assistant Director, Quality Review, of the Joint Commission on Accreditation of Hospitals, U.S.A. He has done fieldwork in demography on chimpanzees in Tanzania, medical anthropological research in the Puna of Argentina, and research on social change among the Iban of Sarawak. His dissertation is on physician reactions to social change in the U.S. He is a permanent member of the American Psychiatric Association's Task Force on the Problem-Oriented Medical Record.

ANTONIO QUINTANILLA (1927–   ) was born in Peru. He studied social sciences and medicine, received his M.D. degree in Lima in 1957, and did postgraduate studies in New York and Chicago. He has taught at the Catholic University of Lima, the Planning Institute of Lima, and the University of Arequipa Medical School. At present he is Associate Professor of Medicine at Northwestern University, Chicago.

DANA RAPHAEL received her B.S. and Ph.D. (1966) from Columbia University in anthropology. She is the author of *The tender gift* (Prentice-Hall, 1973), a work on mothering and lactation. Her research interests include social networks, supportive behavior in animals and human beings, and malnutrition and starvation during the perinatal period. She was formerly a full-time consultant for Columbia University International Institute for the Study of Human Reproduction, where she is working on a comprehensive field guide *The anthropology of human reproduction* (in press). She is Adjunct Professor in Anthropology at Fairfield University in Connecticut where she lives, married and with three children, and is currently Director of the Human Lactation Center.

DALE W. RITTER (1919–) received his B.A. from the University of California at Los Angeles in 1942 and his M.D. from the California School of Medicine in 1946. He finished a residency in obstetrics and gynecology at the Los Angeles County General Hospital in 1952. He is a Diplomate of the American Board of Obstetrics and Gynecology and a Fellow of both the American College of Obstetrics and Gynecology and the American College of Surgery. An interest in anthropology and archaelogy, and a remote American Indian ancestry, led to the special study of petroglyphs and pictographs of the Western United States. Publications have been made in both the field of medicine and archaeology.

ERIC W. RITTER (1944–) was born in Los Angeles. He received his B.A. in Anthropology from the University of Arizona in 1966, his M.A. in Anthropology from the University of California, Davis, in 1968, and is at present completing his Ph.D. in Anthropology at this latter institution. He has also been an Instructor in Anthropology at U.C. Davis (1971–1972) and has worked seasonally as an archaeologist for the California Department of Parks and Recreation (1963–1974). His publications include works on archaeology, ethnography, paleoecology, and geomorphology, emphasizing western North America. At present he is an archaeologist with the United States Department of the Interior, Bureau of Land Management in southern California.

BELA J. RÖMER (1912–) received his M.A. at the University of Zagreb and his Ph.D. in Ethnology at the University of Debrecen. His special interests include food ethnology, technology of folk food, and geophagy.

G. A. SCHAD. No biographical data available.

WILLIAM STABLEIN (1933–) is an associate in the University Seminar on Oriental Thought and Religion at Columbia University, New York. After completing his B.A. at the University of Washington in Seattle, he studied Indic Languages and Culture at Columbia University where he also taught in the Oriental Humanities Program. In 1967 he was granted a Fulbright-Hayes Fellowship to study tantric Buddhism in Kathmandu, Nepal, where his interest in ethnography and medicine led to the establishment of the Karma Clinic. After completing fieldwork for his doctoral dissertation, in 1971 he made a survey of Buddhist-Sanskrit manuscripts in India and Nepal for the Institute for Advanced Studies of World Religions. His present research is the elucidation of Nepalese and Tibetan Buddhist rituals as a medical-cultural system and how this system can serve as a cross-cultural model for health delivery.

KENNETH I. TAYLOR (1934–   ) was born in Glasgow, Scotland. He received his B.Sc. in Architecture from the University of Strathclyde in 1961, and his M.S. and Ph.D. degrees in Anthropology from the University of Wisconsin, Madison, in 1967 and 1972, respectively. As a Ford Foundation Consultant, he taught one semester in the Graduate Program in Social Anthropology of the Federal University of Río de Janeiro (Museu Nacional) in 1972, and since August 1972 has been Assistant Professor at the University of Brasília. He has done fieldwork among Eskimos in northwest Greenland and Kodiak Island, Alaska, and with the Sanumá Indians of north Brazil. He is currently Coordinator of the Perimetral-Yanoama Project of the Fundação Nacional do Índio (FUNAI), a program of assistance and supervision of Indian-white contact in connection with the construction of the Perimetral Norte highway. His special interests are ethnoscience and structuralism, and food prohibitions and shamanism.

MICHIO TSUNOO (1920–   ) was born in Tokyo and received his M.D. from Nippon Medical School. He was a Research Fellow in Billings Hospital, at the University of Chicago, during 1962–1964 and 1967–1968. He has been a Professor of Pharmacology and Head of the Center for Clinical Pharmacology in Nippon Medical School since 1969.

LUIS ALBERTO VARGAS (1941–   ) was born in Mexico City. He received his M.A. in Anthropology at the Escuela Nacional de Antropología in Mexico, his M.D. from the Universidad Nacional Autónoma de México and a Doctorat de troisième cycle en biologie animale, option anthropologie, from the University of Paris. He is currently Secretary and Research Associate at the Instituto de Investigaciones Antropológicas de la UNAM in Mexico City. He is interested in and does research in problems of medical anthropology and human biology in Mexico.

CLYDE WOODS (1932–   ) received a B.A. in Social Science and an M.S. in Sociology at California State University, San Jose, and then completed the Ph.D. in Anthropology at Stanford University in 1968. In the same year, he joined the faculty of the Department of Anthropology at the University of California, Los Angeles. Dr. Woods has had extensive research experience in the United States, Mexico, and Guatemala. His major interests are in behavioral anthropology, sociocultural change, medical anthropology, and peasant societies. He has previously published a number of articles, chapters, and book reviews and recently completed an introductory textbook on culture change (Wm. C. Brown, Dubuque, Iowa, 1975).

Index of Names

Index of Subjects